LANGE

SMART CHARTS

PHARMACOLOGY

Second Edition

Catherine E. Pelletier-Dattu, MD, FACEP, FAAEM

Department of Emergency Medicine
Drexel University College of Medicine
Philadelphia, Pennsylvania

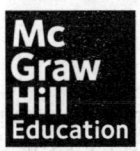

New York   Chicago   San Francisco   Athens   London   Madrid   Mexico City
Milan   New Delhi   Singapore   Sydney   Toronto

Lange Smart Charts: Pharmacology, Second Edition

1 2 3 4 5 6 7 8 9 0 QTN/QTN 20 19 18 17 16 15

ISBN 978-0-07-177436-9
MHID 0-07-177436-X

NOTICE

Medicine is an ever-changing science. As new research and clinical experience broaden our knowledge, changes in treatment and drug therapy are required. The author and the publisher of this work have checked with sources believed to be reliable in their efforts to provide information that is complete and generally in accord with the standards accepted at the time of publication. However, in view of the possibility of human error or changes in medical sciences, neither the author nor the publisher nor any other party who has been involved in the preparation or publication of this work warrants that the information contained herein is in every respect accurate or complete, and they disclaim all responsibility for any errors or omissions or for the results obtained from use of the information contained in this work. Readers are encouraged to confirm the information contained herein with other sources. For example and in particular, readers are advised to check the product information sheet included in the package of each drug they plan to administer to be certain that the information contained in this work is accurate and that changes have not been made in the recommended dose or in the contraindications for administration. This recommendation is of particular importance in connection with new or infrequently used drugs.

This book was set in Goudy by Aptara, Inc.
The editors were Michael Weitz and Peter J. Boyle.
The production supervisor was Richard Ruzycka.
Project management was provided by Amit Kashyap, Aptara.
Quad Graphics Taunton was the printer and binder.

This book was printed on acid-free paper.

Cataloging-in-publication data for this book is on file at the Library of Congress.

McGraw-Hill Education books are available at special quantity discounts to use as premiums and sales promotions, or for use in corporate training programs. To contact a representative please visit the Contact Us pages at www.mhprofessional.com.

To my loving husband, Mohamed, and wonderful children, Anil and Leila:
So sorry about the hours that this project has taken from our family.
Thanks for your patience and support. Love you all so much.

CONTENTS

Preface vii

How to Use This Book ix

Abbreviations xi

Pharmacologic Suffixes xv

Medications That Inhibit and Up-Regulate Cytochrome P450 Enzymes xvii

1. Pharmacology Basics 1

2. Antimicrobial Medications 13

3. Autonomic Nervous System Structure and Medications 79

4. Psychiatric Medications 109

5. Drugs Affecting Neurologic Function 135

6. Medications Affecting Cardiac and Renal Function 197

7. Respiratory Drugs 265

8. Gastrointestinal Drugs 277

9. Drugs Affecting the Endocrine System 289

10. Oncologic Drugs 323

11. Immunomodulators 349

12. Drugs Used to Treat Inflammation 365

13. Toxicology 381

14. Alternative Medications 387

Index 397

PREFACE

Lange Smart Charts: Pharmacology is written specifically for students in the field of medicine. The book not only highlights the information that students need to learn for course examinations and for the pharmacology component of the USMLE Step 1 boards, but also makes it easier to study and remember this material.

The unique approach of this book is immediately apparent. **Tables** and **diagrams** are used exclusively to present well-selected information clearly and concisely. This chart method gives an instant picture of how the various facts are connected, thereby making study time productive and successful. The special feature **Terms to Learn** introduces each chapter and provides the reader with the minimum essentials needed for a quick understanding of the high-yield facts—the information most often targeted on examinations and boards. **Mnemonics** are also included throughout the book to make immediate recall easier.

The material presented in *Pharmacology Smart Charts* is detailed enough for review in pharmacology courses, yet concise enough for board review. The selection and organization of information is designed to promote efficient use of study time by reducing the amount of re-reading required to master this subject area.

As this text's largest market is the United States, I have only included medications currently sold in the United States and their brand names. Also, I have attempted to include the current U.S. boxed warnings for each drug in the adverse effects/side effects column as well as the most common side effects and the "quintessential" side effects that tend to be on examinations.

Many thanks to Dr. Nisarg Patel for his assistance with the second edition of this text.

HOW TO USE THIS BOOK

Layout of the book	The book is composed entirely of tables and diagrams to facilitate comparison and clarify relationships among drugs, drug classes, and drug mechanisms.
Using *Lange Smart Charts: Pharmacology* in conjunction with your pharmacology course	For optimal benefit, start using this book early in the year to follow along with the content of your pharmacology course. *Lange Smart Charts: Pharmacology* is designed to make the most of your studying time. Each chapter is introduced by an **outline** of the classes of drugs that are the focus of study. This is followed by **Terms to Learn,** which provides an understanding of drug classification, the pharmacodynamics and pharmacokinetics of drugs, and relevant diseases. **Diagrams** of drug categories allow quick memorization and **illustrations** clarify difficult concepts. **Tables** make it easy to associate the drugs and drug categories with the relevant high-yield facts that appear most often on the boards and on pharmacology examinations, including pharmacokinetics, mechanisms of action and resistance, clinical uses, and side effects. **Mnemonics** and other learning aids in each chapter promote quick recall of details.
Using *Lange Smart Charts: Pharmacology* as a pharmacology review for the USMLE Step 1.	Begin by reviewing each of the chapter outlines, the Terms to Learn, and the drug classification diagrams. Use the tables to fill in the details. Learn the mnemonics to improve your recall. Find your weaknesses by using a pharmacology question book and then review these topics in the relevant chapters. With this approach, you should be able to review pharmacology in a matter of days.

ABBREVIATIONS

A

AC Adenylate cyclase
ACE Angiotensin-converting enzyme
Ach Acetylcholine
ACS Acute coronary syndrome
ACTH Adrenocorticotropic hormone
ADH Antidiuretic hormone
ADHD Attention-deficit hyperactivity disorder
ADP Adenosine diphosphate
ANS Autonomic nervous system
AP Action potential
ATP Adenosine triphosphate
ATPase Adenosine triphosphatase
AV Atrioventricular

B

BBB Blood brain barrier
BP Blood pressure
BPH Benign prostatic hypertrophy
BMT Bone marrow transplant

C

CA Cancer
CAD Coronary artery disease
CABG Coronary artery bypass graft
cAMP Cyclic adenosine monophosphate
CF Cystic fibrosis

cGMP Cyclic guanosine monophosphate
CHF Congestive heart failure
CMV Cytomegalovirus
CNS Central nervous system
CO Cardiac output
COMT Catechol-*o*-methyltransferase
COPD Chronic obstructive pulmonary disease
COX Cyclooxygenase
CPR Cardiopulmonary resuscitation
CRH Corticotropin-releasing hormone
CSF Cerebrospinal fluid
CTZ Chemoreceptor trigger zone
CV Cardiovascular
CVA Cerebrovascular accident
CVS Cardiovascular system

D

DA Dopamine
DAG Diacylglycerol

E

EC Extracellular
ECF Extracellular fluid
EEG Electroencephalogram
ENT Ear, nose, and throat
EPI Epinephrine
EPS Extrapyramidal side effects

F
FDA Food and Drug Administration

G
G+ Gram-positive
G− Gram-negative
G6PD Glucose-6-phosphate dehydrogenase
GERD Gastroesophageal reflux disease
GFR Glomerular filtration rate
GI Gastrointestinal
GTP Guanosine triphosphate
GU Genitourinary

H
5-HT Serotonin
Hb Hemoglobin
HDL High-density lipoprotein
HIT Heparin induced thrombocytopenia
HIV Human immunodeficiency virus
HMG-CoA Hepatic hydroxymethylglutaryl coenzyme A
HR Heart rate
HSV Herpes simplex virus

I
IBD Inflammatory bowel disease
IC Intracellular
IDDM Insulin dependent diabetes mellitus
IHSS Idiopathic hypertrophic subaortic stenosis
IL Interleukin
IM Intramuscular
IP$_3$ Inositol 1, 4, 5-triphosphate
ISA Intrinsic sympathomimetic activity
IV Intravenous

L
LDL Low-density lipoprotein
LFT Liver function tests
Lp(a) Lipoprotein little A antigen
LTU Long-term use

M
MI Myocardial infarction
MAO Monoamine oxidase
MOA Mechanism of action
MRSA Methicillin-resistant Staphylococcus aureus
MSA Membrane stabilizing activity

N
nACh Nicotinic acetylcholine receptors
NE Norepinephrine
NIDDM Non–insulin dependent diabetes mellitus
NM Neuromuscular
NMJ Neuromuscular junction
NO Nitrous oxide
NRTI Nucleoside reverse transcriptase inhibitor
NSAID Nonsteroidal anti-inflammatory drug
NSR Normal sinus rhythm
NT Neurotransmitter

O
OA Osteoarthritis
OR Operating room
OTC Over the counter

P
PABA Para-aminobenzoic acid
PCI Percutaneous
PCP Pneumocystis carinii pneumonia

PDE Phosphodiesterase
PID Pelvic inflammatory disease
pK$_a$ Negative logarithm of acid ionization constant
PO Oral administration
PSVT Paroxysmal supraventricular tachycardia
PTT Partial thromboplastin time
PUD Peptic ulcer disease
PVD Peripheral vascular disease

R

RA Rheumatoid arthritis
RAS Reticular activating system
REM Rapid eye movement
RTA Renal tubular acidosis

S

SA Sinoatrial
SC Subcutaneous
SIADH Syndrome of inappropriate antidiuretic hormone (secretion)
SLE Systemic lupus erythematosus
SOA Site of action
SSRI Selective serotonin reuptake inhibitor
SVT Supraventricular tachycardia

T

TB Tuberculosis
TCA Tricyclic antidepressant
TG Triglyceride

THC Tetrahydrocannabinol
TIA Transient ischemic attack
TNF Tumor necrosis factor
TPR Total peripheral resistance

U

UA Unstable angina
URI Upper respiratory infection
USMLE United States Medical Licensing Examination
UTI Urinary tract infection

V

VLDL Very low-density lipoprotein
VZV Varicella-zoster virus

PHARMACOKINETICS ABBREVIATIONS:

A: Administration or Absorption
B: Biotransformation or plasma protein binding
D: Distribution
DOA: Duration of action
E: Excretion
M: Metabolism
OOA: Onset of action
R: Redistribution
$t^{1}/_{2}$: Half-life

PHARMACOLOGIC SUFFIXES

Suffix	Class	Clinical Use	Example
-afil	Phosphodiesterase inhibitors	Erectile dysfunction, pulmonary HTN	Sildenafil
-ane	Inhaled anesthetics	Anesthesia	Halothane
-artan	Angiotensin receptor blockers	Hypertension	Losartan
-azepam, -zolam	Benzodiazepinea	Anxiety	Lorazepam, midazolam
-azine	Phenothiazines	Antipsychotic	Chlorpromazine
-azole	Azole antifungals	Antifungal	Ketoconazole
-barbital	Barbituates	Anxiety	Phenobarbital
-caine	Local anesthetics	Anesthesia	Lidocaine
-cillin	Penicillin antibiotics	Antibiotic	Ticarcillin
-cycline	Tetracyclines	Antibiotic	Doxycycline
-etine	Selective serotonin reuptake inhibitors	Depression	Fluoxetine
-feb, -fene	Selective estrogen response modifiers	Osteoporosis, breast cancer	Tamoxifen, clomifene
-floxacin	Fluoroquinolones	Antibiotics	Levofloxacin
-fungin	Echinocandins	Antifungal	Caspofungin
-grastim, gramostim	Granulocyte colony stimulating factors	Blood dyscrasias	Filgrastim, sargramostim
-ide	Loop diuretics	Hypertension	Furosemide

Continued

Suffix	Class	Clinical Use	Example
-ipine	Dihydropyridine calcium channel blockers	Hypertension	Nifedipine
-ipramine	Tricyclic antidepressants	Depression	Desipramine
-ium, -uronium	Nondepolarizing paralytics	Anesthesia	Vecuronium, atracurium
-lukast	LTD$_4$ receptor antagonist	Asthma	Montelukast
-navir	Protease inhibitor	Antiviral	Saquinavir
-olol	Beta blocker	Hypertension	Propranolol
-oxin	Cardiac glycoside	Arrhythmias	Digoxin
-phylline	Methylxanthine	Bronchodilator	Theophylline
-pril	ACE inhibitor	Hypertension	Lisinopril
-quine	Quinolone derivatives	Antimalarial	Chloroquine
-statin	HMG-CoA reductase inhibitors	Hyperlipidemia	Simvastatin
-tecan	Topoisomerase I inhibitor	Chemotherapy	Topotecan
-terol	β_2 agonist	Bronchodilator	Albuterol
-tidine	Second generation antihistamine	Allergies	Cimetidine
-tine	Allylamine antifungals	Antifungal	Terbinafine
-toposide	Topoisomerase II inhibitor	Chemotherapy	Etoposide
-triptan	5-HT$_{1B/1D}$ agonist	Migraines	Imi
-tropin	Pituitary hormone	Hormone deficiency	Somatotropin
-vaptan	Vasopressin receptor antagonist	Hypertension	Tolvaptan
-zosin	α_1 antagonist	Hypertension, BPH	Terazosin

MEDICATIONS THAT INHIBIT AND UP-REGULATE CYTOCHROME P450 ENZYMES

Human liver P450s (CYPs), and some of the drugs metabolized (substrates) inducers, and selective inhibitors. Note: Some P450 substrates can be potent competitive inhibitors and/or mechanism-based inactivators.

CYP	Substrates	Inducers	Inhibitors
1A2	Acetaminophen, antipyrine, caffeine, clomipramine, duloxetine, melatonin, phenacetin, ramelteon, tacrine, tamoxifen, theophylline, warfarin	Smoking, charcoal-broiled foods, cruciferous vegetables, lansoprazole, omeprazole	Galangin, furafylline, fluvoxamine
2A6	Coumarin, tobacco nitrosamines, nicotine (to cotinine and 2′–hydroxynicotine)	Efavirenz, rifampin, phenobarbital	Tranylcypromine, menthofuran, methoxsalen
2B6	Artemisinin, bupropion, clopidogrel, cyclophosphamide, efavirenz, ifosfamide, ketamine, S-mephobarbital, S-mephenytoin (N-demethylation to nirvanol), methadone, nevirapine, propofol, selegiline, sertraline, ticlopidine	Phenobarbital, cyclophosphamide	Clopidogrel, paroxetine, phencyclidine, sertraline, thiotepa, ticlopidine
2C8	Taxol, all-trans-retinoic acid	Rifampin, barbiturates	Gemfibrozil, montelukast, trimethoprim, quercetin, rosiglitazone, pioglitazone
2C9	Celecoxib, diclofenac, flurbiprofen, hexobarbital, ibuprofen, losartan, phenytoin, tolbutamide, trimethadione, sulfaphenazole, S-warfarin, ticrynafen	Barbiturates, carbamazepine, rifampin	Fluconazole, fluvoxamine, sulfaphenazole, tienilic acid
2C18	Tolbutamide, phenytoin	Phenobarbital	

Continued

CYP	Substrates	Inducers	Inhibitors
2C19	Diazepam, S-mephenytoin, naproxen, nirvanol, omeprazole, propranolol	Barbiturates, rifampin	N3-benzylnirvanol, N3-benzylphenobarbital, fluconazole, nootkatone, ticlopidine
2D6	Atomoxetine, bufuralol, bupranolol, clomipramine, clozapine, codeine, debrisoquine, desipramine, dextromethorphan, encainide, flecainide, fluoxetine, guanoxan, haloperidol, hydrocodone, 4 –methoxy-amphetamine, metoprolol, mexiletine, nebivolol, oxycodone, perphenazine, paroxetine, phenformin, propafenone, propoxyphene, risperidone, selegiline (deprenyl), sparteine, tamoxifen, tolterodine, thioridazine, timolol, tricyclic antidepressants, venlafaxine	Unknown	Bupropion, fluoxetine, paroxetine, quinidine
2E1	Acetaminophen, chlorzoxazone, enflurane, halothane, ethanol (a minor pathway)	Ethanol, isoniazid	Clomethiazole, disulfiram, diethyldithiocarbamate, diallyl sulfide, 4 –methylpyrazole
3A4[1]	Acetaminophen, alfentanil, amiodarone, aprepitant, astemizole, buspirone, cisapride, cocaine, conivaptan, cortisol, cyclosporine, dapsone, darunavir, dasatinib, diazepam, dihydroergotamine, dihydropyridines, diltiazem, erythromycin, ethinyl estradiol, everolimus, felodipine, fluticasone, gestodene, indinavir, lidocaine, lopinavir, lovastatin, macrolides, maraviroc, methadone, miconazole, midazolam, mifepristone, nifedipine, nisoldipine, paclitaxel progesterone, quetiapine, quinidine, rapamycin, ritonavir, saquinavir, sildenafil, simvastatin, sirolimus, spironolactone, sulfamethoxazole, sufentanil, tacrolimus, tamoxifen, terfenadine, testosterone, tetrahydrocannabinol, tolvaptan, tipranavir, triazolam, troleandomycin, vardenafil, verapamil	Avasimibe, barbiturates, carbamazepine, glucocorticoids, pioglitazone, phenytoin, rifampin, St. John's wort	Amprenavir, azamulin, boceprevir, clarithromycin, conivaptan, diltiazem, erythromycin, fluconazole, grapefruit juice (furanocoumarins), indinavir, itraconazole, ketoconazole, lopinavir, mibefradil, nefazodone, nelfinavir, posaconazole, ritonavir, saquinavir, telaprevir, telithromycin, troleandomycin, verapamil, voriconazole

Reproduced, with permission, from AJ, Katzung BG, Trevor AJ: *Basic & Clinical Pharmacology.* 13th ed. New York: McGraw-Hill Education; 2013.

CHAPTER 1
PHARMACOLOGY BASICS

I. PHARMACODYNAMICS

Dose-Response Curves

Comparison of Dose-Response Curves

Response Curves: Agonists and Antagonists

II. PHARMACOKINETICS

Drug Movement within the Body

Drug Solubility

Administration

Distribution and Binding

Metabolism

Elimination

Important Equations

Therapeutic Values

Dosing

TERMS TO LEARN

Agonist	A drug that activates its receptor upon binding.
Bioavailability	The percentage of administered dose that reaches the systemic circulation.
Chemical Antagonist	A drug that counters the effects of another by binding the drug and preventing its action.
Competitive Antagonist	A pharmacologic antagonist that can be overcome by increasing the dose of agonist.
EC_{50}	In graded dose-response curves, the concentration or dose that produces 50% of the maximum possible response; in quantal dose-response curves, the dose that causes the specified response in 50% of the population.
ED_{50}	Dose required to produce the desired effect in 50% of subjects.
Effector	Component of the biologic system that accomplishes the biologic effect after being activated by the receptor; often a channel or enzyme.
Efficacy	The maximum effect a drug can bring about, regardless of dose.
Graded Dose-Response Curve	A graph of the increasing responses to increasing doses of a drug.
Inert Binding Site	A component of the biologic system to which a drug binds without changing any function.
Irreversible Antagonist	A pharmacologic antagonist that cannot be overcome by increasing the dose of the agonist.
K_d	The concentration of drug that results in binding to 50% of the receptors.
LD_{50}	Dose that is lethal to 50% of subjects.
Partial Agonist	A drug that binds to its receptor but produces a smaller effect at full dosage than a full agonist.
pH	Inverse log of the hydrogen ion concentration, denotes the acidity or alkalinity of a substance.
Pharmacodynamics	The actions of the drug on the body.
Pharmacokinetics	The action of the body on the drug.
Pharmacologic Antagonist	A drug that binds to its receptor without activating it.

Pharmacology	The study of substances that interact with living systems through chemical reactions.
Physiologic Antagonist	A drug that counters the effects of another by binding to a different receptor and causing opposing effects.
pK_a	Inverse log of the ionization constant of an acid.
Potency	The dose or concentration required to bring about 50% of a drug's maximal effect.
Quantal Dose-Response Curve	A graph of the fraction of a population that shows a specified response to increasing doses of a drug.
Receptor	A component of the biologic system to which a drug binds to bring about a change in function of the system.
Receptor Site	The specific region of the receptor molecule at which the drug binds.
Spare Receptors	Receptors that do not have to bind drug in order for the maximum effect to be produced; ie, K_d greater than the EC_{50}; thought to exist if the maximal response is obtained at less than maximal receptor occupation levels.
TI_{50}	Drug dose that indicates the ratio of desired to undesired effects.

I. Pharmacodynamics

DOSE-RESPONSE CURVES

Type of Curve	Characteristics
Graded dose-response curve	• Unit and time are constant • Dose and effect are variable
Quantal dose-response curve	• Effect and time are constant • Dose and unit are variable • Yields safety information
Time action dose-response curve	• Unit is constant (ie, the same patient is used) • Dose, time, and effect are variable • Yields the time of onset of the action of the drug, the peak effect of the drug, and the duration of effect of the drug

COMPARISON OF DOSE-RESPONSE CURVES

Dose-Response Curve	Unit	Dose	Time	Effect
Graded	Constant	Variable	Constant	Constant
Quantal	Variable	Variable	Constant	Constant
Time Action	Constant	Variable	Variable	Variable

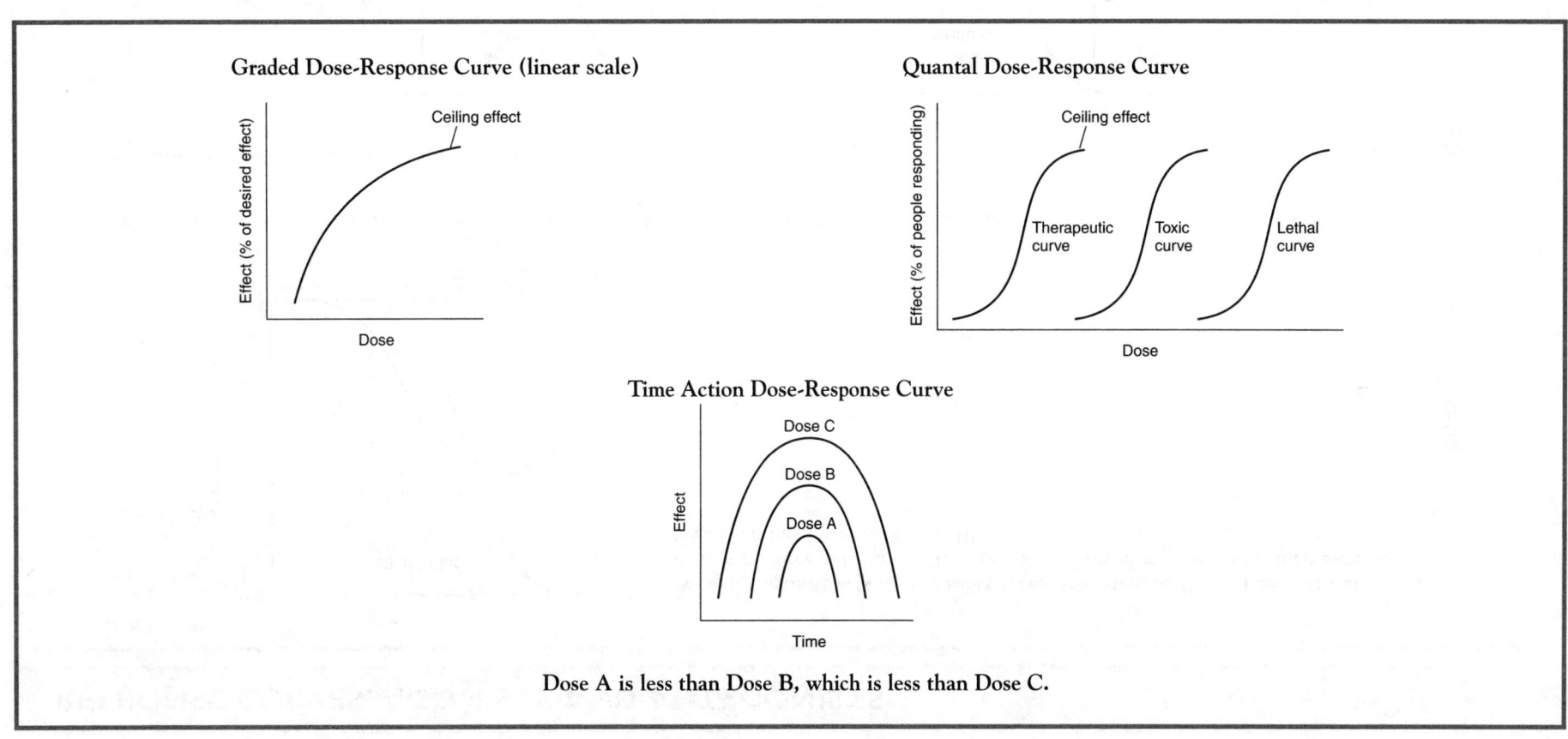

Dose A is less than Dose B, which is less than Dose C.

RESPONSE CURVES: AGONISTS AND ANTAGONISTS

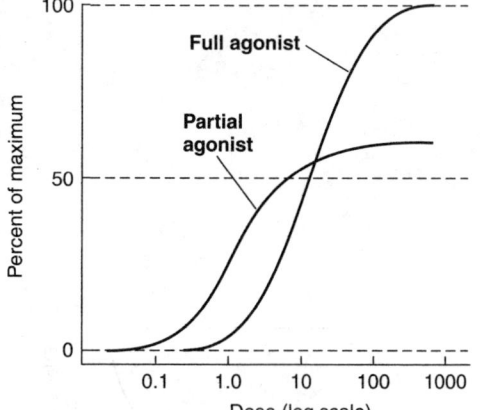

A partial agonist acts on the same receptor system as the full agonist but cannot produce as large an effect, no matter how much the dose is increased because it has lower maximal efficacy.

Reproduced, with permission, from Trevor AJ, Katzung BG, Masters SB: *Katzung & Trevor's Pharmacology Examination & Board Review*, 6th ed, p 14. Originally published by Appleton & Lange. © 2002 by the McGraw-Hill Companies, Inc.

A competitive agonist shifts the agonist curve to the right (A); an irreversible antagonist shifts the agonist curve downward (B).

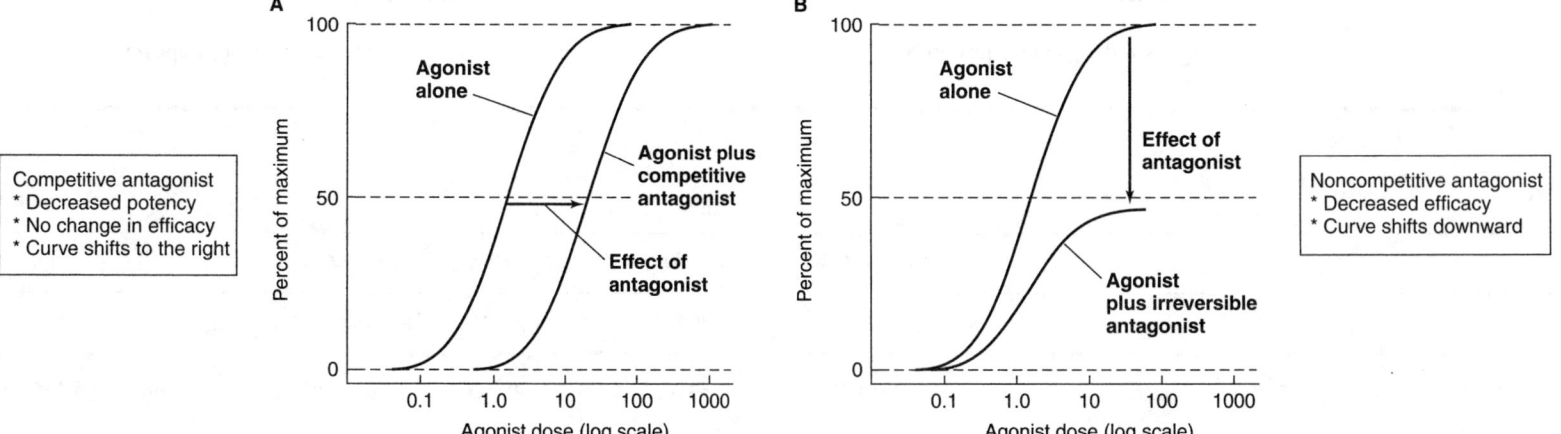

Reproduced, with permission, from Trevor AJ, Katzung BG, Masters SB: *Katzung & Trevor's Pharmacology Examination & Board Review*, 6th ed, p 15. Originally published by Appleton & Lange. © 2002 by the McGraw-Hill Companies, Inc.

II. Pharmacokinetics

DRUG MOVEMENT WITHIN THE BODY

Type of Movement	Requirements
Passive diffusion	Requires no energy
Facilitated diffusion	Requires specific transport mechanisms; no energy required
Active transport	Links energy consuming movement of substances to energy producing mechanisms

DRUG SOLUBILITY

- The movement of a drug within the body depends on the ionization state of the drug molecule. The Henderson-Hasselbalch equation can be used to determine the ionization state of a molecule at a specific pH:

$$pH = pK_a + \log \frac{\text{unprotonated form}}{\text{protonated form}}$$

- Aqueous solubility of a drug is proportional to the molecule's charge.
- Lipid solubility is *inversely* proportional to a molecule's charge.
- The pK_a value is specific to each molecule.

ADMINISTRATION

Route	Significant Features
Oral (PO)	Convenient; subject to first-pass metabolism by liver, which alters bioavailability
Intravenous (IV)	Rapid; 100% bioavailability
Intramuscular (IM)	Allows for larger amounts to be administered; higher bioavailability than PO; avoids first-pass metabolism
Subcutaneous (SC)	Slower absorption than IM; larger volumes of administration not possible
Buccal	Between the cheeks and gums; absorption without first-pass metabolism
Sublingual (SL)	Below the tongue; absorption without first-pass metabolism
Rectal (PR)	Less first-pass metabolism than PO administration
Inhalation	Allows for drug delivery directly to respiratory tissues; allows for rapid absorption due to large surface area of alveoli
Topical	Method of administration for local effect; slowest absorption rate
Transdermal (TD)	Skin application to achieve systemic effects

DISTRIBUTION AND BINDING

Distribution of a drug is determined by several factors:

- Blood flow to the organ
- The solubility of a drug
- The level of binding of drug (ie, to proteins within the blood)

Inert binding sites are locations on endogenous molecules that bind a drug, yielding no resultant effects. Examples of such binding sites include the plasma binding proteins, albumin, and α_1-acid glycoprotein.

METABOLISM

Functions	• Terminate drug activity • Activate drug activity (in which case, the drug administered is termed a prodrug)
Metabolic Reactions Phase 1	• Reactions that convert the parent drug to a more polar or reactive product • Reactions include: oxidation, reduction, deamination, and hydrolysis
Phase 2	• Conjugation reactions that link a polar group to the drug molecule to increase its water solubility • Polar moieties include glucuronate, acetate, gluathione, glycine, sulfate, and methyl
Sites of Metabolism	• Most drugs are metabolized by the liver. • The kidneys are another important site of metabolism. • The enzymes of degradation for a small number of drugs are spread widely throughout other tissues, including the blood and the wall of the GI tract.

ELIMINATION

Elimination determines the duration of action for most drugs, and it may take two forms:

- First order—The rate of elimination is proportional to the drug concentration, resulting in a constant half-life of elimination.

- Zero order—The rate of elimination is constant regardless of drug concentration, and the plasma concentration of the drug decreases linearly.

Comparison of First-Order and Zero-Order Elimination

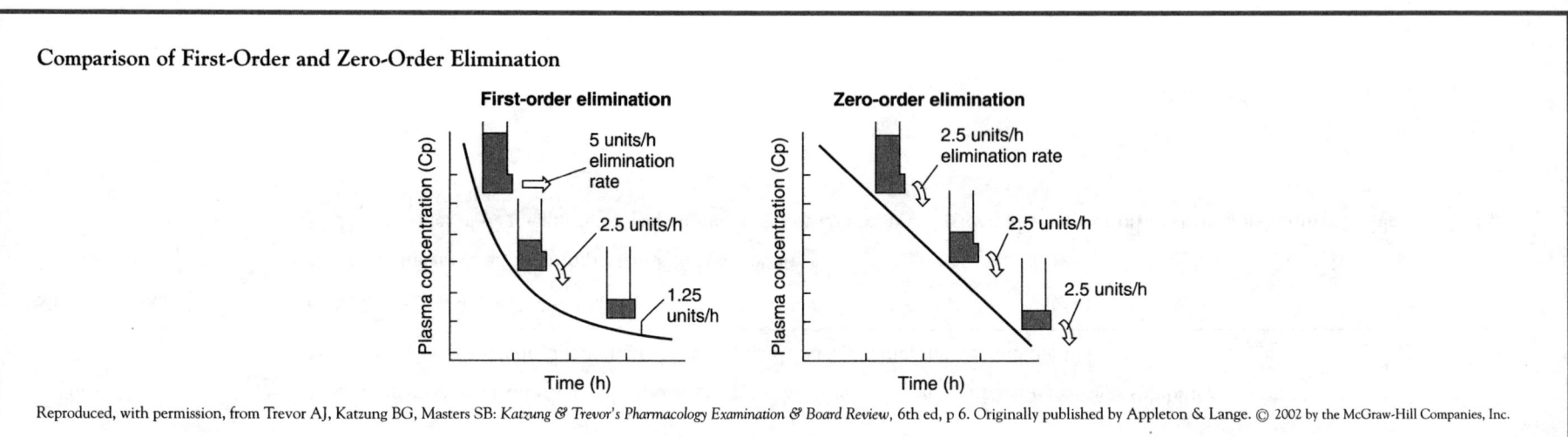

Reproduced, with permission, from Trevor AJ, Katzung BG, Masters SB: *Katzung & Trevor's Pharmacology Examination & Board Review*, 6th ed, p 6. Originally published by Appleton & Lange. © 2002 by the McGraw-Hill Companies, Inc.

IMPORTANT EQUATIONS

Determination	Description	Equation
Clearance (CL)	Relates the rate of elimination to the concentration of drug within the plasma	$CL = \dfrac{\text{Rate of elimination of a drug}}{\text{Plasma concentration of the drug}}$
Volume of distribution (V_d):	Relates the amount of drug in the body to the concentration of drug in the plasma	$V_d = \dfrac{\text{Amount of drug in the body}}{\text{Plasma concentration of the drug}}$
pH	The inverse log of the hydrogen ion concentration	$pH = pK_a + \log \dfrac{(\text{unprotonated form})}{(\text{protonated form})}$
Half-life	The length of time required for 50% of a drug to be cleared from the system. (The equation applies to drugs eliminated by first-order kinetics.)	$t_{1/2} = \dfrac{0.693 \times V_d}{CL}$
Renal dose	The adjusted dose of a drug administered to patients with decreased renal function; takes into account the patient's renal function via creatinine clearance.	$\text{Corrected dose} = \text{average dose} \times \dfrac{\text{patient's creatinine clearance}}{100\ \text{mL / min}}$

THERAPEUTIC VALUES

Therapeutic Index (TI_{50})	• Numerical indication of the safety of a drug • The higher the value, the safer the drug • $TI_{50} = LD_{50} / ED_{50}$ • LD_{50}: the dose that is lethal in 50% of the population • ED_{50}: the dose that is effective in 50% of the population
Therapeutic Window	• The area between the minimum therapeutic concentration (trough) and the minimum concentration to produce toxicity (peak). • For some drugs, these values vary greatly from patient to patient and must be titrated for each patient. • For drugs with small therapeutic windows, smaller doses with more frequent dosing are preferred.

DOSING

Type of Dose	Description	Equation
Maintenance Dose	The regimen used to achieve plasma concentration of a drug within the therapeutic window; a steady state, this value is equal to the elimination rate.	$\text{Dosing rate} = \dfrac{\text{clearance} \times \text{desired plasma concentration}}{\text{bioavailability}}$
Loading Dose	The dose required to achieve therapeutic plasma concentrations quickly.	$\text{Loading dose} = \dfrac{\text{volume of distribution} \times \text{desired plasma concentration}}{\text{bioavailability}}$

CHAPTER 2
ANTIMICROBIAL MEDICATIONS

I. CELL WALL SYNTHESIS INHIBITORS

Antibiotic Mechanisms of Action

Summary of Penicillins

Classification of Penicillins

Penicillins and β-Lactamase–Resistant Penicillins

Extended-Spectrum Penicillins

Combination Preparations of Penicillins

Classification of Cephalosporins

Summary of Cephalosporins

Effectiveness of Cephalosporins Against G– and G+ Organisms

First-Generation Cephalosporins

Second-Generation Cephalosporins

Third-, Fourth-, and Fifth-Generation Cephalosporins

Other β-Lactams

Other Cell Wall Synthesis Inhibitors: Non–β-Lactams

II. 30S ANTIBACTERIAL AGENTS

Aminoglycosides

Tetracyclines

III. 50S ANTIBACTERIAL AGENTS

Macrolides, Clindamycin, and Chloramphenicol

IV. OTHER ANTIBACTERIAL AGENTS

Classification of Other Antibacterial Agents

Antibacterial Synergy of Sulfonamides and Trimethoprim

Sulfonamides, Trimethoprim, and Fluoroquinolones

Miscellaneous Antibiotics

V. ANTIVIRAL AGENTS

Classification of Antiviral Agents

Major Sites of Drug Action on Viral Replication

Tricylic Amines, Guanosine Analog, Glycoproteins, and Pyrophosphonate Derivative

Nucleoside Analogues

Nucleotide Analogue

Nucleoside Reverse Transcriptase Inhibitors

Non–Nucleoside Reverse Transcriptase Inhibitors

Protease Inhibitors

VI. ANTIFUNGAL AGENTS

Mechanisms of Action and Classification of Antifungal Agents

Antifungals: Drug Facts

VII. ANTIPROTOZOAL AGENTS

Therapeutic Classification of Antiprotozoal Agents

Antiprotozoals: Drug Facts

VIII. ANTIHELMINTHIC AGENTS

Antihelminthics: Drug Facts

IX. ANTIMYCOBACTERIAL AGENTS

Available Agents for Tuberculosis and Leprosy Plus Atypical Mycobacterial Agents

Antimycobacterials: Drug Facts

Blackwater Fever	Syndrome of hemolytic anemia, hemoglobinuria, and renal failure associated with massive parasitemia.
Cinchonism	Poisoning syndrome associated with quinine, quinidine, and *Cinchona*; symptoms include tinnitus, deafness, headache, blurry vision, and nausea.
Disulfiram Reaction	Syndrome that occurs due to coingestion of alcohol and disulfiram; disulfiram blocks aldehyde dehydrogenase, leading to accumulation of acetaldehyde; symptoms include nausea, headache, flushing, and hypotension.
G6PD Deficiency	Lack of enzyme important in the oxidation/reduction capabilities of the red blood cell; deficiency leads to hydrogen peroxide accumulation, which causes hemolysis. Hemolysis often associated with drugs that produce oxidative stress (eg, sulfonamides).
Gray Baby Syndrome	May be caused by deficiency of a hepatic enzyme required for the degradation of chloramphenicol or impaired renal function; syndrome is characterized by circulatory collapse, cyanosis (gray color), acidosis, abdominal distention, coma, and death.
Lassa Fever	A hemorrhage febrile illness associated with arenavirus infection.
Mazzotti Reaction	Syndrome of fever, urticaria, tender lymphadenopathy, arthralgias, abdominal pain, edema, hypotension, and tachycardia seen with treatment of microfilariasis with Ivermectin, Praziquantel, and Albendazole.
Methemoglobinemia	Accumulation of methemoglobin, which is a form of hemoglobin with a low oxygen affinity. Methemoglobinemia results in pseudocyanosis, tissue hypoxia, and death.
Stevens-Johnson Syndrome	Immunologic reaction characterized by lesions of the skin and mucous membranes; involves both the mouth and eyes.
Superinfection	A novel infection in addition to a pre-existing one.
Trachoma	Chronic inflammation of the conjunctiva caused by *Chlamydia trachomatis*.

I. Cell Wall Synthesis Inhibitors

ANTIBIOTIC MECHANISMS OF ACTION

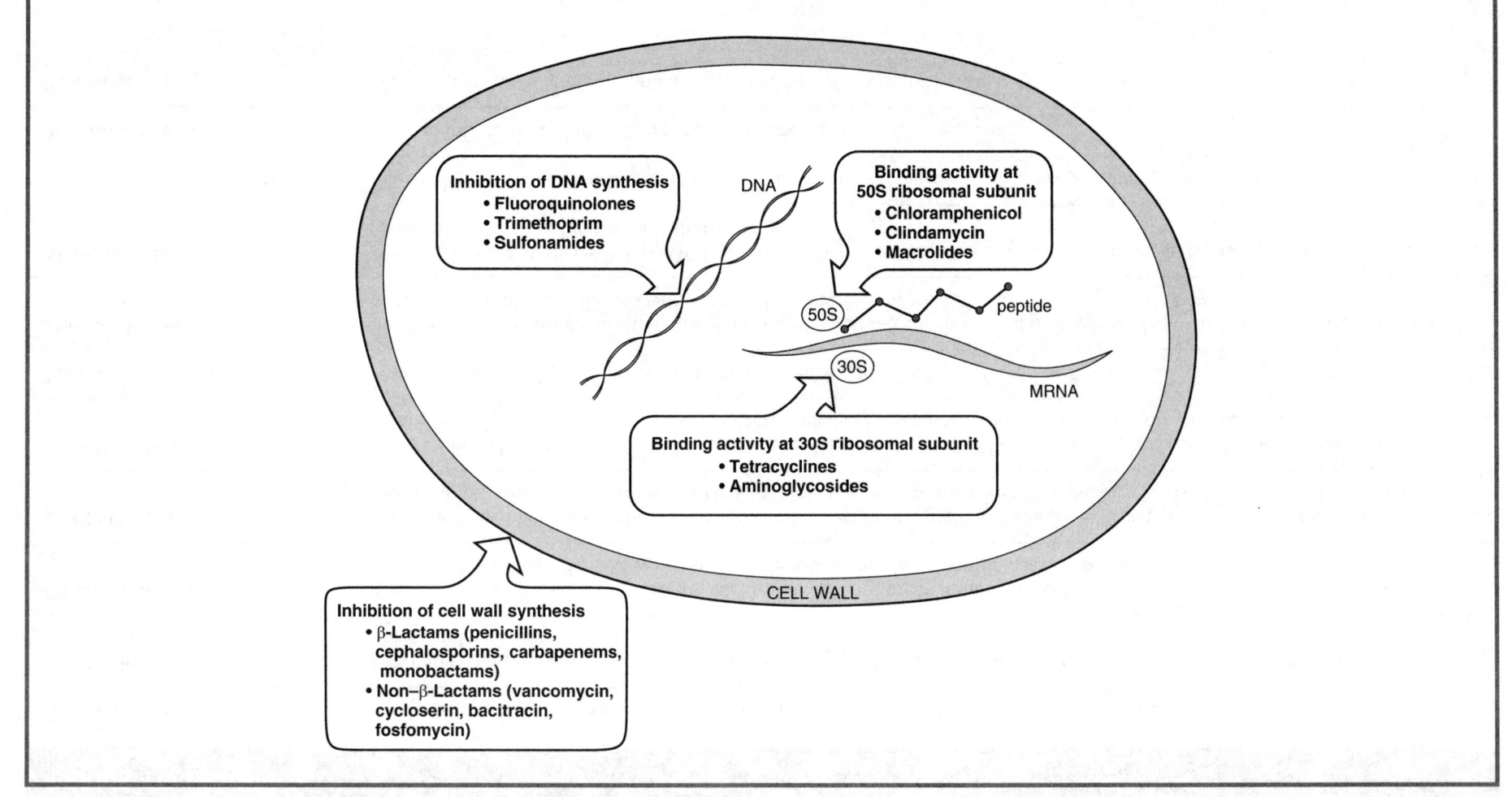

SUMMARY OF PENICILLINS

Types	Class	Pharmacokinetics	Mechanisms of Action and of Resistance	Clinical Uses and Spectrum of Activity	Drawbacks and Side Effects
Penicillin G and penicillin V	• Derivatives of 6-aminopenicillanic acid • Contain a β-lactam ring	• **A:** PO absorption inhibited by coingestion with meals • **M:** Polar compounds, so not extensively metabolized • **E:** Most are excreted in urine via glomerular filtration and tubular secretion; prolong effects by administration with Probenecid, which blocks tubular secretion	**MOA:** • Bactericidal • Inhibit cell wall synthesis by these three steps: 1. Bind drug to specific receptors in the bacterial cell wall 2. Inhibit transpeptidase enzymes that cross-link linear peptidoglycan chains that form bacterial cell walls 3. Activate autolytic enzymes causing lesions in the bacterial cell wall **Resistance:** • β-Lactamase produced by bacteria causes enzymatic hydrolysis of the β-lactam ring, which results in loss of antibacterial activity	• Narrow spectrum • β-Lactamase susceptible • Streptococci, meningococci, G+ bacilli, spirochetes	• Most staphylococci are drug resistant **Allergic reactions:** • Ranges from urticaria to hemolytic anemia and anaphylaxis • Assume cross-reactivity throughout class • 10% of persons who are allergic to penicillin are also allergic to cephalosporins **GI disturbances:** • Nausea and diarrhea caused by oral medications via direct irritation or overgrowth of G+ organisms or yeast • Ampicillin implicated in pseudomembranous colitis **Cation toxicity:** • Possible toxic effects of Na^+ or K^+ when high doses of penicillin salts are used in patients with CV or renal disease
Nafcillin, oxacillin, cloxacillin, and dicloxacillin				• Very narrow spectrum • β-Lactamase resistant • β-Lactamase producing staphylococci (except MRSA)	
Ampicillin and amoxicillin				• Wider spectrum • β-Lactamase susceptible • Similar therapeutic spectrum to narrow spectrum penicillins; also covers enterococci, *Salmonella*, *Proteus*, *Listeria monocytogenes*, and *Moraxella catarrhalis* • Action enhanced when combined with inhibitors of β-lactamase (ie, clavulanic acid and sulbactam)	
Carbenicillin, piperacillin, and ticarcillin				• β-Lactamase susceptible • Similar therapeutic spectrum to narrow spectrum penicillins; also covers several G− rods (*Pseudomonas*, *Enterobacter*, and some *Klebsiella* species) • Action enhanced when combined with inhibitors of β-lactamase (ie, clavulanic acid and sulbactam)	

CLASSIFICATION OF PENICILLINS

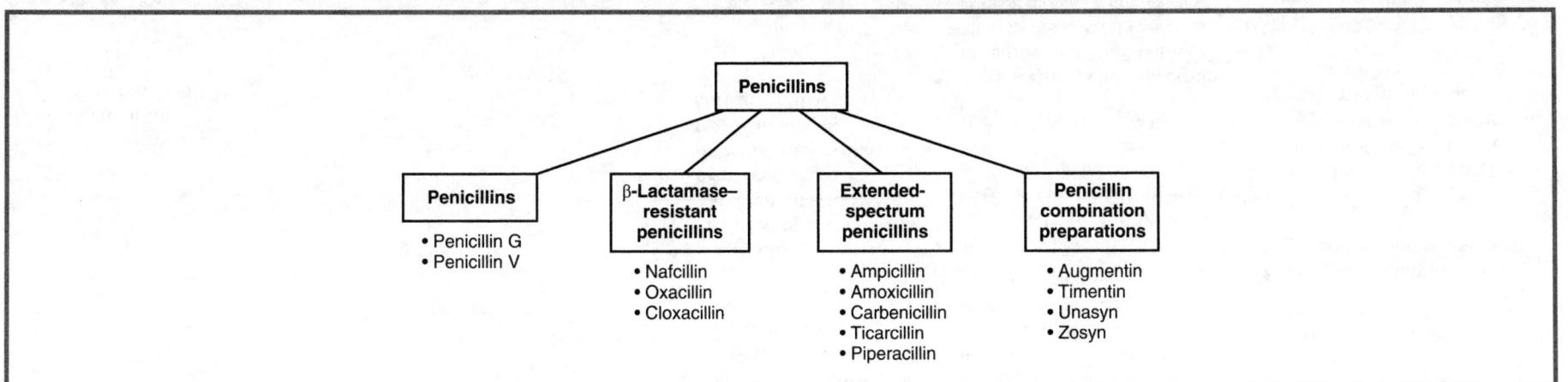

PENICILLINS AND β-LACTAMASE–RESISTANT PENICILLINS

Drug	Pharmacokinetics	Spectrum of Activity	Clinical Uses and General Information	Drawbacks and Side Effects
Penicillin G (Pfizerpen)	• **A:** PO, IM or IV; 20% absorbed following PO administration (80% inactivated) • **B:** Low protein binding • **D:** Limited distribution; crosses BBB (poorly) • **M:** Hepatic • **E:** Rapidly excreted unchanged in urine • Effects prolonged via IM administration of poorly soluble penicillin G salts, which dissolve slowly and enter the blood (ie, procaine penicillin G or benzathine penicillin G)	• G+ cocci (*Enterococcus, Staphylococcus, Streptococcus*) • G− cocci (*Neisseria*) • G+ bacilli (*Actinomyces, Bacillus, Clostridium, Corynebacterium, Listeria*) • Spirochetes (*Leptospira, Treponema*)	• Infections caused by bacteria listed in Spectrum of Activity column • First antibiotic discovered by Alexander Fleming in 1929 • Erysipelas • Facial space infections • Lyme disease • Neurosyphilis • Lepto spirosis	• Widespread resistance due to β-lactamase • Resistance develops quickly • Lack of PO administration • Broader spectrum preferable (lacks coverage of most G− organisms)
Penicillin V (Apo-Pen-VK, Novo-Pen-VK, Nu-Pen-VK)	• **A:** PO; absorbed in the duodenum (stable in acidic pH) • **B:** High protein binding • **D:** Widely distributed • **M:** Hepatic • **E:** Parent drug and metabolites excreted in urine	• β-Lactamase producing *Staphylococcus* and *Streptococcus* ONLY • Not active against G− organisms • Not active against MRSA	• Infections caused by bacteria listed in Spectrum of Activity column • Streptococcal pharyngitis • Erysipelas • Actinomycosis • Resistant staphylococcal infections	• Poor bioavailability • Narrow spectrum • Requires multiple daily dosing

Continued

PENICILLINS AND β-LACTAMASE–RESISTANT PENICILLINS (Continued)

Drug	Pharmacokinetics	Spectrum of Activity	Clinical Uses and General Information	Drawbacks and Side Effects
Nafcillin	• **A:** IV, IM • **M:** Hepatic • **B:** High protein binding widely distributed • **D:** Crosses the BBB (poor penetration) • **E:** In feces		• Skin and soft tissue infections • Prosthetic joint infections • MSSA endocarditis	• Nephrotoxicity (less than methicillin) • Bone marrow suppression • Hepatotoxicity • Induces P450 enzymes
Oxacillin (Bactocill)	• **A:** IV and IM • **M:** Hepatic metabolism to inactive metabolites • **E:** Metabolites excreted in urine and feces		• Prosthetic joint infections • MSSA infections (pneumonia, scalded skin syndrome, brain abscess, osteomyelitis)	• Nephrotoxicity (less than methicillin) - interstitial nephritis • Hepatotoxicity • Bone marrow suppression
Dicloxacillin	• **A:** PO • **B:** High protein binding • **E:** Unchanged in urine		• Prosthetic joint infection suppressive therapy	• Hepatotoxicity • Bone marrow depression • Nephrotoxicity (interstitial nephritis) • Induces P450 enzymes

EXTENDED-SPECTRUM PENICILLINS

Drug	Pharmacokinetics	Spectrum of Activity	Clinical Uses and General Information	Drawbacks and Side Effects
Ampicillin	• **A:** IV and PO; well absorbed with PO administration • **B:** Low protein binding • **D:** Widely distributed, crosses only inflamed meninges • **E:** Unchanged in urine	• G+ cocci (*Streptococcus, Enterococcus*) • G+ rods (*Clostridium, Listeria*) • G− cocci (*Neisseria*)	• UTI • CAP in children • Neonatal prophylaxis for GBS • Sepsis/meningitis • Often used in combination with β-lactamase inhibitors • Endocarditis (treatment and prophylaxis)	• β-Lactamase sensitive • Not useful for treating G+ infections (use penicillin G) • Hypersensitivity reactions • CDAD
Amoxicillin (Moxatag)	• **A:** PO; better absorption than PO ampicillin • **B:** Low protein binding • **D:** Widely distributed, only crosses inflamed meninges • **E:** Unchanged in urine	• G+ cocci (*Enterococcus, Staphylococcus, Streptococcus*) • G− cocci (*Neisseria*) • G− rods (*Escherichia coli, Haemophilus influenzae, Salmonella, Helicobacter pylori, Proteus*) • Spirochete (*Borrelia*)	• ENT infections • GU infections • Lyme disease • Lower respiratory tract infections • Skin infections • *H. pylori* eradication • Endocarditis prophylaxis • Prosthetic joint infections (treatment and prophylaxis)	

Continued

EXTENDED-SPECTRUM PENICILLINS (Continued)

Drug	Pharmacokinetics	Spectrum of Activity	Clinical Uses and General Information	Drawbacks and Side Effects
Carbenicillin (Geocillin)	• **A:** PO; indanyl ester form for PO administration • **E:** Unchanged in urine	• G+ cocci (*Enterococcus*) • G− rods (*Enterobacter, E. coli, Morganella, Proteus, Providencia, Pseudomonas*)	• UTIs • Prostatitis	• β-Lactamase sensitive • Often combined with an aminoglycoside (cannot be mixed in same IV bag)
Ticarcillin	• **A:** IV • **B:** Low protein binding • **E:** Unchanged in urine	• G+ cocci (*Staphylococcus, Streptococcus, Enterococcus*) • G− cocci (*Neisseria*) • G− rods (non–β-lactamase producing forms of *Branhamella, Citrobacter, Enterobacter, E. coli, H influenzae, Klebsiella, Morganella, Proteus, Providencia, Pseudomonas, Salmonella, Serratia*)	• GU infections • Intra-abdominal infections • Pneumonia • Septicemia • Skin infections • Pseudomonal infections	• Hypersensitivity reactions • Almost exclusively available as combinations with β-lactamase inhibitors (see combination preparations of penicillins)
Piperacillin	• **A:** IV, IM • **B:** Low plasma protein binding • **D:** Widely distributed; does not cross BBB • **E:** Unchanged in urine	• G+ cocci (*Streptococcus, Enterococcus*) • G+ bacilli (*Clostridium*) • G− cocci (*Neisseria*) • G− rods (*Bacteriodes, Citrobacter, Enterobacter, E. coli, H. influenzae, Klebsiella, Proteus, Pseudomonas, Serratia*)	• Prosthetic joint infections • GU infections • Intra-abdominal infections • Pneumonia • Septicemia • Surgical prophylaxis • Pseudomonal keratitis	

COMBINATION PREPARATIONS OF PENICILLINS

Drug	Pharmacokinetics	Spectrum of Activity	Clinical Uses and General Information	Drawbacks and Side Effects
Amoxicillin and clavulinic acid (Augmentin)	• A: PO • See Amoxicillin	• G+ cocci (*Staphylococcus, Streptococcus, Enterococcus*) • G− cocci (*Neisseria*) • G− rods (*Bacteroides Eikenella, Enterobacter, E. coli, Fusobacterium, H. influenzae, Klebsiella, Moraxella, Proteus*)	• Bronchitis • Pneumonia • Otitis • Sinusitis • Skin infections • UTIs	• Clavulinic acid function to make it β-lactamase resistant
Ticarcillin and clavulinic acid (Timentin)	• A: IV • See Ticarcillin	• G+ cocci (*Staphylococcus, Streptococcus, Enterococcus*) • G+ bacilli (*Clostridium*) • G− cocci (*Neisseria*) • G− rods (*Bacteroides, Branhamella, Citrobacter, Enterobacter, E. coli, Fusobacterium, H. influenzae, Klebsiella, Morganella, Proteus, Providencia, Pseudomonas, Salmonella, Serratia*)	• Gynecologic infections • Intra-abdominal infections • Pneumonia • Septicemia • Skin infections • UTIs	• Local reactions at injection site • Tazobactam, sulbactam, and clavulinic acid function to make these β-lactamase resistant
Ampicillin and Sulbactam (Unasyn)	• A: IV or IM • See Ampicillin	• G+ cocci (*Staphylococcus, Streptococcus, Enterococcus*) • G+ rods (*Clostridium*) • G− cocci (*Neisseria*) • G− rods (*Bacteroides, E. coli, H. influenzae, Klebsiella, Moraxella, Proteus, Providencia*)	• Gynecologic infections • Intra-abdominal infections • Skin infections	
Piperacillin and Tazobactam (Zosyn)	• A: IV • See Piperacillin	• G+ cocci (*Staphylococcus, Streptococcus, Enterococcus*) • G+ rods (*Clostridium*) • G− cocci (*Neisseria*) • G− rods (*Bacteroides, Fusobacterium, Klebsiella, Moraxella, Morganella, Proteus, Pseudomonas, Serratia*)	• Gynecologic infections • Intra-abdominal infections • Pneumonia • Skin infections	

CLASSIFICATION OF CEPHALOSPORINS

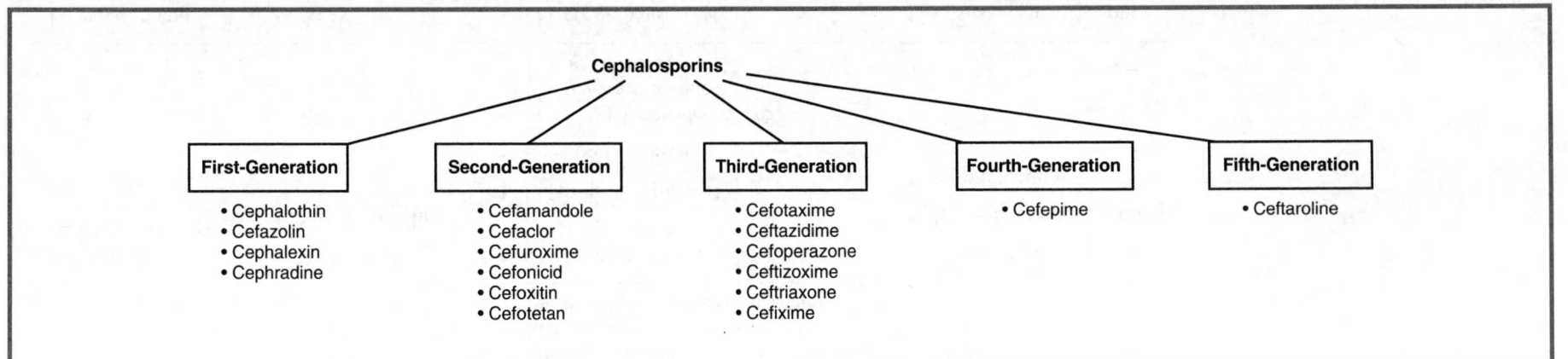

Cephalosporins

First-Generation	Second-Generation	Third-Generation	Fourth-Generation	Fifth-Generation
• Cephalothin	• Cefamandole	• Cefotaxime	• Cefepime	• Ceftaroline
• Cefazolin	• Cefaclor	• Ceftazidime		
• Cephalexin	• Cefuroxime	• Cefoperazone		
• Cephradine	• Cefonicid	• Ceftizoxime		
	• Cefoxitin	• Ceftriaxone		
	• Cefotetan	• Cefixime		

SUMMARY OF CEPHALOSPORINS

Type*	Pharmacokinetics	Mechanisms of Action and of Resistance	Spectrum of Activity	Clinical Uses and General Information	Drawbacks and Side Effects
First-generation	• **A:** IV and PO • **D:** Most first- and second-generation cephalosporins do not cross BBB, even with inflamed meninges • **M:** Cephalosporins with side chains may undergo hepatic metabolism • **E:** Majority excreted unchanged in urine via active tubular secretion; EXCEPT cefoperazone and ceftriaxone, which are mainly excreted in bile	**MOA:** • Bactericidal • Bind to site on organism cell wall • Inhibit cell wall synthesis **Resistance:** • Less resistance than seen with penicillins because cephalosporins have a more stable β-lactam ring • Via production of β-lactamase • Via decreased membrane permeability to cephalosporins • Via mutation in the binding site on cell membrane	• Best for G+ cocci • Susceptible to β-lactamase	• Surgical prophylaxis	**Allergic reactions:** 5–15% of persons allergic to penicillin are also allergic to cephalosporins • Anaphylaxis (contraindicated in patients with penicillin anaphylaxis) • Fever • Skin rash • Nephritis • Granulocytopenia • Hemolytic anemia **Other reactions:** • MTT side chain blocks Vitamin K epoxide reductase (likely cause of thrombocytopenia) and aldehyde dehydrogenase (causes disulfiram like reaction) • Local irritation (at injection site) and thrombophlebitis • Increase nephrotoxicity of aminoglycosides when administered together
Second-generation			• Extended G− coverage • Less activity against G+ organisms than first generation	• Parenteral administration required (except for cefaclor)	
Third-generation			• Exquisitely active against G− bacilli • Not useful for G+ infections	• All administered parenterally (except for cefixime) • Almost all cross BBB • Generally reserved for serious infections (ie, bacterial meningitis)	
Fourth-generation			• G+ activity of first-generation • Best for G− organisms • More resistant to β-lactamases produced by G− organisms	• Better for infections caused by β-lactamase–producing G− organisms including *Enterobacter*, *Haemophilus*, *Neisseria* • In general, to prevent resistance, administer cephalosporins with other agents such as aminoglycosides. • Generally, cephalosporins are used prophylactically	
Fifth-generation			• G− and G+ coverage • MRSA coverage	• As the generation increases, so does the potency and spectrum, especially against G− species (decreases somewhat against G+ species)	

*All contain the β-lactam ring.

EFFECTIVENESS OF CEPHALOSPORINS AGAINST G− AND G+ ORGANISMS

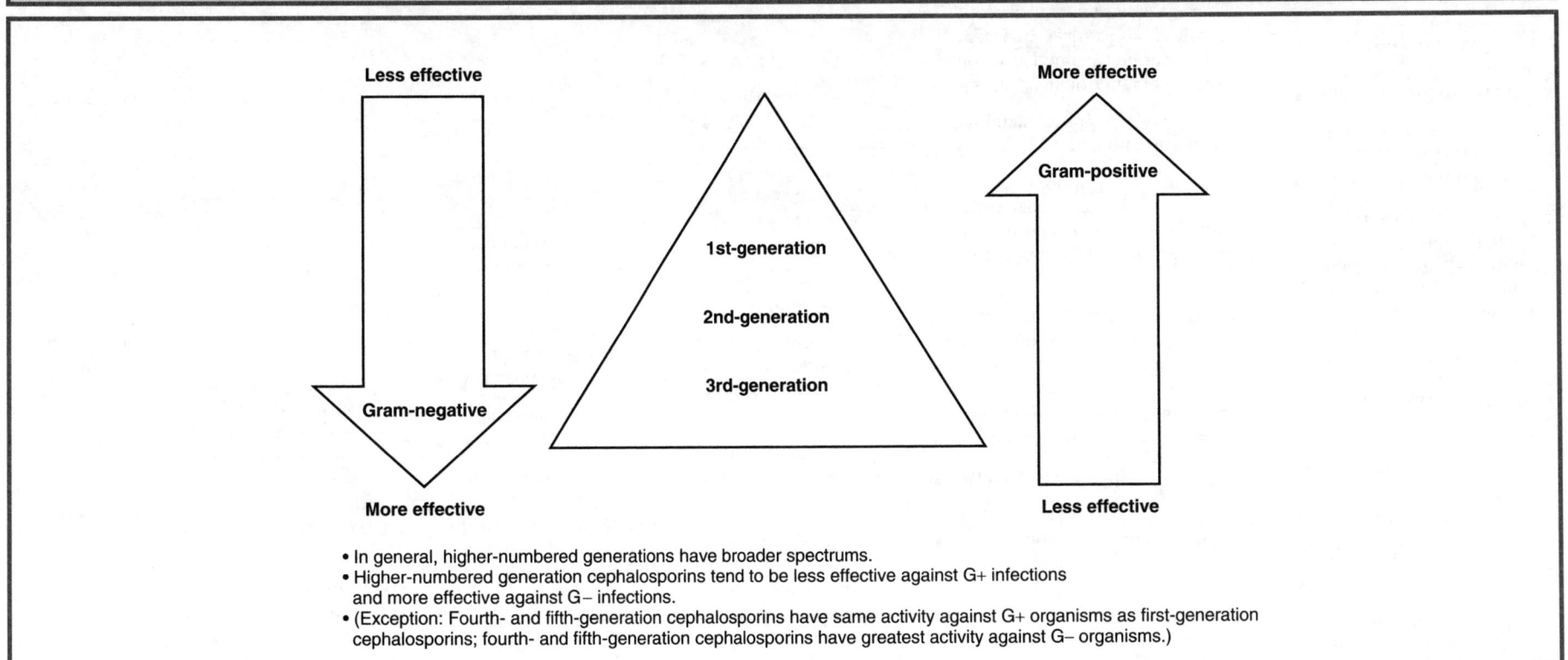

- In general, higher-numbered generations have broader spectrums.
- Higher-numbered generation cephalosporins tend to be less effective against G+ infections and more effective against G− infections.
- (Exception: Fourth- and fifth-generation cephalosporins have same activity against G+ organisms as first-generation cephalosporins; fourth- and fifth-generation cephalosporins have greatest activity against G− organisms.)

FIRST-GENERATION CEPHALOSPORINS

Drug	Pharmacokinetics	Spectrum of Activity	Clinical Uses and General Information	Drawbacks and Side Effects
Cephalothin (Keflin)	• **A:** IM • $t_{1/2}$: 30–60 minutes • **E:** In urine	• Best generation cephalosporins for G+ infections • Susceptible to β-lactamases	• Surgical prophylaxis • Pneumonia • UTI • Cholecystitis	**Allergic reactions:** ∼10% of persons allergic to penicillins are also allergic to cephalosporins • Anaphylaxis (contraindicated in patients with penicillin anaphylaxis)
Cefazolin (Ancef, Kefzol)	• **A:** IV and IM • **D:** Penetrates well into most tissues; does not cross BBB • $t_{1/2}$: 1.4–2 hours • **E:** Unchanged in urine		• Surgical prophylaxis • Pneumonia • UTI	• Fever • Skin rash • CDAD **Other reactions:** • Local irritation (at injection site) and thrombophlebitis • Increase nephrotoxicity of aminoglycosides when administered together
Cephalexin (Keflex)	• **A:** PO • $t_{1/2}$: 0.9–1.5 hours • **E:** Unchanged in urine		• ENT infections • GU infections • Skin and soft tissue infections	
Cephradine (Anspor, Velosef)	• **A:** PO, IV, and IM • $t_{1/2}$: 1.3 hours • **E:** Unchanged in urine		• UTI • Skin and soft tissue infections • Pneumonia • Prostatitis	

SECOND-GENERATION CEPHALOSPORINS

Drug	Pharmacokinetics	Spectrum of Activity	Clinical Uses and General Information	Drawbacks and Side Effects
Cefamandole (Mandol) (no longer available in the United States)	• A: IV and IM • $t_{1/2}$: 0.5–1.2 hours • E: Unchanged in urine	• More G− coverage than first-generation cephalosporins • Less G+ coverage than first-generation cephalosporins	• Surgical prophylaxis • Skin and soft tissue infections • Pneumonia	**Allergic reactions:** 5–15% of persons allergic to penicillin are also allergic to cephalosporins • Anaphylaxis (contraindicated in patients with penicillin anaphylaxis)
Cefaclor (Ceclor)	• A: PO • $t_{1/2}$: 0.6–0.9 hour • E: Unchanged in urine		• Pharyngitis • Tonsillitis • Otitis • Pneumonia • UTI • Skin and soft tissue infections	• Fever • Skin rash • CDAD • Pseudomembranous colitis **Other reactions:**
Cefuroxime (Ceftin, Zinacef)	• A: PO, IM, IV • D: Only second-generation drug to cross BBB • $t_{1/2}$: 1.2–1.9 hours • E: Unchanged in urine		• Pharyngitis • Tonsillitis • UTI • Skin and soft tissue infections • Bronchitis • Gonorrhea • Lyme disease	• MTT side chain: causes hypo-prothrombinemia and inhibits aldehyde dehydrogenase (can cause disulfiram-like reaction with alcohol ingestion); seen with cefamandole and cefotetan • Local irritation (at injection site) and thrombophlebitis
Cefonicid (Monocid)	• A: IV and IM • $t_{1/2}$: 3.5–4.5 hours • E: Unchanged in urine		• Surgical prophylaxis • UTI	• Increase nephrotoxicity of aminoglycosides when administered together

Cefoxitin (Mefoxin)	• **A:** IM and IV • $t_{1/2}$: 0.7–1.1 hours • **E:** Majority excreted unchanged in urine	• Surgical prophylaxis (especially for abdominal surgery and for mixed anaerobic infections such as those found in peritonitis and diverticulitis)	• Aspiration pneumonia • PID • Complicated intra-abdominal infections
Cefotetan (Cefotan)	• **A:** IM and IV • $t_{1/2}$: 3–4.6 hours • **E:** Unchanged in urine	• Surgical prophylaxis • UTI • Skin and soft tissue infections • PID	

THIRD-, FOURTH-, AND FIFTH-GENERATION CEPHALOSPORINS

Drug	Pharmacokinetics	Spectrum of Activity	Clinical Uses and General Information	Drawbacks and Side Effects
Cefotaxime (Claforan)	• **A:** IM and IV • **D:** Widely distributed; crosses BBB • $t_{1/2}$: 1 hour • **M:** Partial hepatic • **E:** Parent drug and metabolites excreted in urine	• Exquisitely active against G− bacilli • Not useful for G+ infections	• Surgical prophylaxis • Septicemia • Gonorrhea • GU infections • Lower respiratory tract infections	**Allergic reactions:** 5–15% of persons allergic to penicillin are also allergic to cephalosporins • Anaphylaxis (contraindicated in patients with penicillin anaphylaxis) • Skin rash • CDAD
Ceftazidime (Tazicef, Fortaz)	• **A:** IM and IV • **D:** Widely distributed; crosses BBB • $t_{1/2}$: 1.4–2 hours • **E:** Unchanged in urine		• UTIs • Pneumonia • Bone and joint infections • Intra-abdominal infections • Septicemia • Skin and soft tissue infections	• Pseudomembranous colitis • Granulocytopenia **Other reactions:** • MTT side chain: causes hypoprothrombinemia and inhibits aldehyde dehydrogenase (can cause disulfiram-like reaction with alcohol ingestion); seen with cefoperazone
Cefoperazone (not available in the United States)	• **A:** IM and IV • **D:** Widely distributed; does not cross BBB • $t_{1/2}$: 1.6–2.4 hours • **E:** Majority excreted unchanged in feces; remainder unchanged in urine		• Severe infections (including pyelonephritis)	• Local irritation (at injection site) and thrombophlebitis • Increase nephrotoxicity of aminoglycosides when administered together
Ceftizoxime (Cefizox)	• **A:** IM and IV • $t_{1/2}$: 1.4–1.7 hours • **E:** Unchanged in urine		• PID • Lower respiratory tract infections • UTI • Gonorrhea	

Ceftriaxone (Rocephin)	• **A:** IM and IV • $t_{1/2}$: 4.3–8.7 hours • **E:** Unchanged in feces and urine		• Meningitis • Lower respiratory tract infections • Skin and soft tissue infections • Surgical prophylaxis • UTIs • Gonorrhea • PID • Intra-abdominal infections	
Cefixime (Suprax)	• **A:** PO • **D:** Widely distributed • $t_{1/2}$: 3–4 hours • **E:** Majority excreted unchanged in urine		• Bronchitis • Otitis media • Pharyngitis • Tonsillitis • UTI • Gonorrhea	

Fourth-Generation

Cefepime (Maxipime)*	• **A:** IM and IV • **D:** Widely distributed; crosses BBB • **M:** Minimal hepatic • $t_{1/2}$: 2 hours • **E:** Majority excreted unchanged in urine	• Same activity against G+ organisms as first-generation cephalosporins • Greatest activity against G− organisms • Good activity against *Pseudomonas*, Enterobacteriaceae, *Staphylococcus aureus*, and *Streptococcus pneumoniae*	• Intra-abdominal infections • Skin and soft tissue infections • UTI • Pneumonia • Neutropenic fever (monotherapy)	• Hypersensitivity reactions • CDAD • Pseudomembranous colitis

Fifth-Generation

Ceftaroline (Teflaro)	• **A:** IV • **M:** Metabolized in plasma • **E:** Majority excreted in urine	• As above with MRSA coverage	• Skin and soft tissue infections • Pneumonia	

*Indicates only fourth-generation cephalosporin in the table.

OTHER β-LACTAMS

Drug	Pharmacokinetics	Spectrum of Activity	Clinical Uses and General Information	Drawbacks and Side Effects
Carbapenem				
Imipenem (Primaxin)	• **A:** IV • **D:** Penetrates tissues well; crosses BBB • **M:** Inactivated in renal tubules (coadministered with cilastatin, which inhibits this enzymatic inactivation) • **E:** In urine	• G− rods • G+ organisms • Anaerobes	• Reserved for infections resistant to other medications • Less susceptible to β-lactamase inactivation • Combined with cilastatin to decrease renal metabolism/inactivation • Lower respiratory tract infections • Bone and joint infections • Intra-abdominal infections • GU infections • Skin and soft tissue infections	• CNS toxicity (ie, seizures, confusion) • Hypersensitivity reactions • CDAD • Pseudomembranous colitis
Meropenem (Merrem)	• **A:** IV • **D:** Penetrates tissues well; crosses BBB • **E:** Unchanged in urine	• Similar spectrum to imipenem • Greater activity against G− aerobes • Less effective against G+ organisms	• Reserved for infections resistant to other medications • Less susceptible to β-lactamase inactivation • Neonatal meningitis • Not metabolized by renal tubule enzymes therefore does not require cilastatin coadministration • Intra-abdominal infections • Less risk of CNS toxicity than imipenem • Skin and soft tissue infections	

| Ertapenem (Invanz) | • **A:** IM, IV
• **M:** Hepatic (minimal)
• **E:** Primarily excreted unchanged in urine | • Similar spectrum to imipenem | • Reserved for infections resistant to other medications
• Complicated intra-abdominal infections
• Complicated skin and soft structure infections
• Complicated UTI
• Acute pelvic infections
• Community-acquired pneumonia | |

Monobactam

| Aztreonam (Azactam) | • **A:** IM and IV
• **E:** Majority excreted unchanged in urine | • G− rods (including pseudomonas) | • Relatively resistant to β-lactamase inactivation
• Can be used in patients who are allergic to penicillin
• UTI
• Severe systemic illnesses
• Meningitis | • Skin rashes
• Elevation of serum aminotransferases
• CDAD
• Pseudomembranous colitis
• Neutropenia |

OTHER CELL WALL SYNTHESIS INHIBITORS: NON–β-LACTAMS

Drug	Pharmacokinetics	Mechanisms of Action and of Resistance	Spectrum	Clinical Uses	Drawbacks and Side Effects
Vancomycin (Vancocin)	• **A:** IV and PO; PO form poorly absorbed • **D:** Widely distributed; crosses inflamed meninges • **E:** 90% excreted unchanged in urine	**MOA:** • Binds to end of nascent protein • This inhibits transglycosylase, which elongates the protein • Thus, elongation and cross-linking are prevented **Resistance:** • Via modification at binding site on peptidoglycan	• G+ organisms	• Used for serious infections caused by drug-resistant G+ organisms • Infections caused by MRSA • Infections caused by penicillin-resistant pneumococci • Oral forms for the treatment of CDAD or *S. aureus* enterocolitis	• Chills • Fever • Phlebitis • Ototoxicity • Nephrotoxicity • Red man syndrome: flushing, erythema, and pruritis which seems to be a rate-dependent infusion reaction
Cycloserine (Seromycin)	• **A:** PO • **D:** Widely distributed • **E:** Majority excreted unchanged in urine	**MOA:** • Structural analog of D-alanine • Inhibits incorporation of D-alanine into pentapeptide side chain of peptidoglycan	• G+ organisms • G− organisms	• Infections caused by *Mycobacterium tuberculosis* that is resistant to other first-line agents	• CNS toxicity (eg, tremors, psychosis, seizures)
Bacitracin	• **A:** Topical, ophthalmic • **E:** Small absorbed amounts are excreted in urine	**MOA:** • Interferes with late stage of cell wall synthesis	• G+ organisms	• Superficial skin infections • Ophthalmologic infections	• Nephrotoxic (thus, systemic use is not indicated)
Fosfomycin (Monurol)	• **A:** PO and IV (only PO approved in the United States) • **E:** Majority excreted unchanged in urine	**MOA:** • Interferes with early stage of cell wall synthesis **Resistance:** • Via inadequate transport of the drug into the cell	• G+ organisms (*Enterococcus faecalis*) • G− organisms (*E. coli*)	• Uncomplicated UTIs	• Diarrhea

II. 30S Antibacterial Agents

AMINOGLYCOSIDES

Drug	Pharmacokinetics		Mechanisms of Action and of Resistance	Spectrum of Activity	Clinical Uses and General Information	Drawbacks and Side Effects
Streptomycin	• A: IM	• A: Poor PO absorption due to ionization, IM and IV well absorbed • D: Widely distributed, crosses inflamed meninges only • E: Urine	**MOA:** • Bactericidal • Binds to 30S ribosomal subunit • Causes abnormal peptide synthesis • Synergistic action with β-lactams **Resistance:** • Via genetic change leading to impaired drug entry into the cell • Via mutation at the binding site on the 30S ribosomal subunit • Via enzymatic degradation by organism	• Aerobic G-rods • Limited activity against facultative anaerobes in the presence of oxygen • Transportation across the cytoplasmic membrane can be inhibited by acidic, hyperosmolar, and anaerobic environments	• Tuberculosis (second-line agent) • Plague • Tularemia • Streptococcal and enterococcal endocarditis • UTIs • Brucellosis • Buruli ulcers • Chancroid granuloma inguinale	• Drug resistance is fairly widespread (therefore they are often used with second- and third-generation cephalosporins) • Optic nerve toxicity (seen with streptomycin) • Allergic skin reactions (most seen with neomycin) • Neuromuscular blockade—rare (decreased Ach release at NMJ can cause respiratory paralysis)
Gentamicin	• A: IM, IV				• Similar uses as above • Hospital-acquired pneumonia • PID • Cholangitis • Complicated diverticulitis	• Cannot be physically mixed with β-lactams due to acid/base neutralization reaction • Nephrotoxicity of the proximal tubular cells (increased with concurrent use of cephalosporins)
Tobramycin (Tobi, Tobi Podhaler)	• A: IM, IV, inhaled				• Infections from organisms resistant to other aminoglycosides • Inhaled form used to treat infections in cystic fibrosis patients	• Ototoxicity (occurs in fetus as well) (worsened with concurrent use of loop diuretics)

Continued

AMINOGLYCOSIDES (Continued)

Drug	Pharmacokinetics	Mechanisms of Action and of Resistance	Spectrum of Activity	Clinical Uses and General Information	Drawbacks and Side Effects
Neomycin (Neo-Fradin)	• **A:** PO, topical			• Preoperative bowel sterilization • Treatment of hepatic encephalopathy and chronic hepatic insufficiency • Topical use for skin infections • Most nephrotoxic, so systemic use is contraindicated	☞ **AMINO** **A**–Allergic skin reactions (mostly with Neomycin) **M**–Mixing with β-lactams causes inactivation secondary to neutralization reaction **I**–Induction of resistance fairly common (often mixed with second- and third-generation cephalosporins) **N**–Nephrotoxicity, Neurotoxicity **O**–Ototoxicity, Optic nerve toxicity
Amikacin	• **A:** IM, IV			• Hospital-acquired pneumonia • Meningitis	
Netilmicin (Netromycin)				• Infections from organisms resistant to other aminoglycosides	
Kanamycin				• Peritonitis following surgical contamination • Systemic infections	
Paromomycin	• **A:** PO			• Acute and chronic intestinal amebiasis • Hepatic coma	

TETRACYCLINES

Drug	Pharmacokinetics		Mechanisms of Action and of Resistance	Spectrum of Activity	Clinical Uses	Drawbacks and Side Effects
Tetracycline (Sumycin)	• **A:** PO, topical	• **A:** Good PO absorption (impaired when consumed with foods containing Ca, Fe, or Al); IV (can inhibit platelet aggregation); IM (tends to be painful) • **D:** Extremely good distribution; crosses healthy meninges and placenta • **E:** Enterohepatic cycling; glomerular filtration with urinary excretion EXCEPT doxycycline which undergoes inactivation in the GI tract excretion in feces	**MOA:** • Bacteriostatic • Enter organism via diffusion or via active transport pump • Bind (reversibly) to 30S ribosomal subunit • Inhibit protein synthesis **Resistance:** • Via impaired transport pump (decreased influx or increased efflux) • Via mutation at the ribosomal subunit binding site • Via enzymatic inactivation	• G+ organisms • G− organisms • Coverage of many atypical pathogens	• Drugs of choice for infections caused by atypical pathogens including: – Brucella – Borrelia (burgdorferi, recurrentis) – Burkholderia pseudomallei – Calymmatobacterium granulomatis – Chlamydia – Coxiella burnetii – Entamoeba histolytica – Leptospira – Mycoplasma pneumoniae – Mycobacterium marinum – Plasmodium – Rickettsia – Treponema – Vibrio (cholerae, vulnificus) • Demeclocycline can be used to treat SIADH by inhibiting the action of ADH at the renal tubule • Doxycycline useful in patients with renal failure due to its fecal excretion	• Bony structure dysplasia and discoloration; also occurs in fetus • Photosensitivity • GI irritation; eg, nausea, vomiting, and diarrhea • Alters normal flora; can precipitate pseudomembranous colitis caused by C. difficile • Hepatotoxicity, usually in pregnant women • Nephrotoxicity • Vestibular reactions; eg, vertigo, dizziness, nausea, and vomiting
Oxytetracycline (Terramycin)	A: PO, IM					
Demeclocycline (Declomycin)	A: PO					
Minocycline (Minocin, Solodyn, Dynacin)	A: PO					
Doxycycline (Vibramycin, Adoxa, Doryx Monodox, Doxy morgidox, Avidoxy ocudox, Oracea Alodox, Oraxyl)	A: PO, IV					

III. 50S Antibacterial Agents

MACROLIDES, CLINDAMYCIN, AND CHLORAMPHENICOL

Drug	Pharmacokinetics	Mechanisms of Action and of Resistance	Spectrum of Activity and Clinical Uses	Drawbacks and Side Effects
Macrolides				
Erythromycin (Erythrocin, EryPed, EES)	• **A:** PO, Ophthalmic, Topical • **M:** Hepatic (P450) • **E:** Parent drug and metabolites excreted primarily in feces	**MOA:** • Bacteriostatic • Binds to the 23S rRNA of the 50S subunit and blocks protein synthesis **Resistance:** • Develops primarily by mutations in the binding site on the 50S subunit	• Legionnaire's disease • Lymphogranuloma venereum • Nongonococcal urethritis • Pertussis • Streptococcal pharyngitis/tonsillitis	• GI distress (abdominal cramping, diarrhea, nausea) • QT prolongation (esp with erythromycin) • Inhibits cytochrome P450 enzymes
Clarithromycin (Biaxin)	• **A:** PO • **M:** Hepatic (P450) • **E:** Parent drug and metabolites excreted in urine; metabolites excreted in feces		• Similar spectrum as erythromycin plus *H. influenzae*, *Bordetella*, and *M. catarrhalis* • Bronchitis • Sinusitis • Treatment and prevention of disseminated *Mycobacterium avium* infections • Treatment of disseminated *M. intracellulare* • *H. pylori* in patients with PUD • Pharyngitis • Tonsillitis • Pneumonia • Uncomplicated skin and soft tissue infections	• Inhibits cytochrome P450 enzymes

Azithromycin (Zithromax, Z-Pak, Zmax)	• **A:** PO, IV • **M:** Hepatic • **E:** Parent drug and metabolites excreted in feces		• Sinusitis • *Chlamydia trachomatis* • Pneumonia • Disseminated M. *avium* disease	
Fidaxomicin (Dificid)	• **A:** PO • **M:** Intestinal hydrolysis • **E:** Parent drug and metabolites excreted in feces		• CDAD	

Miscellaneous 50S Antibacterial Agents

Clindamycin (Cleocin)	• **A:** PO, IV, IM • **M:** Hepatic • **E:** Metabolites excreted in urine and feces	**MOA:** • Inhibits bacterial protein synthesis similarly to macrolides **Resistance:** • Via methylation of the binding site on the 50S ribosomal subunit • Via enzymatic inactivation	• Amnionitis • Canine bite wounds • Gangrenous pyomyositis • PID • GAS pharyngitis • Prosthetic joint infections • Toxic shock syndrome	• CDAD
Chloramphenicol	• **A:** IV • **M:** Hepatic (P450) • **E:** Parent drug and metabolites excreted in urine	**MOA:** • Bacteriostatic • Inhibits activity of bacterial 50S ribosomal subunit **Resistance:** • Via enzymatic inactivation	• Very broad spectrum of activity (G+ and G−) • Serious systemic infections • Pediatric meningitis	• Blood dyscrasias (aplastic anemia, granulocytopenia, thrombocytopenia) • Gray syndrome • Inhibits cytochrome P450 enzymes

Continued

MACROLIDES, CLINDAMYCIN, AND CHLORAMPHENICOL (Continued)

Drug	Pharmacokinetics	Mechanisms of Action and of Resistance	Spectrum of Activity and Clinical Uses	Drawbacks and Side Effects
Linezolid (Zyvox)	• **A:** IV • **M:** Hepatic • **E:** Parent drug and metabolites excreted primarily in urine	**MOA:** • Bacteriostatic for staphlycocci and enterococci • Bactericidal for streptococci • Binds to 50S ribosomal subunit thus inhibiting protein synthesis **Resistance:** • Via mutation of the 23 subunit of the 50S ribosomal subunit	• Pneumonia • Skin and soft structure infections • VRE infections	• Headache • Diarrhea • Blood dyscrasias (anemia, leukopenia, thrombocytopenia)
Quinupristin and dalfopristin (Synercid)	• **A:** IV • **M:** Hepatic • **E:** Parent drug and metabolites excreted primarily in feces	**MOA:** • Bacteriostatic for vancomycin-resistant *Enterococcus faecium* (VREF) • Bactericidal for staphylcoccus (MSSA and MRSA) • Binds to two different sites of the 50S ribosomal subunit thus inhibiting protein synthesis	• Skin and soft structure infections	• Arthralgia • Myalgias • Hyperbilirubinemia

IV. Other Antibacterial Agents

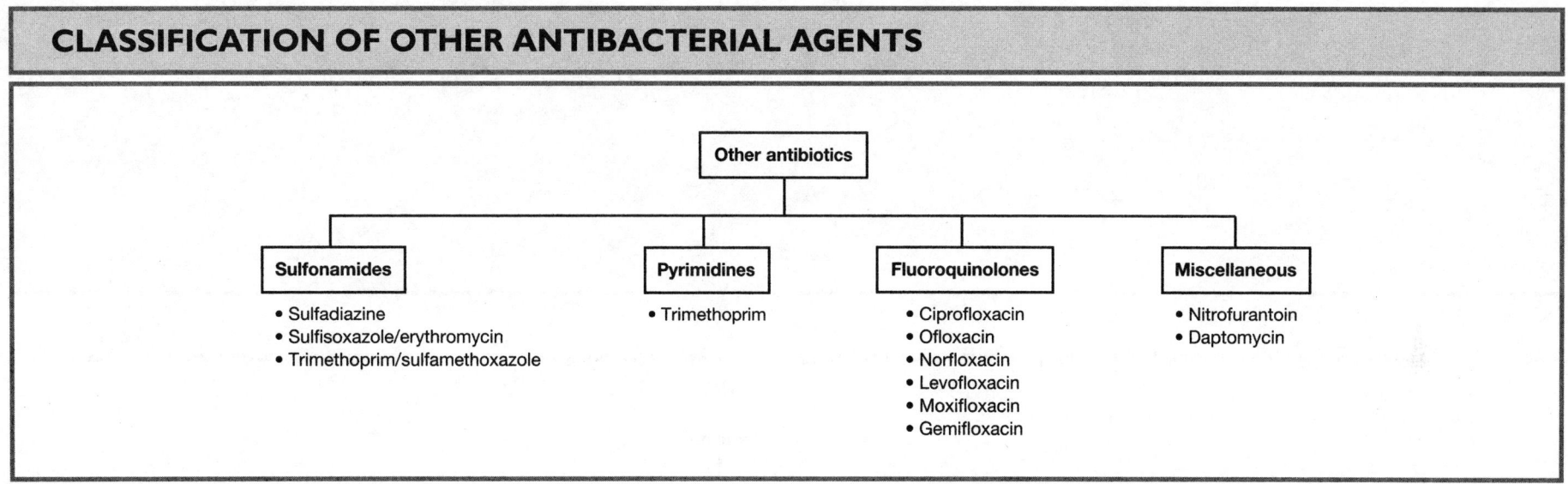

CLASSIFICATION OF OTHER ANTIBACTERIAL AGENTS

Other antibiotics

Sulfonamides
- Sulfadiazine
- Sulfisoxazole/erythromycin
- Trimethoprim/sulfamethoxazole

Pyrimidines
- Trimethoprim

Fluoroquinolones
- Ciprofloxacin
- Ofloxacin
- Norfloxacin
- Levofloxacin
- Moxifloxacin
- Gemifloxacin

Miscellaneous
- Nitrofurantoin
- Daptomycin

ANTIBACTERIAL SYNERGY OF SULFONAMIDES AND TRIMETHOPRIM

Inhibition of two successive steps in tetrahydrofolic acid formation results in antibacterial synergy.

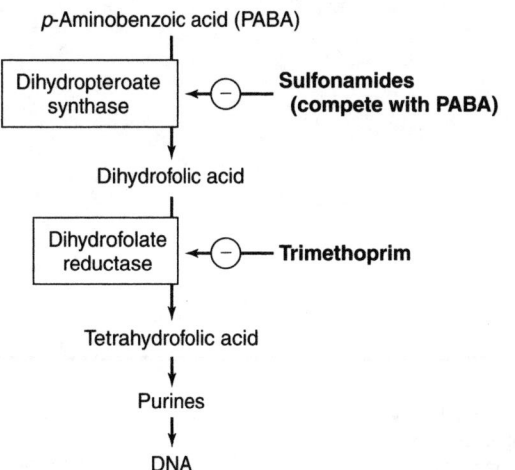

Reproduced, with permission, from Trevor AJ, Katzung BG, Masters SB: *Katzung & Trevor's Pharmacology Examination & Board Review,* 6th ed, p 404. Originally published by Appleton & Lange. © 2002 by the McGraw-Hill Companies, Inc.

SULFONAMIDES, TRIMETHOPRIM, AND FLUOROQUINOLONES

Drugs	Pharmacokinetics	Mechanisms of Action and of Resistance	Clinical Uses	Drawbacks and Side Effects
Sulfonamides				
Sulfadiazine	• **A:** PO • **M:** Hepatic (P450) • **E:** Parent drug and metabolites excreted in urine	**MOA:** • Bacteriostatic • Structural analogs of PABA • Competitively inhibits the conversion of PABA to folic acid by dihydropteroate synthase • Lack of folic acid inhibits bacterial growth by interfering with microbial DNA synthesis	• Rheumatic fever prophylaxis • *Toxoplasma gondii* encephalitis	• Crystalluria • Rash • Hepatitis • Pancreatitis • Inhibits cytochrome P450 enzymes
Sulfisoxazole/ erythromycin (ESP, Eryzole, Pediazole)	• **A:** PO • **M:** Hepatic (P450) • **E:** Parent drug and metabolites excreted in urine	**Resistance:** • Via microbial overproduction of PABA • Via loss of cell permeability to sulfonamides • Via structural changes that occur in bacterial dihydropteroate synthase	• OM (pediatric)	• Rash • Hepatotoxicity • Inhibits cytochrome P450 enzymes
Trimethoprim/ sulfamethoxazole (Bactrim)	• **A:** PO, IV • **M:** Hepatic (P450) (both components) • **E:** Parent drug and metabolites excreted in urine (both components)		• UTIs • Traveler's diarrhea • *Shigellosis* • Sepsis • Treatment and prophylaxis of *Pneumocystis jirovecii* • PNA • *Nocardiosis* • Acute exacerbation of chronic bronchitis	• Hemolysis in patients with G6PD deficiency • Rash • Hepatotoxicity • Nephrotoxicity • Pancreatitis • Kernicterus in infants • Inhibits cytochrome P450 enzymes

Continued

SULFONAMIDES, TRIMETHOPRIM, AND FLUOROQUINOLONES (Continued)

Drugs	Pharmacokinetics	Mechanisms of Action and of Resistance	Clinical Uses	Drawbacks and Side Effects
Trimethoprim (TMP, Prismol)	• **A:** PO • **M:** Hepatic (P450) (minor) • **E:** Primarily excreted unchanged in urine	**MOA:** • Bacteriostatic (weakly bactericidal when combined with sulfonamides) • Inhibits dihydrofolate reductase • Inhibits bilateral growth by interfering with microbial DNA synthesis • Synergistic with sulfonamides **Resistance:** • Via reduced cell permeability • Via overproduction of dihydrofolate reductase • Via microbial modification of enzyme with decreased drug binding	• Acute OM	• GI: nausea, vomiting, and diarrhea • Rash • Hematologic: megaloblastic anemia, leukopenia, neutropenia • Inhibits cytochrome P450 enzymes

Second-Generation

Ciprofloxacin (Cipro)	• **A:** IV, PO • **M:** Minor hepatic (P450) metabolism • **E:** Excreted primarily unchanged in urine	**MOA:** • Bactericidal • Prevents DNA unwinding required for transcription and translation by inhibiting DNA gyrase **Resistance:** • Via alteration of membrane permeability into the bacterial cell • Via microbial modification of DNA gyrase structure	• Anthrax • Bone and joint infections • Febrile neutropenia • Gonococcal infections • Infectious diarrhea • Lower respiratory tract infections • Nosocomial PNA • Prostatitis • Sinusitis • Skin and soft structure infections • Typhoid fever	• CNS: headache, tremor, confusion • GI: abnormal LFTs, hepatotoxicity, nausea, diarrhea • MS: tendinitis, increased tendon rupture • Neuro: exacerbation of myasthenia gravis • CV: QT prolongation • Inhibits cytochrome P450 enzymes
Ofloxin (Floxin)	• **A:** PO • **E:** Excreted primarily unchanged in urine		• Cervicitis/urethritis • Exacerbation of chronic bronchitis • PID • Prostatitis • Skin and soft structure infection • UTI	
Norfloxacin (Noroxin)	• **A:** IV, PO • **M:** Hepatic • **E:** Metabolites and parent drug excreted in urine and feces		• Prostatitis • Gonococcal infections • UTI	

Continued

SULFONAMIDES, TRIMETHOPRIM, AND FLUOROQUINOLONES (Continued)

Drugs	Pharmacokinetics	Mechanisms of Action and of Resistance	Clinical Uses	Drawbacks and Side Effects
Third-Generation				
Levofloxacin (Levaquin)	• **A:** IV, PO • **M:** Minor hepatic metabolism • **E:** Excreted primarily unchanged in urine		• Anthrax • Bacterial rhinosinusitis • Exacerbation of chronic bronchitis • Plague • PNA • Prostatitis • Skin and soft structure infection • UTI	
Fourth-Generation				
Moxifloxacin (Avelox)	• **A:** IV, PO • **M:** Hepatic • **E:** Metabolites and parent drug excreted in urine and feces		• Bacterial rhinosinusitis • CABP • Complicated intra-abdominal infections • Exacerbation of chronic bronchitis • M. *genitalium* infections • Skin and soft structure infection	
Gemifloxacin (Factive)	• **A:** PO • **M:** Hepatic (minor) • **E:** Metabolites and parent drug excreted in feces and urine		• Exacerbation of chronic bronchitis • CABP	
Quinolones	**General Antimicrobial Action**			
First-Gen Second-Gen Third-Gen Fourth-Gen	N/A (no longer available) G− (including *Pseudomonas*); S. *aureus* (no MRSA or pneumococcus coverage); some atypical coverage G− (including *Pseudomonas*); G+ (including pneumococcus and S. *aureus* [no MRSE coverage]); more atypical coverage than second-gen Third-gen coverage, better coverage of pneumococcus but less pseudomonal coverage			

MISCELLANEOUS ANTIBIOTICS

Drugs	Pharmacokinetics	Mechanisms of Action and of Resistance	Clinical Uses	Drawbacks and Side Effects
Nitrofurantoin (Macrobid, Furadantin, Macrodantin)	• **A:** PO • **M:** Metabolized in tissues • **E:** Parent drug and metabolites excreted primarily in urine	• Bacteriostatic • Bactericidal in urine at therapeutic doses • Metabolites alter or inactivate ribosomal subunits in bacteria interfering with protein synthesis, metabolism, and cell wall synthesis	• Prophylaxis and treatment of UTI	• Brown urine discoloration
Daptomycin (Cubicin)	• **A:** IV • **E:** Primarily excreted unchanged in urine	• Bactericidal • Binds to bacterial cell membranes causing depolarization which inhibits synthesis of protein, DNA, and RNA	• Complicated skin and soft structure infections MRSA/MSSA bacteremia or native valve endocarditis	• Diarrhea • Vomiting • Hypokalemia

V. Antiviral Agents

CLASSIFICATION OF ANTIVIRAL AGENTS

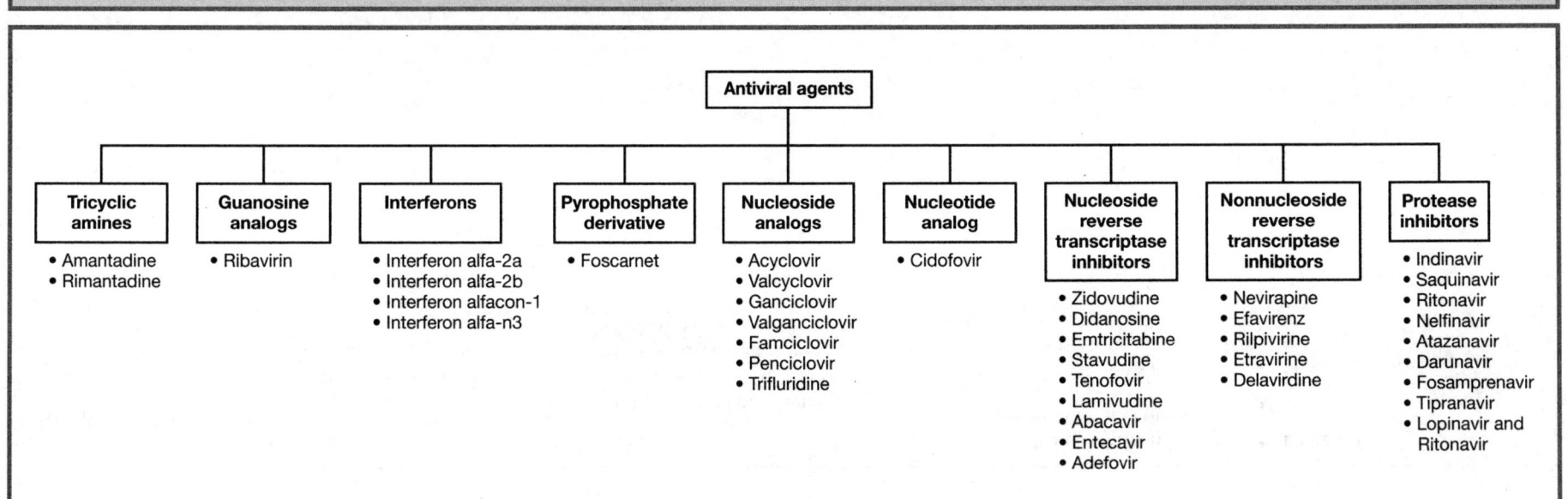

Antiviral agents

Tricyclic amines
- Amantadine
- Rimantadine

Guanosine analogs
- Ribavirin

Interferons
- Interferon alfa-2a
- Interferon alfa-2b
- Interferon alfacon-1
- Interferon alfa-n3

Pyrophosphate derivative
- Foscarnet

Nucleoside analogs
- Acyclovir
- Valcyclovir
- Ganciclovir
- Valganciclovir
- Famciclovir
- Penciclovir
- Trifluridine

Nucleotide analog
- Cidofovir

Nucleoside reverse transcriptase inhibitors
- Zidovudine
- Didanosine
- Emtricitabine
- Stavudine
- Tenofovir
- Lamivudine
- Abacavir
- Entecavir
- Adefovir

Nonnucleoside reverse transcriptase inhibitors
- Nevirapine
- Efavirenz
- Rilpivirine
- Etravirine
- Delavirdine

Protease inhibitors
- Indinavir
- Saquinavir
- Ritonavir
- Nelfinavir
- Atazanavir
- Darunavir
- Fosamprenavir
- Tipranavir
- Lopinavir and Ritonavir

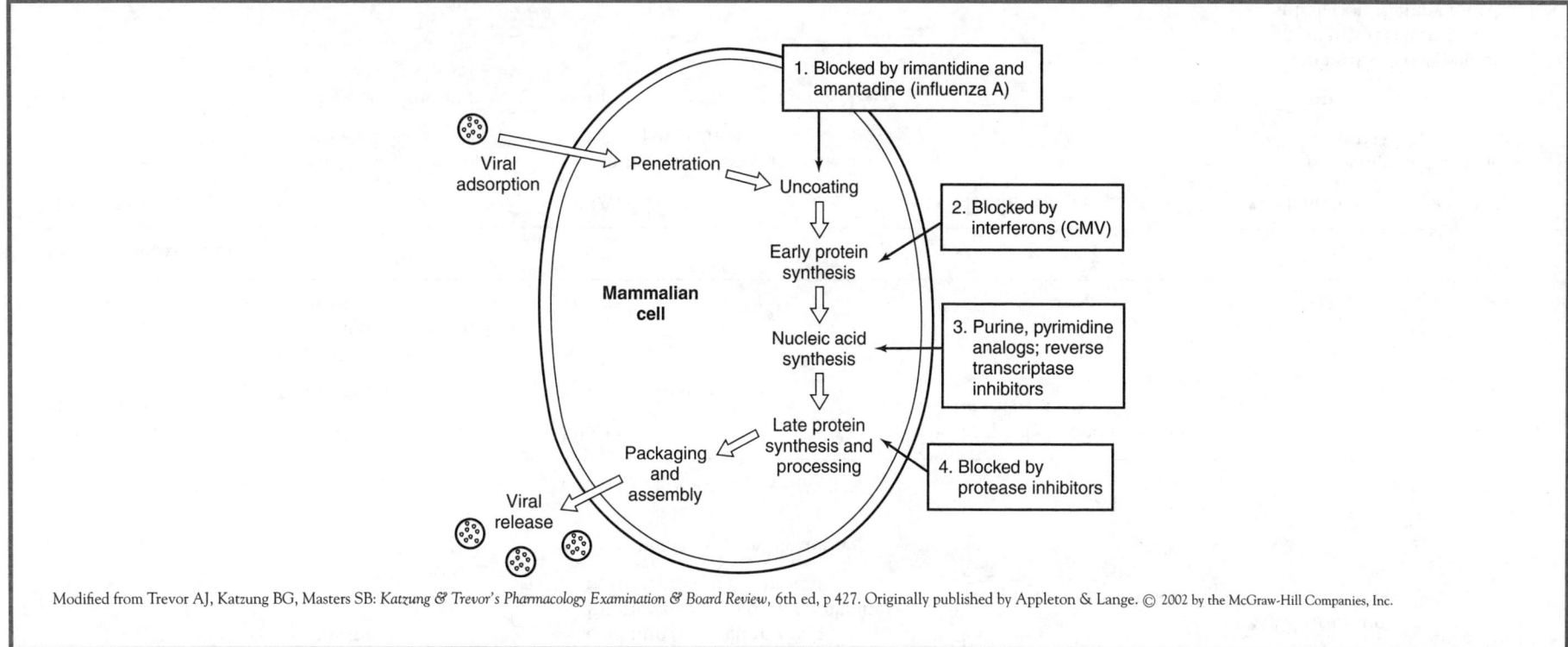

1. Blocked by rimantidine and amantadine (influenza A)

2. Blocked by interferons (CMV)

3. Purine, pyrimidine analogs; reverse transcriptase inhibitors

4. Blocked by protease inhibitors

Viral adsorption — Penetration — Uncoating — Early protein synthesis — Nucleic acid synthesis — Late protein synthesis and processing — Packaging and assembly — Viral release

Mammalian cell

Modified from Trevor AJ, Katzung BG, Masters SB: *Katzung & Trevor's Pharmacology Examination & Board Review*, 6th ed, p 427. Originally published by Appleton & Lange. © 2002 by the McGraw-Hill Companies, Inc.

TRICYLIC AMINES, GUANOSINE ANALOG, NEURAMINIDASE INHIBITORS, INTERFERONS, AND PYROPHOSPHONATE DERIVATIVE

Drug	Pharmacokinetics	Mechanisms of Action and of Resistance	Clinical Uses	Drawbacks and Side Effects
Tricyclic Amines				
Amantadine	• **A:** PO • **E:** Excreted unchanged in urine	**MOA:** • Prevents release of viral nucleic acid into host cell through interference with transmembrane portion of viral M2 protein • Prevents viral assembly during replication • Causes DA release in the CNS	• Prophylaxis and treatment of influenza A • Parkinson's disease • Treatment of drug-induced EPS	• Agitation • Ataxia • GI irritation
Rimantadine (Flumadine)	• **A:** PO • **M:** Hepatic • **E:** Parent drug and metabolites excreted in urine	**MOA:** • Blocks viral uncoating	• Prophylaxis and treatment of influenza A	
Guanosine Analogs				
Ribavirin	• **A:** PO, inhaled • **M:** Hepatic and intracellular • **E:** Parent drug and metabolites excreted in urine	**MOA:** • Inhibits viral RNA-dependent RNA polymerase • Inhibits capping of viral mRNA	• Treatment of hepatitis C	• Hemolytic anemia • Monotherapy to be avoided in hepatitis C • Teratogen • Respiratory decompensation in infants receiving inhalation therapy for RSV

Neuraminidase Inhibitors

Zanamivir (Relenza)	• **A:** Inhaled • **E:** Excreted unchanged in urine	**MOA:** • Inhibit influenza neuraminidase	• Prophylaxis for influenza A and B • Treatment of influenza A and B (useful only 48 hours from onset of symptoms)	• Headache
Oseltamivir	• **A:** PO • **M:** Hepatic • **E:** Primarily excreted as metabolites excreted in urine			• Nausea • Diarrhea • Neuropsychiatric disturbances

Interferons

Interferon alfa-2a	• **A:** SC	**MOA:** • Bind to cell wall causing multiple intracellular reactions resulting in antiviral, immunoregulatory, and antiproliferative effects	• Chronic hepatitis B • Chronic hepatitis C	• Neuropsychiatric disturbances • Aggravation of autoimmune illnesses • Aggravation of ischemic conditions • Aggravation of infectious conditions • Flu-like symptoms • Bone marrow suppression • Increased toxicity when combined with Ribavirin (except interferon alfa-2b)
Interferon alfa-2b (Intron-A)	• **A:** IM, IV, SC, intralesional		• Chronic hepatitis B • Chronic hepatitis C • Hairy cell leukemia • Follicular lymphoma • Malignant melanoma • Kaposi's sarcoma • Condylomata acuminata	
Interferon alfacon-1 (Infergen)	• **A:** SC		• Chronic hepatitis C	
Interferon alfa-n3 (Alferon N)	• **A:** Intralesional		• Condylomata acuminata	• Flu-like symptoms

Continued

TRICYLIC AMINES, GUANOSINE ANALOG, NEURAMINIDASE INHIBITORS, INTERFERONS, AND PYROPHOSPHONATE DERIVATIVE (Continued)

Drug	Pharmacokinetics	Mechanisms of Action and of Resistance	Clinical Uses	Drawbacks and Side Effects
Pyrophosphonate Derivative				
Foscarnet (Foscavir)	• **A:** IV • **E:** Primarily excreted unchanged in urine	**MOA:** • Pyrophosphate analog • Directly inhibits viral RNA and DNA polymerases and HIV reverse transcriptase by interacting with the pyrophosphate binding site **Resistance:** • Via point mutations in the DNA polymerase gene	• CMV retinitis in HIV patients • Acyclovir-resistant HSV infections in immunocompromised patients	• Fever • Headache • Nausea • Renal impairment • Seizures related to electrolyte imbalances • Hypokalemia • Hypomagnesemia • Hypocalcemia • Hypophosphatemia

NUCLEOSIDE ANALOGUES

Drug	Pharmacokinetics	Mechanisms of Action and of Resistance	Clinical Uses	Drawbacks and Side Effects
Acyclovir (Zovirax)	• **A:** PO, IV • **E:** Primarily excreted unchanged in urine	**MOA:** • First phosphorylation by viral thymidine kinase • Second and third phosphorylations by host cell kinases • Triphosphate form incorporated into viral DNA	• Genital HSV infections • Herpes zoster • Varicella zoster • HSV encephalitis • Mucocutaneous HSV infections	• Malaise • Headache • Nephrotoxicity
Valcyclovir (Valtrex)	• **A:** PO • **M:** Hepatic and intestinal metabolism to acyclovir • **E:** Primarily excreted as metabolites in urine	**Resistance:** • Via alteration in viral thymidine kinase • Via alteration in DNA polymerase • Cross resistance across class	• Herpes zoster • Treatment and suppression of Herpes labialis • Genital herpes • Varicella	• Headache • Nausea
Ganciclovir (Cytovene)	• **A:** IV • **E:** Primarily excreted unchanged in urine	**MOA:** • First phosphorylation by viral thymidine kinase • Second and third phosphorylations by host cell kinases • Triphosphate form incorporated into viral DNA	• CMV retinitis • Prevention of CMV infection in immunocompromised patients	• Blood dyscrasias (anemia, thrombocytopenia, leukopenia) • Nausea • Fever • Diarrhea • Teratogenic • Carcinogenic • Inhibition of spermatogenesis
Valganciclovir (Valcyte)	• **A:** PO • **M:** Hepatic and intestinal metabolism to gancicyclovir • **E:** Primarily excreted as metabolites in urine	**Resistance:** • Via mutation of CMV DNA polymerase • Via alteration in viral kinase		

Continued

NUCLEOSIDE ANALOGUES (Continued)

Drug	Pharmacokinetics	Mechanisms of Action and of Resistance	Clinical Uses	Drawbacks and Side Effects
Famciclovir (Famvir)	• **A:** PO • **M:** Prodrug that undergoes hepatic metabolism to penciclovir • **E:** Primarily excreted as metabolites	• Phosphorylated form competes with deoxyguanosine triphosphate to inhibit HSV-2 polymerase	• Herpes zoster • Treatment and prevention of genital herpes • Prevention of recurrent herpes labialis	• Headache • Nausea
Penciclovir (Denavir)	• **A:** Topical		• Herpes labialis	• Localized erythema
Trifluridine (Viroptic)	• **A:** Ophthalmic	• Inhibits viral thymidylate synthetase • Phosphorylated form incorporated into viral DNA	• Herpes keratitis • Herpes keratoconjunctivitis	• Ocular pain

NUCLEOTIDE ANALOGUE

Drug	Pharmacokinetics	Mechanisms of Action and of Resistance	Clinical Uses	Drawbacks and Side Effects
Cidofovir (Vistide)	• **A:** IV • **E:** Primarily excreted unchanged in urine	• Phosphorylated form selectively inhibits viral DNA synthesis	• CMV retinitis in HIV patients	• Nephrotoxicity • Neutropenia • Teratogenic • Carcinogenic

NUCLEOSIDE REVERSE TRANSCRIPTASE INHIBITORS

Drug	Pharmacokinetics	Mechanisms of Action and of Resistance	Clinical Uses	Drawbacks and Side Effects
Zidovudine/AZT (Retrovir)	• **A:** PO, IV • **M:** Hepatic (P450) • **E:** Primarily excreted as metabolites in urine	**MOA:** • Phosphorylated by host enzymes to form nucleoside analogs that are competitive inhibitors of reverse transcriptase resulting in chain termination	• Treatment of HIV infection • Prevention of maternal–fetal HIV transmission • Treatment of neonate within 24 hours of delivery for 6 weeks to prevent HIV transmission	• Bone marrow suppression (esp neutropenia and anemia) • Headache • Nausea • Myopathy/myositis
Didanosine/DDI (Videx)	• **A:** PO • **E:** Primarily excreted unchanged in urine		• Treatment of HIV infection	• Peripheral neuropathy • Pancreatitis • Diarrhea • Hyperuricemia
Emtricitabine (Emtriva)				• Headache • Diarrhea • Hyperpigmentation • Exacerbation of hepatitis B infection following cessation of therapy
Stavudine (Zerit)				• Headache • Nausea • Pancreatitis
Tenofovir (Viread)			• Treatment of HIV infection • Treatment of hepatitis B infection	• Hypercholesterolemia • Exacerbation of hepatitis B infection following cessation of therapy

Continued

NUCLEOSIDE REVERSE TRANSCRIPTASE INHIBITORS (Continued)

Drug	Pharmacokinetics	Mechanisms of Action and of Resistance	Clinical Uses	Drawbacks and Side Effects
Lamivudine (Epivir)				• Headache • Fatigue • Nausea • Exacerbation of hepatitis B infection following cessation of therapy • HIV resistance in patients being treated for chronic hepatitis B infection • Avoid use of HBV dosing for HIV
Entecavir (Baraclude)			• Treatment of hepatitis B	• Exacerbation of hepatitis B • Development of HIV resistance
Abacavir (Ziagen)	• **A:** PO • **M:** Hepatic • **E:** Primarily excreted as metabolites in urine		• Treatment of HIV infection	• Hypersensitivity reactions
Adefovir (Hepsera)	• **A:** PO • **M:** Prodrug converted in intestine • **E:** Parent drug and metabolite excreted in urine	• Phosphorylated by host enzymes to form nucleotide analogs that are competitive inhibitors of reverse transcriptase resulting in chain termination	• Treatment of hepatitis C	• Exacerbation of hepatitis B • Development of HIV resistance • Nephrotoxicity

Entire class carries box warning for rare occurrences of fatal lactic acidosis and severe hepatomegaly with steatosis.

NON–NUCLEOSIDE REVERSE TRANSCRIPTASE INHIBITORS

Drug	Pharmacokinetics	Mechanisms of Action and of Resistance	Clinical Uses and General Information	Drawbacks and Side Effects
Nevirapine (Viramune)	• **A:** PO • **M:** Hepatic (P450) • **E:** Primarily excreted as metabolites in urine	**MOA:** • Bind to and inhibit reverse transcriptase	• Treatment of HIV infection	• Hepatotoxicity • Rash • Hypercholesterolemia • Induce cytochrome P450 enzymes
Efavirenz (Sustiva)	• **A:** PO • **M:** Hepatic (P450) • **E:** Primarily excreted as metabolites in urine and unchanged in feces	**Resistance:** • Via mutation in the *pol* gene which encodes for reverse transcriptase		• Rash • Hypercholesterolemia • Hypertriglyceridemia • Induce cytochrome P450 enzymes
Rilpivirine (Edurant)	• **A:** PO • **M:** Hepatic • **E:** Primarily excreted as metabolites in feces			• Hypercholesterolemia • Hepatotoxicity
Etravirine (Intelence)	• **A:** PO • **M:** Hepatic • **E:** Primarily excreted unchanged in feces			• Rash • Hypercholesterolemia • Hyperglycemia
Delavirdine (Rescriptor)	• **A:** PO • **M:** Hepatic • **E:** Primarily excreted as metabolites in urine and feces			• Headache • Depression • Nausea • Vomiting

PROTEASE INHIBITORS

Drug	Pharmacokinetics	Mechanisms of Action and of Resistance	Clinical Uses	Drawbacks and Side Effects
Indinavir (Crixivan)	• **A:** PO • **M:** Hepatic (P450) • **E:** Primarily excreted as metabolites in feces	**MOA:** • Inhibit viral protease that cleaves precursor proteins • Prevent maturation of new virus **Resistance:** • Via mutation in the *pol* gene which encodes for reverse transcriptase • Confers cross resistance to class members	• Treatment of HIV infection	• Nephrolithiasis • Nausea • Abdominal pain • Hyperbilirubinemia • Hyperglycemia • Inhibits cytochrome P450 enzymes
Saquinavir (Invirase)				• Nausea • Hyperglycemia • Inhibits cytochrome P450 enzymes
Ritonavir (Norvir)				• Fatigue • Multiple medication interactions • Hypertriglyceridemia • Hypercholesterolemia • Diarrhea • Rash • Induces cytochrome P450 enzymes
Nelfinavir (Viracept)				• Diarrhea • Hyperglycemia • Inhibits cytochrome P450 enzymes

Atazanavir (Reyataz)		• Hypercholesterolemia • Hypertriglyceridemia • Hyperglycemia • Rash • Nausea • Inhibits cytochrome P450 enzymes
Darunavir (Prezista)		• Nausea • Diarrhea • Hypercholesterolemia • Hyperglycemia • Rash • Inhibits cytochrome P450 enzymes
Lopinavir and Ritonavir (Kaletra)		• Hypercholesterolemia • Hypertriglyceridemia • Rash • Diarrhea • Vomiting • Inhibits cytochrome P450 enzymes
Fosamprenavir (Lexiva)	• **A:** PO • **M:** Prodrug converted to amprenavir by gut epithelium which then undergoes hepatic (P450) metabolism • **E:** Primarily excreted as metabolites in feces	• Hypertriglyceridemia • Hyperglycemia • Diarrhea • Rash
Tipranavir (Aptivus)	• **A:** PO • **M:** Hepatic (P450) • **E:** Primarily excreted unchanged in feces (when coadministered with Ritonavir)	• Hypertriglyceridemia • Hypercholesterolemia • Diarrhea • Rash • When combined with Ritonavir, increased risk of hepatotoxicity and intracranial hemorrhage

VI. Antifungal Agents

MECHANISMS OF ACTION AND CLASSIFICATION OF ANTIFUNGAL AGENTS

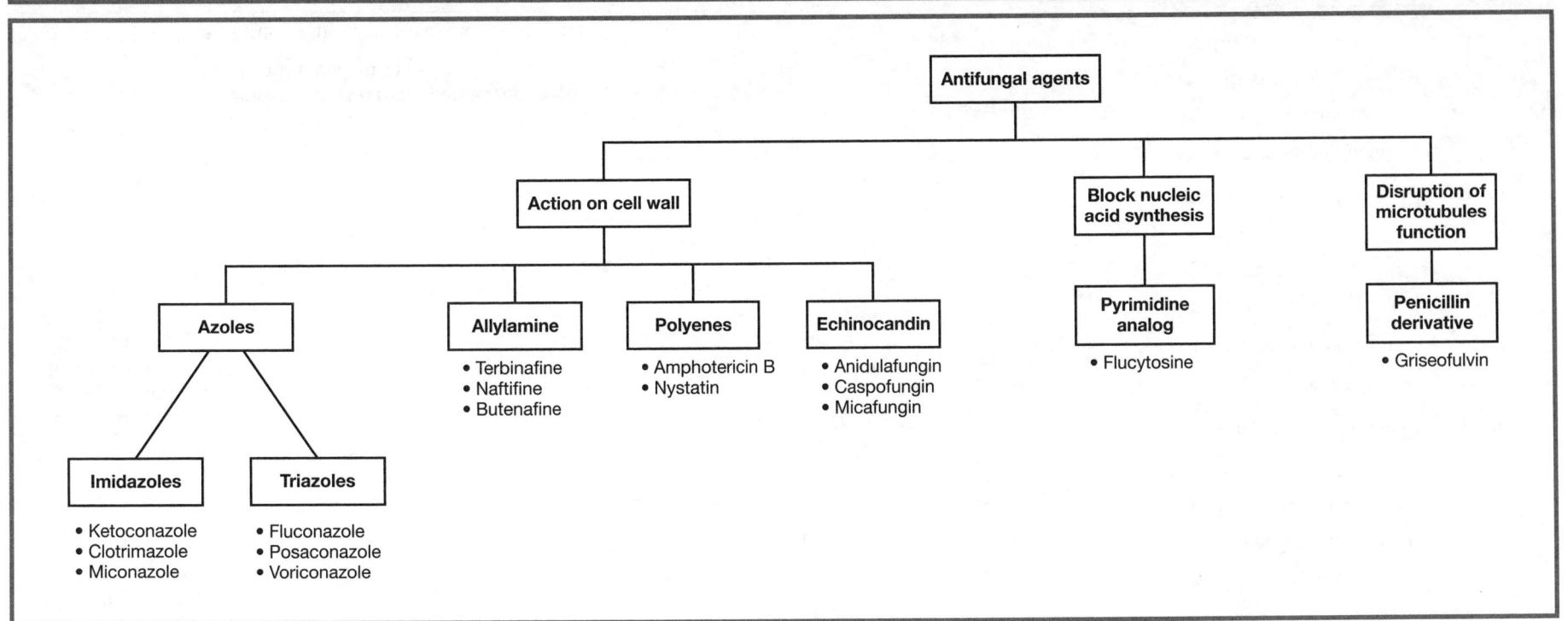

ANTIFUNGALS: DRUG FACTS

Drug	Pharmacokinetics	Mechanisms of Action and of Resistance	Spectrum of Activity	Clinical Uses	Adverse Effects
Polyenes					
Amphotericin B	• **A:** IV • **M:** Unclear • **E:** Primarily excreted as metabolites in urine	**MOA:** • Binds to sterols (primarily ergosterol) in fungal cell membrane forming cytotoxic pores **Resistance:** • Via decreased membrane concentration of ergosterol • Via modification of sterol-binding site	• *Candida albicans* • *Candida krusei* • *Cryptococcus neoformans* • *Aspergillus fumigatus* • *Histoplasma capsulatum* • *Blastomyces dermatitidis* • *Penicillium marneffei* • *Coccidioides immitis* • *Sporothrix schenckii*	• Aspergillosis • Prophylaxis for BMT • Candidemia • Disseminated candidiasis • Endocarditis • Oropharyngeal/esophageal candidiasis • Meningitis • Cryptococcal meningitis and pneumonia • Osteoarticular candidiasis • Sporotrichosis • Urinary tract candidiasis	• Use should be limited to potentially life threatening infections • Infusion reactions (hypotension, nausea, vomiting) • Hypokalemia
Nystatin (Nyamyc, Nystop, Bio-Statin)	• **A:** Topical, PO • **E:** Excreted unchanged in feces		• Several candidal species	• Mucocutaneous candidiasis	• GI distress with oral forms

Continued

ANTIFUNGALS: DRUG FACTS (Continued)

Drug	Pharmacokinetics	Mechanisms of Action and of Resistance	Spectrum of Activity	Clinical Uses	Adverse Effects
Echinocandins					
Anidulafungin (Eraxis)	• **A:** IV • **M:** Hydrolysis • **E:** Parent drug and metabolites excreted in feces and urine	**MOA:** • Inhibits synthesis of $\beta(1,3)$-D-glucan, an essential component of fungal cell wall	• Several candidal species • Aspergillus	• Esophageal candidiasis • Candidemia	• GI distress • Infusion reactions (hypotension, rash, angioedema) • Hepatotoxicity
Caspofungin (Cancidas)				• Invasive aspergillosis • Esophageal candidiasis • Candidemia	
Micafungin (Mycamine)	• **A:** IV • **M:** Hepatic • **E:** Metabolites excreted primarily in feces			• Esophageal candidiasis • Candidemia • Prophylaxis for candidal infections	
Allylamines					
Terbinafine (Lamisil, Terbinex)	• **A:** Topical, PO • **M:** Hepatic (P450) • **E:** Metabolites excreted in urine	**MOA:** • Inhibits squalene epoxidase which limits production of ergosterol as well as toxic accumulation of intracellular squalene	• Dermatophytes • Several candidal species	• Onychomycosis • Tinea capitis • Tinea cruris • Tinea corporis • Tinea pedis • Tinea versicolor • Cutaneous candidiasis	• Headache • Local irritation

Naftifine (Naftin)	• **A:** Topical		• Dermatophytes	• Tinea cruris • Tinea corporis • Tinea pedis	• Local irritation
Butenafine (Lotrimin, Mentax)				• Tinea cruris • Tinea corporis • Tinea pedis • Tinea versicolor	
Azoles					
Clotrimazole (Lotrimin, Desenex, Alevazol)	• **A:** Topical, PO • **M:** Hepatic (P450) • **E:** Metabolites excreted in feces	**MOA:** • Inhibits fungal P450 system limiting production of ergosterol (essential cell wall component)	• Several candidal species • Dermatophytes	• Oropharyngeal candidiasis • Cutaneous candidiasis • Vulvovaginal candidiasis • Dermatophytoses • Superficial mycoses	• Negligible • Inhibits cytochrome P450 enzymes
Fluconazole (Diflucan)	• **A:** IV, PO • **M:** Hepatic (P450) (minimal) • **E:** Primarily excreted unchanged in urine		• Several candidal species (no coverage of C. krusei) • Dermatophytes • Cryptococcus neoformans • Blastomycosis • Coccidioidomycosis • Histoplasmosis • Paracoccidioidomycosis	• Coccidioidomycosis (treatment and prophylaxis) • Candidiasis • Systemic candidal infections	• GI distress • Hepatotoxicity • Alopecia • Inhibits cytochrome P450 enzymes

Continued

ANTIFUNGALS: DRUG FACTS (Continued)

Drug	Pharmacokinetics	Mechanisms of Action and of Resistance	Spectrum of Activity	Clinical Uses	Adverse Effects
Ketoconazole	• **A:** IV, PO, topical • **M:** Hepatic (P450) • **E:** Parent drug and metabolites primarily excreted in feces		• Blastomycosis • Chromomycosis • Coccidioidomycosis • Histoplasmosis • Paracoccidioidomycosis • Several candidal species • Dermatophytes	• Systemic mycoses	• Hepatotoxicity • Numerous drug interactions (some precipitate cardiac arrhythmias) • Headache • Dizziness • GI distress • Inhibits cytochrome P450 enzymes
Miconazole (Monistat, Oravig)	• **A:** Topical, PO • **M:** Hepatic • **E:** Metabolites excreted in urine		• Several candidal species • Dermatophytes	• Oropharyngeal candidiasis	• GI distress
Posaconazole (Noxafil)	• **A:** IV, PO • **M:** Hepatic (minimal) • **E:** Primarily excreted unchanged in feces		• Several candidal species • Mucorales • Aspergillus species	• Cryptococcal • Treatment and prophylaxis of candidal infections • Treatment and prophylaxis of invasive aspergillosis	• GI distress

Voriconazole (Vfend)	• **A:** PO, IV • **M:** Hepatic (P450) • **E:** Metabolites excreted in urine		• Several candidal species • Aspergillus species • *Scedosporium apiospermum* • Fusarium species	• Invasive aspergillosis • Esophageal candidiasis • Candidemia • Disseminated candidiasis • Serious *Scedosporium* infections • Serious *Fusarium* infections	• Vision changes • Neurotoxicity (hallucinations) • Rash • Periostitis • Alopecia • Cardiac toxicity • Inhibits cytochrome P450 enzymes
Penicillin Derivative					
Griseofulvin (Griseofulvin, Gris-PEG)	• **A:** PO • **M:** Hepatic • **E:** Metabolites excreted in urine, feces, and sweat	**MOA:** • Interferes with microtubule function to inhibit fungal cell at mitosis **Resistance:** • Decrease in energy-dependent transport of drug into dermatophyte	• Dermatophytes	• Tinea capitis • Tinea cruris • Tinea corporis • Tinea pedis • Tinea unguium	• Hepatotoxicity • Induces cytochrome P450 enzymes
Pyrimidine Analog					
Flucytosine (Ancobon)	• **A:** PO • **E:** Primarily excreted unchanged in urine	• Competes with uracil in fungal DNA inhibiting RNA and protein synthesis	• *Cryptococcus neoformans* • *Candida albicans*	• Adjunctive therapy for systemic cryptococcal and candidal infections (encephalitis, UTI, endocarditis, pulmonary septicemia)	• Bone marrow toxicity • Hepatotoxicity • Narrow therapeutic window so monitor renal function closely

VII. Antiprotozoal Agents

THERAPEUTIC CLASSIFICATION OF ANTIPROTOZOAL AGENTS

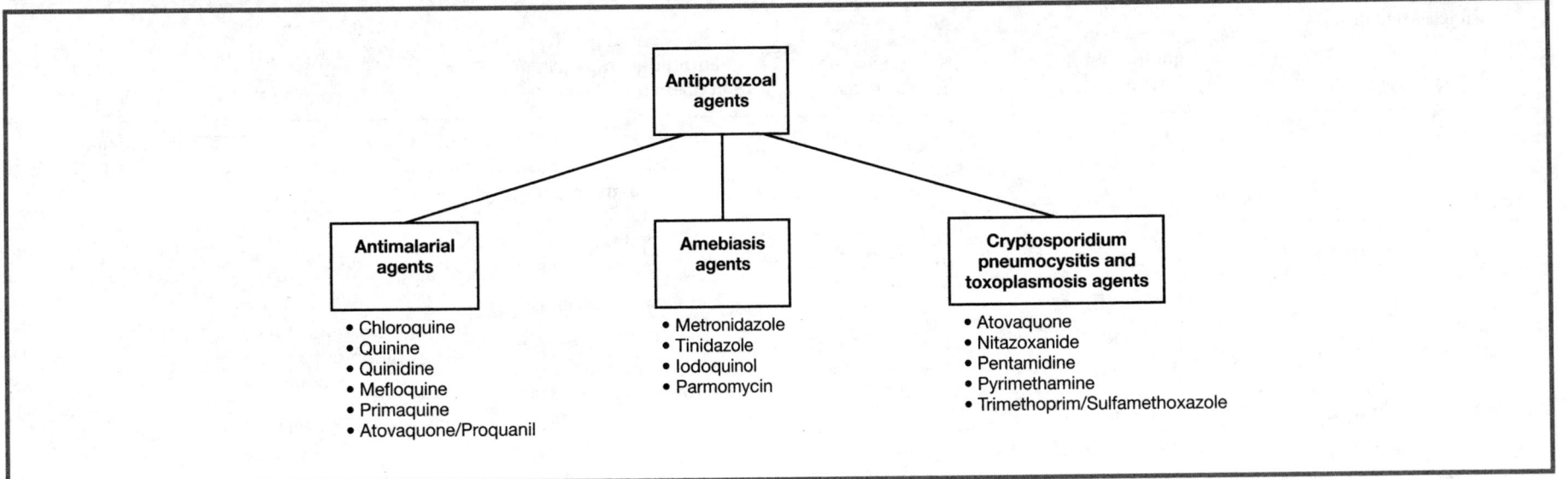

Antiprotozoal agents

Antimalarial agents
- Chloroquine
- Quinine
- Quinidine
- Mefloquine
- Primaquine
- Atovaquone/Proquanil

Amebiasis agents
- Metronidazole
- Tinidazole
- Iodoquinol
- Parmomycin

Cryptosporidium pneumocysitis and toxoplasmosis agents
- Atovaquone
- Nitazoxanide
- Pentamidine
- Pyrimethamine
- Trimethoprim/Sulfamethoxazole

ANTIPROTOZOALS: DRUG FACTS

Drug	Pharmacokinetics	Mechanisms of Action and of Resistance	Clinical Uses and General Information	Drawbacks and Side Effects
Antimalarial Agents **Quinoline Derivatives**				
Chloroquine (Aralen)	• **A:** PO • **M:** Hepatic (P450) • **E:** Parent drug and metabolites excreted in urine	**MOA:** • Prevents polymerization of heme into hemozoin leading to toxic intracellular accumulation of cytotoxic heme after parasite-metabolized hemoglobin **Resistance:** • Increased efflux of medication from cells	• Treatment and prophylaxis of malaria caused by *Plasmodium vivax, P. malariae, P. ovale, P. falciparum* • Extraintestinal amebiasis	• GI distress • Pruritis • Alopecia • Retinopathies • QT prolongation • Cardiomyopathy • Inhibits cytochrome P450 enzymes
Quinine (Qualaquin)	• **A:** PO • **M:** Hepatic (P450) • **E:** Parent drug and metabolites excreted in urine	**MOA:** • Prevents polymerization of heme into hemozoin leading to toxic intracellular accumulation of cytotoxic heme after parasite-metabolized hemoglobin	• Treatment of uncomplicated malaria due to chloroquine-resistant *P. falciparum* • Treatment of uncomplicated malaria due to chloroquine-resistant *P. vivax*	• Avoid for off label treatment of leg cramps due to significant side effects • Cinchonism • Inhibits cytochrome P450 enzymes
Quinidine	• **A:** IV form for malaria, PO • **M:** Hepatic (P450) • **E:** Parent drug and metabolites excreted in urine		• Treatment of severe malaria • Pharmacologic conversion and maintenance of sinus rhythm in patients with atrial fibrillation/ flutter	• Increased risk of mortality in patients with arrhythmias especially with underlying structural heart disease • GI distress • Ligh-theadedness • Cinchonism • Inhibits cytochrome P450 enzymes

Continued

ANTIPROTOZOALS: DRUG FACTS (Continued)

Drug	Pharmacokinetics	Mechanisms of Action and of Resistance	Clinical Uses and General Information	Drawbacks and Side Effects
Mefloquine	• **A:** PO • **M:** Hepatic (P450) • **E:** Parent drug and metabolites primarily excreted in feces	**MOA:** • Unknown	• Treatment and prophylaxis for malaria secondary to *P. vivax* and *P. falciparum*	• Vomiting • Dizziness • CNS disturbances (seizures, psychosis) • Contraindicated for prophylaxis in patients with psychiatric disorders • Inhibits cytochrome P450 enzymes
Primaquine	• **A:** PO • **M:** Hepatic (P450) to active metabolite • **E:** Primarily excreted as metabolites in urine		• Treatment and prevention of relapse of malaria due to *P. vivax*	• Hemolytic anemia in G6PD deficiency • Methemoglobinemia • Inhibits cytochrome P450 enzymes
Antifolates				
Atovaquone and proguanil (Malarone)	• **A:** PO • **M:** Hepatic (proguanil) • **E:** Atovaquone excreted unchanged in feces, proguanil metabolites excreted in urine	• Atovaquone inhibits the mitochondrial electron transport chain • Proguanil metabolite inhibits dihydrofolate reductase	• Prevention and treatment of acute malaria due to *P. falciparum*	• GI distress • Headache • Pruritis
Amebiasis Agents				
Metronidazole (Flagyl, Metro)	• **A:** PO, IV, topical • **M:** Hepatic (P450) • **E:** Parent drug and metabolites excreted primarily in urine	• Causes loss of helical DNA structure and strand breakage leading to decreased protein synthesis	• Amebiasis • Amebic liver abscess • Bacterial vaginosis/vaginitis • Intra-abdominal infections • Trichomoniasis • Surgical prophylaxis	• Headache • GI distress • Metallic taste • Possible carcinogen • Disulfiram reaction with alcohol consumption • Inhibits cytochrome P450 enzymes

Iodoquinol (Yodoxin)	• **A:** PO • **E:** Excreted unchanged in feces	• Unknown MOA	• Intestinal amebiasis due to *Entamoeba histolytica*	• Peripheral neuropathy • Visual dysfunction
Tinidazole (Tindamax)	• **A:** PO • **M:** Hepatic (P450) • **E:** Parent drug and metabolites excreted primarily in urine	• Damages DNA and prevents additional DNA production	• Intestinal amebiasis • Amebic liver abscess • Bacterial vaginosis • Giardiasis • Trichomoniasis	
Paromomycin (Humatin)	• **A:** PO • **E:** Excreted unchanged in stool	• Interferes with bacterial 30S ribosomal subunit leading to decreased protein synthesis	• Hepatic coma • Intestinal amebiasis	• GI distress

Cryptosporidium, Pneumocystis, and Toxoplasmosis Agents

Atovaquone (Mepron)	• **A:** PO • **E:** Excreted unchanged in feces	• Inhibits the mitochondrial electron transport chain	• Prevention and treatment of *Pneumocystis jirovecii* pneumonia	• GI distress • Headache • Pruritis • Rash
Nitazoxanide (Alinia)	• **A:** PO • **M:** Hepatic • **E:** Metabolites excreted in urine and feces	• May be due to disruption of the enzyme-dependent electron transport system portion of anaerobic metabolism	• Treatment of diarrhea from *Giardia lamblia* or *Cryptosporidium parvum*	• GI distress • Headache
Pentamidine (Pentam, Nebupent)	• **A:** IM, IV, inhaled • **M:** Unknown • **E:** Metabolites slowly excreted in urine	• Unknown MOA	• Prevention and treatment of *Pneumocystis jirovecii* pneumonia	• Fatigue • Dizziness • Fever • Anorexia • Dyspnea

Continued

ANTIPROTOZOALS: DRUG FACTS (Continued)

Drug	Pharmacokinetics	Mechanisms of Action and of Resistance	Clinical Uses and General Information	Drawbacks and Side Effects
Pyrimethamine (Daraprim)	• **A:** PO • **M:** Hepatic • **E:** Parent drug and metabolites excreted primarily in urine	• Inhibits parasitic dihydrofolate reductase	• Prevention and treatment of toxoplasmosis • Preventions and treatment of toxoplasmosis in HIV patients • Isosporiasis in HIV patients • Prophylaxis and treatment of malaria	• Arrhythmias • Hematologic abnormalities (thrombocytopenia, leukopenia, anemia) • Inhibits cytochrome P450 enzymes
Trimethoprim/ Sulfamethoxazole (Bactrim)	• **A:** PO, IV • **M:** Hepatic (SMX via P450) (both components) • **E:** Parent drug and metabolites excreted in urine (both components)	• Competitively inhibits the conversion of PABA to folic acid by dihydropteroate synthase • Lack of folic acid inhibits bacterial growth by interfering with microbial DNA synthesis	• Treatment and prophylaxis of *Pneumocystis jirovecii* pneumonia in HIV patients • UTIs • Treatment of *Pneumocystis jirovecii* pneumonia • Traveller's diarrhea *Shigellosis* • Sepsis • *Nocardiosis* • Acute exacerbation of chronic bronchitis	• Hemolysis in patients with G6PD deficiency • Rash • Hepatotoxicity • Nephrotoxicity • Pancreatitis • Kernicterus in infants

VIII. Antihelminthic Agents

ANTIHELMINTHICS: DRUG FACTS

Drug	Pharmacokinetics	Mechanisms of Action	Clinical Use	Drawbacks and Side Effects
Antihelminthic Agents				
Albendazole (Albenza)	• **A:** PO • **M:** Hepatic (P450) • **E:** Parent drug and metabolites excreted primarily in urine	• Causes degeneration of cytoplasmic tubules in intestinal and tegumental cells in intestinal hemilinths	• Neurocysticercosis • Hydatid disease of liver, lung, and peritoneum	• Headache • Bone marrow suppression • Elevated transaminases • Mazzotti-type reaction
Ivermectin (Stromectol)	• **A:** PO • **M:** Hepatic (P450) • **E:** Primarily excreted as metabolites in feces	• Binds to glutamate-gated chloride ion channel in parasites leading to hyperpolarization in nerve and muscle cells causing parasitic death	• Onchocerciasis • Strongyloidiasis	• Pruritis • Rash • Lymphadenopathy • Mazzotti-type reaction
Praziquantel (Biltricide)	• **A:** PO • **M:** Hepatic (P450) • **E:** Primarily excreted as metabolites in urine	• Increases cellular membrane permeability to Ca^{2+} causing muscular contraction/paralysis of the parasite leading to dislodgement	• Schistosomiasis • Clonorchiasis • Opisthorchiasis	• Nausea • Abdominal pain • Dizziness • Headache • Mazzotti-type reaction • Inhibits cytochrome P450 enzymes
Pyrantel pamoate (Pamix, Pin-X, Reese's pinworm)	• **A:** PO • **M:** Hepatic (P450) (partial) • **E:** Parent drug and metabolites excreted primarily in urine	• Inhibits cholinesterase and causes Ach release leading to neuromuscular blockade of helminths	• *Enterobius vermicularis*	• Headache • Dizziness • GI distress

IX. Antimycobacterial Agents

AVAILABLE AGENTS FOR TUBERCULOSIS AND LEPROSY PLUS ATYPICAL MYCOBACTERIAL AGENTS

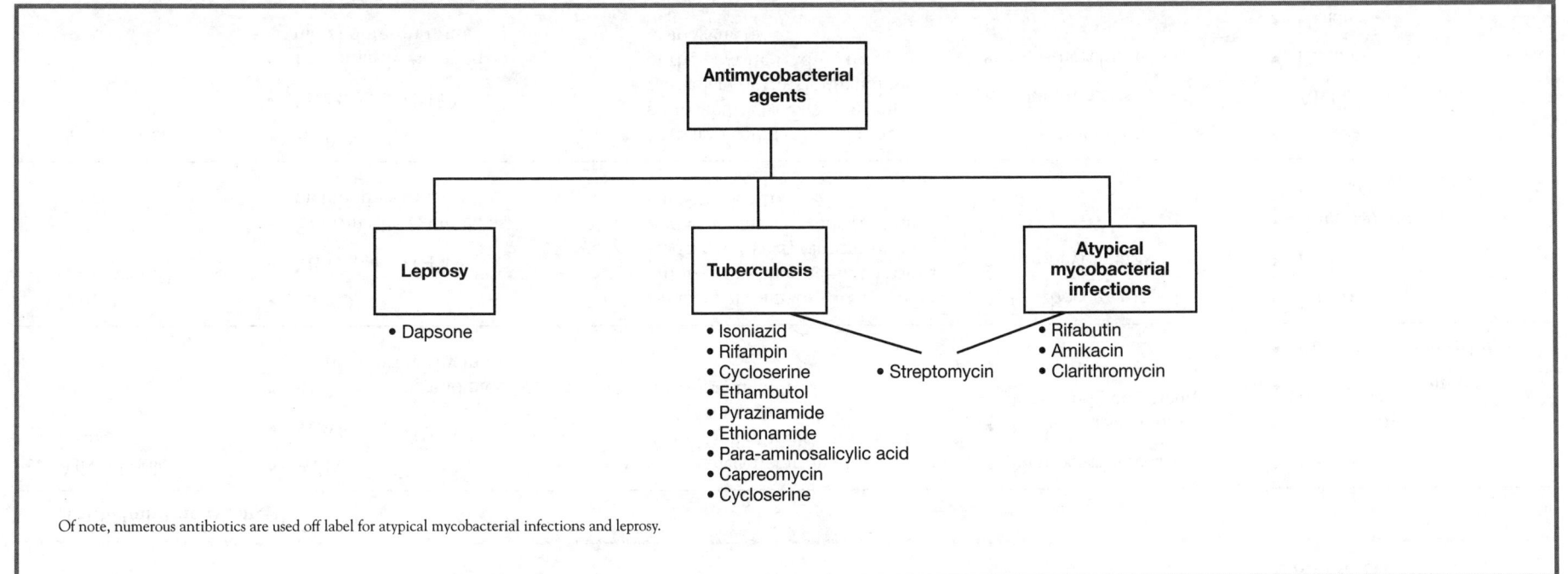

Of note, numerous antibiotics are used off label for atypical mycobacterial infections and leprosy.

ANTIMYCOBACTERIALS: DRUG FACTS

Drug	Pharmacokinetics	Mechanisms of Action and of Resistance	Clinical Uses and General Information	Drawbacks and Side Effects
Isoniazid (INH) ☞ **INH** **I**nhibits mycolic acid synthesis **N**europathy **H**epatotoxicity	• **A:** IM and PO • **M:** Hepatic (P450) acetylation (note that rate of acetylation is genetically determined) • **E:** Metabolites excreted in urine	**MOA:** • Inhibits the synthesis of mycolic acids • Mycolic acids are essential components of the mycobacterial cell wall • Tuberculocidal to intracellular and extracellular organisms **Resistance:** • Via mutation in the gene coding for the enzyme required for drug activation	• Tuberculosis (active and latent) • Tuberculous meningitis (active) • Not effective against *Mycobacterium kansasii* and *Mycobacterium avium–intracellulare* complex • Must be administered with Pyridoxine	• Allergic reactions • Hepatitis • Peripheral neuropathy (increased risk in slow acetylator populations) • Lupus-like syndrome • CNS toxicity (memory loss, insomnia, and seizures) • Hemolysis in patients with G6PD deficiency • Drug resistance emerges rapidly with monotherapy • Inhibits and Induces cytochrome P450 enzymes
Rifampin (Rifadin) ☞ **4 R's for Rifampin:** **R**evs up P450 **R**NA polymerase inhibitor **R**ed/orange bodily fluids **R**apid resistance if used alone	• **A:** IV and PO • **M:** Hepatic (P450) • **E:** Metabolites excreted in feces; parent drug and metabolites excreted in urine	**MOA:** • Inhibits RNA synthesis by binding to the β subunit of DNA-dependent RNA polymerase in susceptible microorganisms • Inhibits protein synthesis by preventing chain initiation • Virtually no effect on mammalian RNA polymerase • Tuberculocidal to intracellular and extracellular organisms **Resistance:** • Via mutation in gene coding for β subunit of DNA-dependent RNA polymerase	• Active and latent tuberculosis	• Causes orange-colored urine, tears, sweat, and contact lenses • Induces cytochrome P450 enzymes • Rashes • Fever • Thrombocytopenia • Nausea and vomiting • Hepatotoxicity • Drug resistance develops rapidly with monotherapy

Continued

ANTIMYCOBACTERIALS: DRUG FACTS (Continued)

Drug	Pharmacokinetics	Mechanisms of Action and of Resistance	Clinical Uses and General Information	Drawbacks and Side Effects
Ethambutol (Myambutol)	• **A:** PO; well absorbed • **M:** Hepatic • **E:** Parent drug and metabolites excreted in urine and feces	**MOA:** • Inhibits arabinosyl transferase, an enzyme in the synthesis of arabinogalactan (a component of mycobacterium cell wall) • Tuberculostatic to intracellular and extracellular organisms **Resistance:** • Via mutation in the gene coding for the arabinosyl transferase	• Active tuberculosis	• Hypersensitivity (rare) • Optic neuritis (precludes use in children too young for visual examinations) • Drug resistance develops rapidly with monotherapy • Red/green color blindness • Hepatotoxicity • Rash
Pyrazinamide	• **A:** PO; well absorbed • **M:** Hepatic • **E:** Majority of metabolites excreted in urine	**MOA:** • Precise MOA unknown • Enzymatic activation to pyrazinoic acid which lowers pH • Tuberculocidal only to intracellular organisms **Resistance:** • Via lack of activating enzymes • Via decreased drug uptake	• Adjunctive treatment of tuberculosis	• Hepatotoxicity • Arthralgias • Hyperuricemia (may precipitate gout) • Myalgia • GI distress • Porphyria • Drug resistance develops rapidly with monotherapy

Streptomycin	• **A:** IM • **E:** Primarily excreted unchanged in urine	**MOA:** • Irreversibly blocks bacterial protein synthesis by binding to the 30S ribosomal subunit • Tuberculocidal only to extracellular organisms (poor for intracellular organisms) **Resistance:** • Via altered structure of ribosomal proteins	• Tuberculosis • Tularemia • Brucellosis • *Mycobacterium avium* complex • Rifampin-resistant *Mycobacterium kansasii* • *Mycobacterium ulcerans* • Plague • Endocarditis (enterococcal or streptococcal)	• Ototoxicity • Nephrotoxicity • Neurotoxicity • Drug resistance precludes monotherapy
Amikacin (Amikin)	• **A:** IM, IV • **E:** Excreted unchanged in urine	**MOA:** • Blocks bacterial protein synthesis by binding to the 30S ribosomal subunit	• Health care-associated pneumonia • *Mycobacterium fortuitum* • *M. chelonae* • *M. abscessus*	• Ototoxic • Nephrotoxic • Neuromuscular blockade • Neurotoxicity
Capreomycin (Capastat)	• **A:** IM, IV • **E:** Majority excreted unchanged in urine	**MOA:** • Peptide synthesis inhibitor	• Treatment of tuberculosis in multi drug-resistant	• Ototoxicity • Nephrotoxicity • Local injection site reactions • Eosinophilia

Continued

ANTIMYCOBACTERIALS: DRUG FACTS (Continued)

Drug	Pharmacokinetics	Mechanisms of Action and of Resistance	Clinical Uses and General Information	Drawbacks and Side Effects
Cycloserine (Seromycin)	• A: PO • M: Hepatic • E: Majority excreted unchanged in urine	MOA: • Cell wall synthesis inhibitor by competition with D-alanine for incoporation into bacterial cell wall	• Treatment of tuberculosis	• Side effects limit clinical usefulness • Peripheral neuropathy • CNS dysfunction (depression and psychosis) • Pyridoxine coadministration can reduce CNS side effects
Ethionamide (Trecator)	• A: PO • M: Hepatic • E: Prodrug that undergoes hepatic metabolism to active and inactive metabolites; metabolites excreted in urine	MOA: • Similar structure to isoniazid • Inhibits the synthesis of mycolic acids • Mycolic acids are essential components of the mycobacterial cell wall	• Adjunctive therapy of tuberculosis	• Side effects limit clinical usefulness • Intense gastric irritation • Adverse neurologic effects • Hepatotoxic • Pyridoxine coadministration can reduce CNS side effects
Para-aminosalicylic Acid/PAS (Paser)	• A: PO; readily absorbed • D: Widely distributed; does not cross BBB • M: Hepatic acetylation • E: Parent drug and metabolites excreted in urine	MOA: • Inhibits folic acid synthesis via competitive inhibition of PABA		• GI irritation • Crystalluria • Peptic ulceration • Hypersensitivity reactions (fever, rash, hepatitis, granulocytopenia) • Primary resistance is common • Resistance limits usefulness

| Clarithromycin (Biaxin) | • **A:** PO
 • **M:** Hepatic (P450)
 • **E:** Parent drug and metabolites excreted in urine; metabolites excreted in feces | **MOA:**
 • Bacteriostatic
 • Binds to the 23S rRNA of the 50S subunit and blocks protein synthesis

 Resistance:
 • Develops primarily by mutations in the binding site on the 50S subunit | • Similar spectrum as erythromycin plus *H. influenza*, *Bordetella*, and M. *catarrhalis*
 • Bronchitis
 • Sinusitis
 • Treatment and prevention of disseminated *Mycobacterium avium* infections
 • Treatment of disseminated M. *intracellulare*
 • *H. pylori* in patients with PUD
 • Pharyngitis
 • Tonsillitis
 • Pneumonia
 • Uncomplicated skin and soft tissue infections | • GI distress (abdominal cramping, diarrhea, nausea)
 • QT prolongation (esp with erythromycin)
 • Inhibits cytochrome P450 enzymes |
| Rifabutin (Mycobutin) | • **A:** PO
 • **M:** Hepatic (P450)
 • **E:** Metabolites excreted in urine and feces | **MOA:**
 • Inhibits RNA synthesis by binding to the β subunit of DNA-dependent RNA polymerase in susceptible microorganisms
 • Inhibits protein synthesis by preventing chain initiation
 • Virtually no effect on mammalian RNA polymerase
 • Tuberculocidal to intracellular and extracellular organisms | • Prevention of MAC infection in AIDS patients | • Drug interactions due to induction of P450 enzymes
 • Brown/orange discoloration of urine
 • Neutropenia
 • Leukopenia
 • Rash
 • Induces cytochrome P450 enzymes |

Continued

ANTIMYCOBACTERIALS: DRUG FACTS (Continued)

Drug	Pharmacokinetics	Mechanisms of Action and of Resistance	Clinical Uses and General Information	Drawbacks and Side Effects
Dapsone	• **A:** PO; well absorbed • **D:** Widely distributed • **M:** Hepatic (P450) • **E:** Parent drug metabolites excreted in urine	**MOA:** • Inhibits folic acid synthesis via competitive inhibition of PABA	• Treatment of leprosy from susceptible strains of M. *leprae* • Treatment of dermatitis herpetiformis	• GI irritation • Drug-induced lupus erythematosus • Agranuclocytosis • Anemia • Fever • Skin rashes • Methemoglobinemia • Hemolysis (especially in patients with G6PD deficiency)

CHAPTER 3

AUTONOMIC NERVOUS SYSTEM STRUCTURE AND MEDICATIONS

I. STRUCTURE

ANS Components

Overview of ANS and Actions of Some Drugs

Effects of ANS on Organ Systems

II. MEDICATIONS

Classification of Cholinergic Agonists

Direct Cholinergic Agonists: Acetylcholine Agonists

Indirect Cholinergic Agonists: Antiacetylcholinesterases

Classification of Muscarinic Antagonists

Muscarinic Antagonists

Classification of Ganglionic Blockers

Ganglionic Blockers

Classification of Sympathomimetics

Catecholamines

Noncatecholamines

Effects of Sympathomimetics on Organ Systems

Classification of Adrenergic Blockers

α-Blockers and Neuronal Blockers

β-Blockers

III. PHARMACOLOGY OF THE EYE

Cholinergic and Adrenergic Drugs for Treating Conditions of the Eye

Eye Receptor Mechanisms

Cholinergic Agents, Miotic Agents

Clinically Important Structures of the Eye and Their Receptors

TERMS TO LEARN

Acetylcholinesterase	Enzyme responsible for the degradation of Ach.
Adrenergic Neuronal Blockers	Medications that prevent NE from exiting the nerve terminal.
Anisocoria	Unequal pupils.
Intrinsic Sympathomimetic Activity (ISA)	Drugs with paradoxical partial β-agonist properties; clinical significance unknown.
Lipid Solubility	Accounts for the CNS side effects of a drug.
Malignant Hypertension	Severely elevated blood pressure associated with CNS, renal, or cardiac symptoms.
Membrane Stabilizing Activity (MSA)	Imparts a local anesthetic quality to β-blockers; may contribute to antiarrhythmic property.
Miosis	Pupillary constriction.
Myasthenia Gravis	Autoimmune disease characterized by increasing muscle weakness with use due to the presence of antibodies to the Ach receptor at the neuromuscular junction.
Mydriasis	Pupillary dilation.
Nonselective α-Adrenergic Blockers	Medications that block α_1- and α_2-adrenergic sites.
Nonselective β-Blockers	Medications that block β_1- and β_2-adrenergic sites.
Pheochromocytoma	Tumor of the adrenal gland that secretes catecholamines.
Plasma Binding	Accounts for the drug interactions.
Postural (orthostatic) Hypotension	A 20 mm Hg drop in systolic blood pressure or 10 mm Hg drop in diastolic blood pressure within 3 minutes of standing due to a defect in the blood pressure control system.
Raynaud's Disease	Vascular disorder characterized by peripheral vasoconstriction.

Selective α-Adrenergic Blockers	Medications that block α_1-adrenergic sites only.
Selective β-Adrenergic Blockers	Medications that block β_1-adrenergic sites only.
Sjögren's Syndrome	Syndrome of dry mouth and dry eyes due to lymphocytic infiltration of the salivary and lacrimal glands; often observed in patients with autoimmune disorders including RA and SLE.
Tourette's Syndrome	Syndrome characterized by motor and verbal tics.
Xerostomia	Dry mouth.

ANS COMPONENTS

Component	Parasympathetic Nervous System	Sympathetic Nervous System
Path of preganglionic cell	CN III, VII, IX, X, and S2–S4	T1–L2
Preganglionic fiber length	Long	Short
Preganglionic myelination	Myelinated	Myelinated
Pre- to postganglionic ratio	One to one (except vagus nerve)	One to many
Preganglionic cell NT	Ach	Ach
Postganglionic cell location	On or near organ	Sympathetic chain next to spinal cord
Postganglionic fiber length	Short	Long
Postganglionic myelination	Unmyelinated	Unmyelinated
Postganglionic cell NT	Ach	NE (except adrenal medulla—EPI; piloerector muscles and sweat glands—Ach)

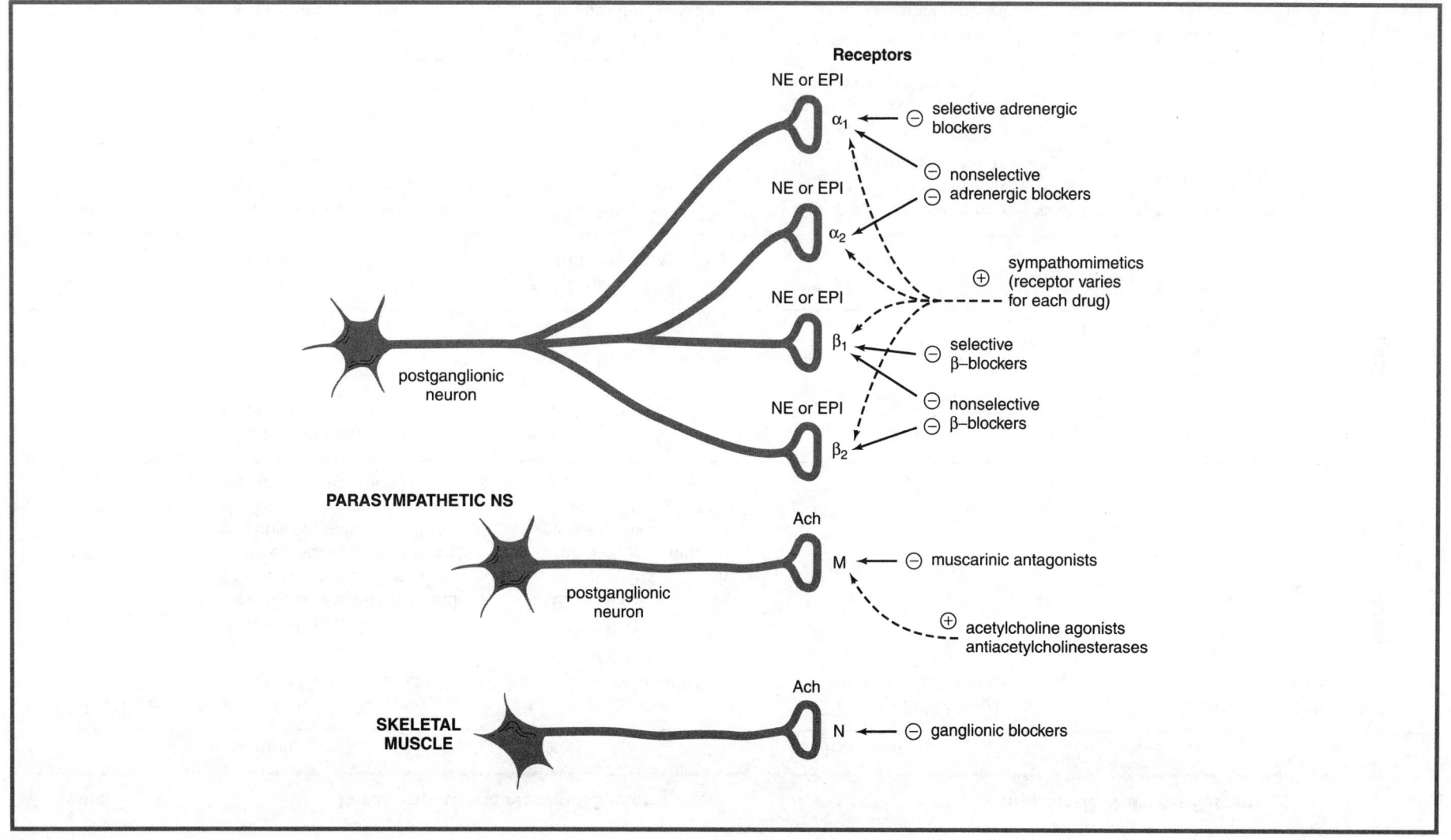

EFFECTS OF ANS ON ORGAN SYSTEMS

Tissue	Parasympathetic Nervous System		Sympathetic Nervous System	
	Mechanism	Effect	Mechanism	Effect
Pupil of the eye	• Ach binds to muscarinic receptors on the sphincter muscle • Ach binds to muscarinic receptor on the ciliary muscle	• Contraction of the sphincter muscle leads to constriction of the pupil • Contraction of ciliary muscle (causes opening of canal of Schlemm, which leads to decreased intraocular pressure) (Note: Contraction of ciliary muscle causes relaxation of the suspensory ligaments, allowing the lens to get rounder and facilitates near vision)	• NE or EPI binds to α₁-receptors on the radial muscles	• Contraction of the radial muscles leads to dilation of the pupil
Bronchi	• Ach binds to muscarinic receptors	• Contracts smooth muscle surrounding bronchi	• NE or EPI binds to α₁-receptors • NE or EPI binds to β₂-receptors	• Increases organic content of secretions • Relaxation of smooth muscles surrounding bronchi
Heart	• Ach binds to muscarinic receptors	• Decrease in heart rate and ionotropy	• NE or EPI binds to β₁-receptors	• Increase in heart rate and ionotropy
Blood vessels	• Ach from exogenous source (no direct parasympathetic innervation of the blood vessels)	• Vasodilation	• NE or EPI binds to α₁-receptors on all blood vessels except those supplying skeletal muscles • NE or EPI binds to β₂-receptors on blood vessels that supply skeletal muscles	• Vasoconstriction • Vasodilation
GI tract	• Ach binds to muscarinic receptors on longitudinal muscles	• Contraction of longitudinal muscles	• NE or EPI on β₂-receptors on longitudinal muscles	• Relaxation of longitudinal muscles

	• Ach binds to muscarinic receptors on sphincter muscles	• Relaxation of sphincter muscles • Both lead to increased peristalsis and bowel movements	• NE or EPI binds to α_1-receptors on sphincter muscles	• Contraction of sphincter muscles • Both effects result in decrease of bowel movement
Bladder	• Ach binds to muscarinic receptors on body of bladder • Ach binds to muscarinic receptors on sphincter of the bladder	• Contraction of body of bladder • Relaxation of the sphincter of the bladder • Both effects result in urination	• NE or EPI binds to β_2-receptors on the body of the bladder • NE or EPI binds to α_1-receptors on the sphincter of the bladder	• Relaxation of the body of the bladder • Contraction of the sphincter of the bladder • Both effects result in decreased urination
Liver	• Impulses via vagus nerve	• Slight glycogen synthesis; weak gallbladder contraction	• NE or EPI binds to β_2-receptors	• Increase in glycogenolysis and gluconeogenesis
Pancreas	• Impulses via vagus nerve Ach release	• Secretion of moderate to large amounts of enzymes into the pancreatic acini	• NE or EPI binds to β_2-receptors on the beta cells • NE or EPI binds to α_2-receptors on the beta cells	• Increase in insulin release (predominant effect) • Decrease in insulin release
Kidney	• Insignificant	• Insignificant	• NE or EPI binds to β_1-receptors	• Renin release
Adipose tissue	• Insignificant	• Insignificant	• NE binds to β_3-receptors on adipocytes	• Increased lipolysis (release of free fatty acids)

II. Medications

CLASSIFICATION OF CHOLINERGIC AGONISTS

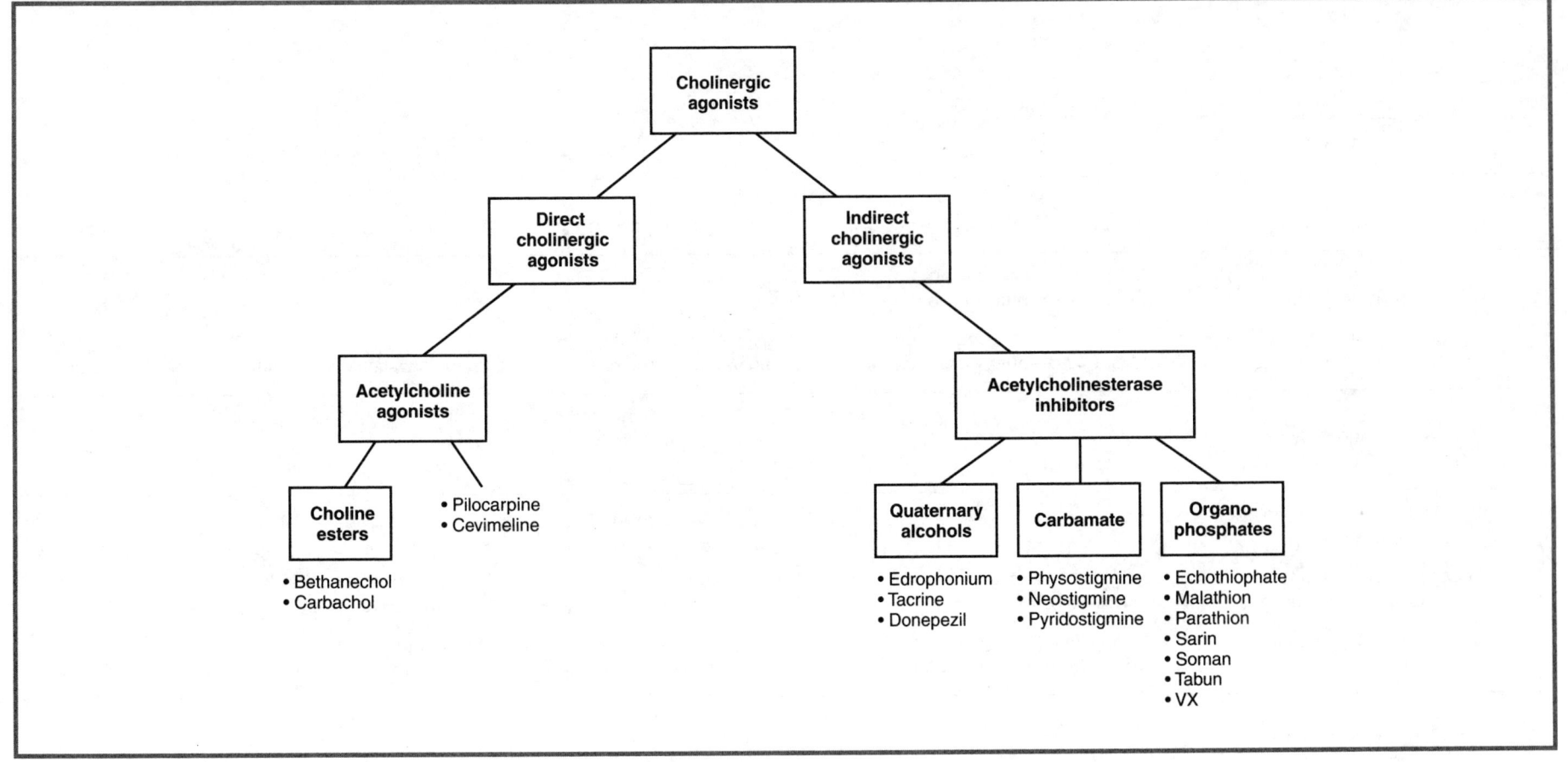

DIRECT CHOLINERGIC AGONISTS: ACETYLCHOLINE AGONISTS

Drug	Pharmacokinetics	Mechanism of Action	Clinical Uses	Drawbacks and Side Effects
Bethanechol (Urecholine)	• **A:** PO • **D:** Poor lipid solubility; does not cross the BBB • **DOA:** Longer duration of action than acetylcholine due to resistance to cholinesterases	• Favors M receptors (especially M_3)	• Treatment of urinary retention	**Contraindications:** • Asthma—increase bronchial constriction and secretions • Hyperthyroidism • Coronary insufficiency—stimulation of M receptors in coronary arteries causes vasoconstriction • Peptic ulcer disease
Carbachol (Isopto Carbachol, Miostat)	• **A:** Ophthalmic drops and intraoptic • **D:** Poor lipid solubility; does not cross the BBB • **DOA:** Longer duration of action than acetylcholine due to resistance to acetylcholinesterase	• More N than M activity	• Wide-angle glaucoma (acts by constricting the ciliary muscle, which opens the meshwork of the canal of Schlemm) • Miosis for surgery	**Muscarinic Poisoning Symptoms = Parasympathetic Overdrive** **Poisoning symptoms:** ☞ **DUMBELS** • Diarrhea • Urination • Miosis • Bronchoconstriction • Excitation (skeletal muscle and CNS) • Lacrimation • Salivation and sweating
Pilocarpine (Isopto Carpine, Salagen)	• **A:** PO and ophthalmic drops; well absorbed • **D:** Good lipid solubility	• Favors M receptors	• Wide-angle glaucoma (acts by constricting the ciliary muscle, which opens the meshwork of the canal of Schlemm) • Used to treat xerostomia in patients with head and neck cancers or Sjögren's syndrome	
Cevimeline (Evoxac)	• **A:** PO • **D:** Moderate lipid solubility • **M:** Hepatic (P450) • **E:** Parent drug and metabolites excreted in urine	• Favors M receptors	• Treatment of xerostomia associated with Sjögren's syndrome	**These symptoms can be reversed with administration of atropine**

INDIRECT CHOLINERGIC AGONISTS: ANTIACETYLCHOLINESTERASES

Drug	Pharmacokinetics	Mechanism of Action	Clinical Uses	Drawbacks and Side Effects
Quaternary Alcohols				
Edrophonium (Enlon, Tensilon)	• **A:** IM and IV • **D:** No CNS effects • **E:** In urine	• Reversibly bind directly to acetylcholinesterase	• Diagnosis of myasthenia gravis	**Poisoning symptoms:** ☞ **DUMBELS** • **D**iarrhea • **U**rination • **M**iosis • **B**ronchoconstriction • **E**xcitation (skeletal muscle and CNS) • **L**acrimation • **S**alivation and sweating • Poisoning can be treated with atropine • Use of tacrine is limited due to hepatotoxicity
Tacrine (Cognex)	• **A:** PO • **D:** Enters the CNS • **M:** Hepatic (P450) • **E:** Not fully elucidated; small amounts excreted in urine		• Treatment of Alzheimer's disease	
Donepezil (Aricept)	• **A:** PO • **M:** Hepatic (P450) • **E:** Parent drug and metabolites excreted in urine			
Carbamates				
Physostigmine	• **A:** IM, IV, and ophthalmic • **M:** Hydrolyzed by cholinesterases, degraded more slowly than Ach • **D:** Crosses the BBB	• Reversibly bind directly to acetylcholinesterase	• Applied topically for wide-angle glaucoma • Treatment of CNS toxicity associated with anticholinergic poisoning	Same as above

Neostigmine (Prostigmin, Bloxiverz)	• **A:** IM, IV, SC, and PO • **M:** Hepatic • **E:** Parent drug and metabolites excreted in urine		• Drug of choice for paralytic atony of the bladder from surgery • Treatment and diagnosis of myasthenia gravis • Reversal of NM blockade	
Pyridostigmine (Mestinon, Regonol)	• **A:** IM, IV, and PO • **M:** Hepatic • **E:** Majority excreted unchanged in urine		• Treatment of myasthenia gravis • Pretreatment to reduce risk of mortality on exposure to "nerve gases" • Reversal of NM blockade	
Organophosphates				
Echothiophate (Phospholine iodide) Malathion (Ovide) Parathion Sarin (GB) Soman (GD) Tabun (GA) VX	• **A:** Well absorbed through skin, lung, gut, and conjunctiva • **M:** Metabolized (especially in insects) by mixed function oxygenases to active form (ie, parathion to paraxin and malathion to malaoxon)	• Irreversibly bind to acetylcholinesterase (exception: malathion, which binds reversibly and is the least toxic of the class)	• Glaucoma (second-line agent) • Treatment of head lice • Used in insecticides • Nerve gases (highly volatile liquids that are among the most toxic synthetic agents known) • Sarin was used in 1995 terrorist attack on Japanese subway	• Poisoning symptoms as above • Poisoning (aside from CNS symptoms) can be treated with atropine • Poisoning can be reversed with pralidoxime (2-PAM) and atropine • Parathion causes most cases of poisoning and death associated with organophosphates

CLASSIFICATION OF MUSCARINIC ANTAGONISTS

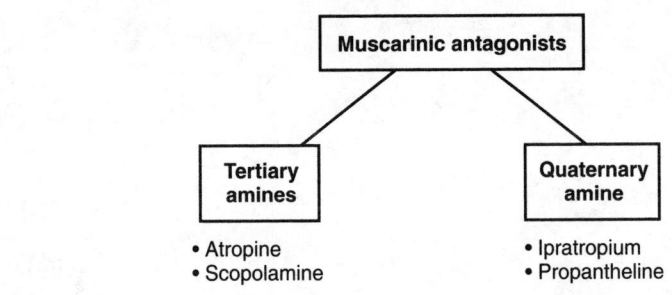

Some members of these classes of drugs also possess antimuscarinic activity: neuromuscular blockers, phenothiazine antipsychotics, antidepressants (tricyclics), and antihistamines.

MUSCARINIC ANTAGONISTS

Drug	Pharmacokinetics	Mechanism of Action	Clinical Uses	Drawbacks and Side Effects	Toxicity of Muscarinic Antagonists
Tertiary Amines					
Atropine (Sal-Tropine, Isopto Atropine)	• **A:** Endotracheal, IM, IV, PO, SC, and ophthalmic drops • **D:** Well distributed; crosses BBB • **M:** Hepatic • **E:** Parent drug and metabolites excreted in urine	• Act as competitive inhibitors • Effects can be overcome by increased concentrations of muscarinic agonists	• Reverse muscarinic or antiacetylcholine sterase poisoning • Mydriasis with cycloplegia • Mydriasis for prolonged periods of time • Bradycardia • Decreases secretions and salivation	**Contraindications:** • Can precipitate acute glaucoma in patients with narrow anterior chamber angle • Can precipitate hyperthermia in infants • Use with caution in the setting of BPH	☞ • Mouth (dry) • Urinary retention • Skin (hot and flushed) • Constipation • Airway dilation and reduction of secretions • Rhythm disturbance (tachycardia) • Intraventricular conduction may be blocked • Nervous system (CNS confusion) • Eyes (mydriasis) OR Adage "dry as a bone, blind as a bat, red as a beet, mad as a hatter"
Scopolamine (Isopto Hyoscine, Hyoscine)	• **A:** IM, IV, PO, SC, ophthalmic, or transdermal patch • **D:** Crosses BBB • **M:** Hepatic • **E:** Metabolites excreted in urine		• Treatment and prevention of motion sickness • Ophthalmologic applications (see Medications for Treating Diseases of the Eye)		

Continued

MUSCARINIC ANTAGONISTS (Continued)

Drug	Pharmacokinetics	Mechanism of Action	Clinical Uses	Drawbacks and Side Effects	Toxicity of Muscarinic Antagonists
Quaternary Amines					
Ipratropium (Atrovent)	• **A:** Inhaled • **D:** Poorly absorbed; does not cross BBB • **E:** Urine		• Bronchodilator in asthma and COPD	• Less risk of side effects due to poor distribution	
Propantheline (Pro-Banthine)	• **A:** PO • **D:** Poorly absorbed; does not cross BBB • **M:** In GI tract and liver • **E:** Parent drug and metabolites excreted in urine		• Decrease acid secretion in patients with PUD		

CLASSIFICATION OF GANGLIONIC BLOCKERS

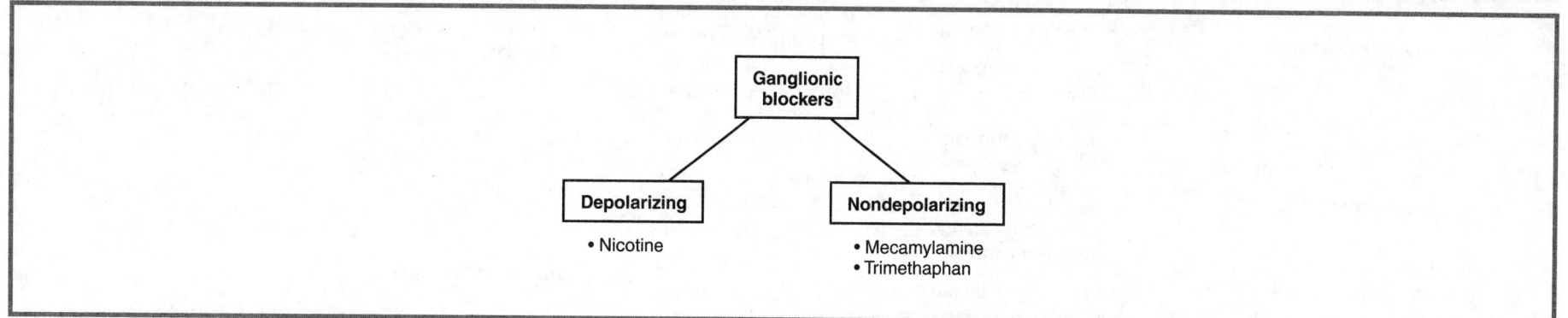

Drug	Pharmacokinetics	Mechanism of Action	Clinical Uses	Drawbacks and Side Effects
Nicotine (Nicoderm, Nicotrol, Nicotrol inhaler, Nicorette)	• A: Inhaler, nasal spray, buccal, or transdermal • M: Liver, kidney, and lungs • E: Parent drug and metabolites excreted in urine	• Blockade via persistent depolarization • Stimulation of autonomic ganglia (parasympathetic and sympathetic) followed by blockade • Stimulation of adrenal medulla • Stimulation of CNS (alerting response, change in respiration)	• Treatment of nicotine addiction to aid in smoking cessation	**Mild:** • Vomiting • Transient increase in salivation • Cold sweat • Disturbed vision • Dizziness • Muscular weakness **Severe:** • Tachycardia and arrhythmia • Respiratory distress • Convulsion • Death
Mecamylamine (Inversine)	• A: PO • E: Unchanged in urine	• Competitive pharmacologic antagonists • Block both parasympathetic and sympathetic systems • These drugs were the first used to treat hypertension; however, their use for this condition is limited due to excessive side effects	• Treatment of moderate to severe hypertension • Treatment of hypertensive emergencies • Possible use in Tourette's syndrome and nicotine addiction	• Extensive side effects have led to limited clinical usefulness of nondepolarizing ganglionic blockers • Postural hypotension • Xerostomia • Blurred vision • Constipation • Severe sexual dysfunction
Trimethaphan (Arfonad)	• A: IV • E: Majority excreted unchanged in urine		• Treatment of hypertensive emergencies • Induction of controlled hypotension to reduce bleeding in the surgical field	

CLASSIFICATION OF SYMPATHOMIMETICS

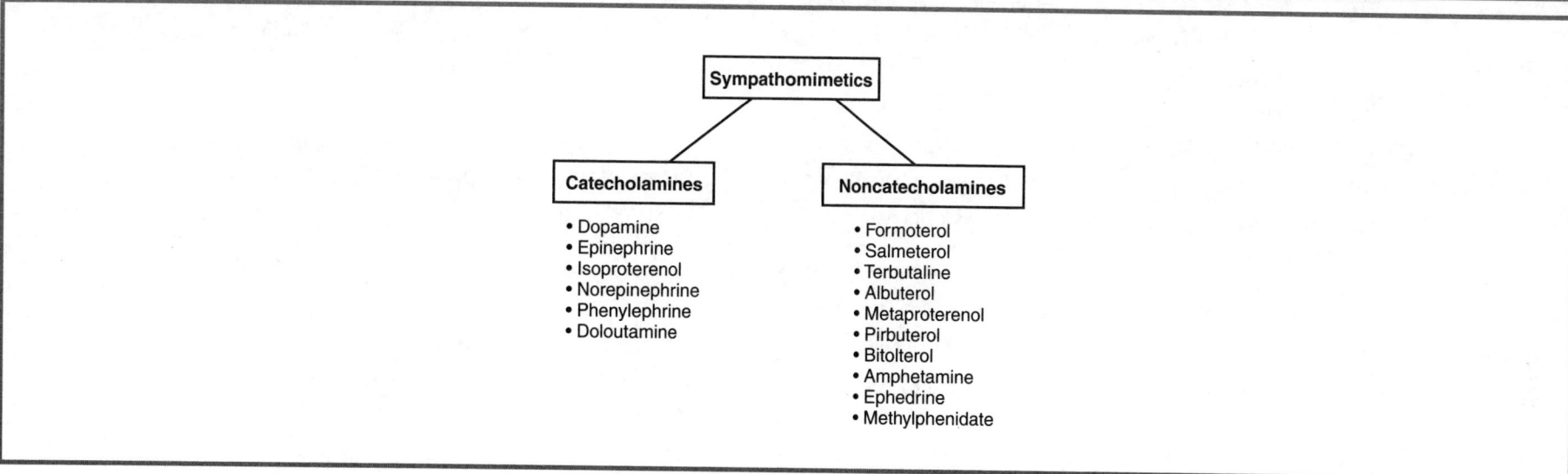

CATECHOLAMINES

Drug	Administration	Mechanism of Action	Clinical Uses	Drawbacks and Side Effects
Dopamine	• **A:** IV • **E:** Metabolites excreted in urine	• Stimulates NE release • $D_1 = D_2 > \beta > \alpha$ activity	• Hemodynamic support • Maintains renal perfusion	• High doses can lead to vasoconstriction through α stimulation • Extravasation can lead to necrosis and tissue loss

Continued

CATECHOLAMINES (Continued)

Drug	Administration	Mechanism of Action	Clinical Uses	Drawbacks and Side Effects
Epinephrine (Adrenalin, Epipen)	**A:** IM, IV, SC, intracardiac, endotracheal, topical, inhaled **E:** Metabolites excreted in urine	• α_1, α_2, β_1 and β_2 agonist • Lower doses selective for β_1 receptors	• Bradycardia/asystolic arrest • Pulseless VF/VT • Combined with local anesthetics to prolong their action and contribute to hemostasis • Mydriasis during ocular surgery • Bronchodilator in asthma • Treatment of anaphylaxis	• HR increases • BP increases • TPR decreases slightly
Phenylephrine	**A:** IM, IV, SC, topical, nasal, PO, ophthalmic **E:** Metabolites excreted in urine	• α_1 and α_2 agonist	• Hypotension/shock • Refractory SVT • Nasal congestion	• HR decreases
Isoproterenol	**A:** IM, IV, inhaled **E:** Metabolites excreted in urine	• β_1 and β_2 agonist	• Bradyarrhythmias • AV nodal block • Refractory torsade de pointes • Bronchodilator	• HR increases • BP decreases (pulse pressure increases) • TPR decreases
Norepinephrine (Levophed)	**A:** IV **A:** Metabolites excreted in urine	• α_1 and α_2 agonist • Some β_1 activity	• Hypotension/shock • Pressor of choice in sepsis	• HR increases (less than others) • BP increases (pulse pressure unchanged) • TPR increases • Extravasation can lead to necrosis and tissue loss
Dobutamine	**A:** IV **E:** Metabolites excreted in urine	• β_1 agonist • Less β_2 and α activity	• Hemodynamic support in cardiovascular compromise	• HR increases • BP can increase or decrease • TPR increases

NONCATECHOLAMINES

Drug	Pharmacokinetics	Mechanism of Action	Clinical Uses	Drawbacks and Side Effects
Terbutaline (Brethine)	• **A:** Inhaled, PO, and SC	• β_2-Agonists	• Bronchodilators for treatment of asthma	• Minimal side effects
Albuterol (Proventil, Ventolin)	• **A:** Inhaled and PO		• Terbutaline used to stop premature contractions in pregnant women	• Skeletal muscle tremor
Metaproterenol (Metaprel, Alupent)			• Salmeterol and formoterol are long-acting β_2 agonists	• Tachycardia
Pirbuterol (Maxair)	• **A:** Inhaled			• Long-acting β_2 agonists have increased risk of asthma-related deaths and should only be used as adjunctive therapy in patients not controlled on a long-term control medication such as glucocorticoids
Bitolterol (Tornolate)				
Salmeterol (Serevent)	• **A:** Inhaled			
Formoterol (Foradil, Perforomist)				
Amphetamine/ Dextroamphetamine (Adderall)	• **A:** PO	• α- and β-Agonist • Causes release of DA, NE, and 5-HT from nerve terminal	• Treatment of ADHD • Treatment of narcolepsy	• Restlessness • Tremor • Insomnia
Ephedrine	• **A:** IM, IV, PO, and SC	• α- and β-Agonist • Causes release of NE	• Bronchodilator for treatment of asthma • Treatment of nasal congestion • Treatment of anesthesia-induced hypotension	• Anxiety • Tachycardia • Adderall is associated with serious cardiovascular events such as sudden deaths in patients with cardiac abnormalities
Methylphenidate (Ritalin, Metadate, Daytrana, Concerta)	• **A:** PO, transdermal	• Blocks reuptake of NE	• Treatment of ADHD • Treatment of narcolepsy (some preparations)	

EFFECTS OF SYMPATHOMIMETICS ON ORGAN SYSTEMS

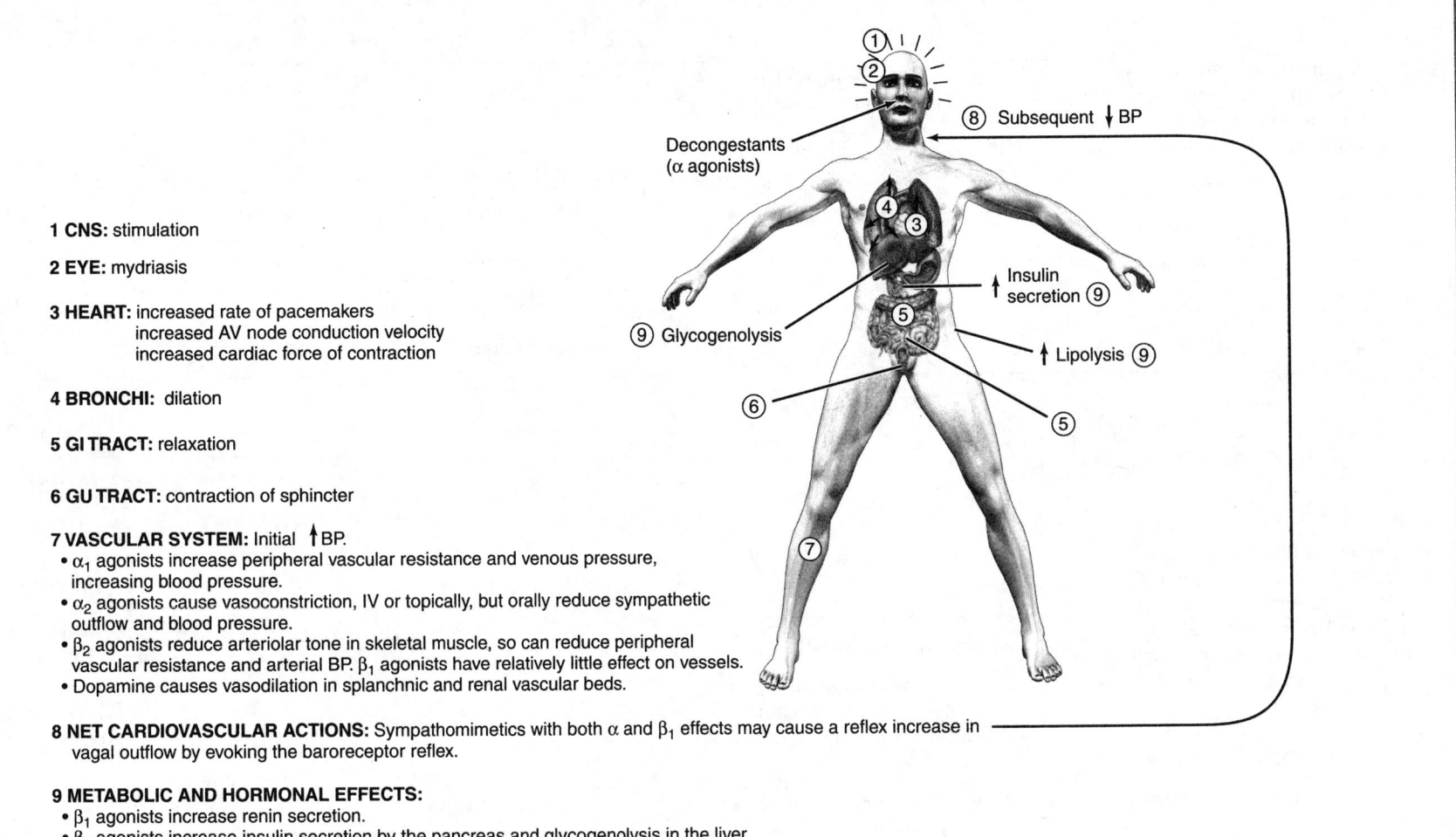

1 CNS: stimulation

2 EYE: mydriasis

3 HEART: increased rate of pacemakers
increased AV node conduction velocity
increased cardiac force of contraction

4 BRONCHI: dilation

5 GI TRACT: relaxation

6 GU TRACT: contraction of sphincter

7 VASCULAR SYSTEM: Initial ↑BP.
- α_1 agonists increase peripheral vascular resistance and venous pressure, increasing blood pressure.
- α_2 agonists cause vasoconstriction, IV or topically, but orally reduce sympathetic outflow and blood pressure.
- β_2 agonists reduce arteriolar tone in skeletal muscle, so can reduce peripheral vascular resistance and arterial BP. β_1 agonists have relatively little effect on vessels.
- Dopamine causes vasodilation in splanchnic and renal vascular beds.

8 NET CARDIOVASCULAR ACTIONS: Sympathomimetics with both α and β_1 effects may cause a reflex increase in vagal outflow by evoking the baroreceptor reflex.

9 METABOLIC AND HORMONAL EFFECTS:
- β_1 agonists increase renin secretion.
- β_2 agonists increase insulin secretion by the pancreas and glycogenolysis in the liver.
- All β agonists appear to stimulate lipolysis.

CLASSIFICATION OF ADRENERGIC BLOCKERS

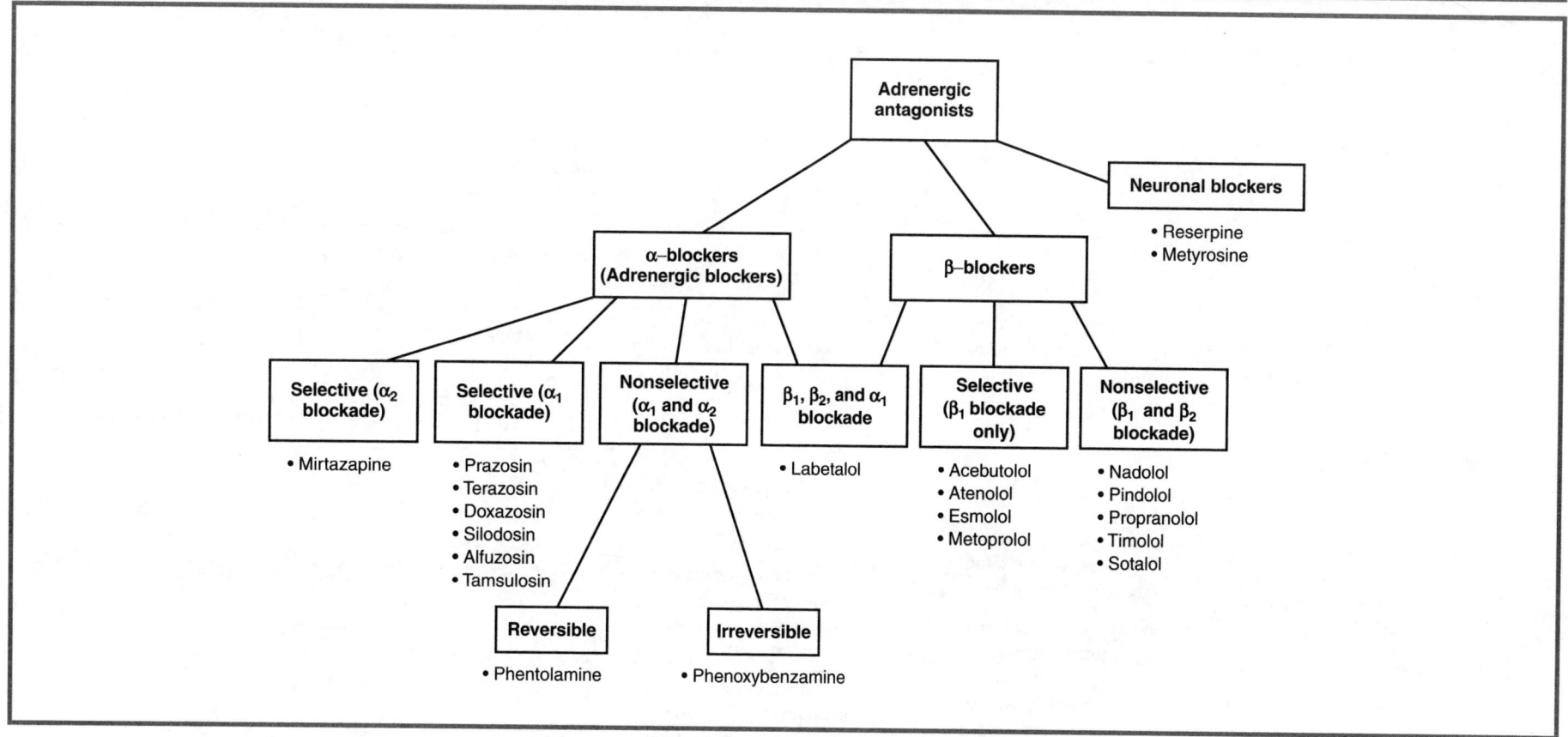

α-BLOCKERS AND NEURONAL BLOCKERS

Drug	Pharmacokinetics	Mechanism of Action	Clinical Uses	Drawbacks and Side Effects
Nonselective α-Adrenergic Blocker (Reversible)				
Phentolamine	• **A:** IV or IM • **M:** Hepatic • **E:** Excreted in urine	• Decreases in TPR and BP through action upon α-receptors in vascular smooth muscle • Orthostatic hypotension via antagonism of sympathetic stimulation of α_1-receptors in venous smooth muscle • Big increase in HR due to decreased autoregulation by α_2-receptor blocking	• Diagnosis of pheochromocytoma • Blocks vasoconstriction in patients with sympathomimetic vasopressor extravasation • Treatment of hypertensive emergencies associated with pheochromocytoma • Reversal of soft tissue anesthesia	• Tachycardia and other arrhythmias • Myocardial ischemia • Orthostatic hypotension • Increased gastric acid production
Nonselective α-Adrenergic Blocker (Irreversible)				
Phenoxybenzamine (Dibenzyline)	• **A:** PO • **DOA:** Long (3–4 days) • **M:** Hepatic • **E:** Metabolites excreted in urine and feces	• Prevention of symptoms of pheochromocytoma via α blockade	• Treatment of symptoms of pheochromocytoma	• Sedation • Orthostatic hypotension

Selective α_1-Adrenergic Blockers

Prazosin (Minipress) Silodosin (Rapaflo) Terazosin (Hytrin) Alfuzosin (Uroxatral) Doxazosin (Cardura) Tamsulosin (Flomax)	• **A:** PO • **M:** Hepatic • **E:** Majority of parent drug and metabolites excreted in feces; remainder in urine (urine > feces with Tamsulosin)	• Relaxation of arterial and venous smooth muscle via α_1 blockade	• Treatment of BPH • Treatment of hypertension	• Exaggerated orthostatic hypotension response to first dose in some patients so should be taken at bedtime

Selective α_2-Adrenergic Blocker

Mirtazapine (Remeron)	"See page 114"			

Neuronal Blockers

Reserpine	• **A:** PO • **M:** Hepatic • **E:** Metabolites excreted in feces > urine	• Blocks reuptake of NE, DA, and 5-HT into vesicle • Results in depletion of DA, NE, and 5-HT from central and peripheral neurons	• Treatment of mild to moderate hypertension	• Diarrhea • Parkinson-like syndrome • Sedation • Severe depression and suicide
Metyrosine (Demser)	• **A:** PO • **E:** Majority excreted unchanged in urine	• Blocks tyrosine hydroxylase • Interferes with DA synthesis • Therefore, there is less NE and EPI secreted by the tumor	• Treatment of pheochromocytoma (especially in patients with metastatic or inoperable disease)	• Crystalluria • Sedation • Diarrhea • EPS

β-BLOCKERS

Drug	Pharmacokinetics			Mechanisms of Clinical Effects	Clinical Uses	Drawbacks and Side Effects
	Selective	Administration	$t_{1/2}$ (hours)			
Acebutolol (Sectral)	Yes, affinity for β_1 sites only	PO	3–4	• Treatment of hypertension via decreased HR, CO, contractility, renin release by kidney, and BP via CNS actions	• Hypertension • Ventricular arrhythmias • Angina	**Contraindications:** • Acute CHF • Cardiogenic shock • Bradycardia
Atenolol (Tenormin)		PO	6–9		• Hypertension • Angina	**Side Effects:**
Esmolol (Brevibloc)		IV	10 min	• Treatment of angina via decreased HR, contractility, heart work, and oxygen consumption	• Acute coronary syndrome • Arrhythmias • Intraoperative NR and BP control	• CNS—depression • CVS—bradycardia and hypotension • Bronchoconstriction therefore use selective blockers cautiously
Metoprolol (Toprol XL, Lopressor)		PO, IV	3–4	• Treatment of hyperthyroidism by blocking thyroxin, which causes β_1 stimulation of the heart	• Hypertension • CHF • Angina • MI • Rate control in a fib/flutter	• PVD and Raynaud's disease-aggravation of symptoms of arterial insufficiency
Betaxolol (Kerlone)	Yes, β_1 affinity	PO	14–22		• Hypertension	
Nebivolol (Bystolic)	Yes, β_1 affinity	PO	12		• Hypertension	
Bisoprolol (Zebeta)	Yes, β_1 affinity	PO	9–12		• Hypertension	

Nadolol (Corgard)	No, affinity for β_1 and β_2 sites	PO	24		• Hypertension
Pindolol		PO	3–4		• Angina
Propranolol (Inderal LA)		PO, IV	3–6	• Treats glaucoma by decreasing production of aqueous humor	• Tachyarrhythmias • Pheochromocytoma • Hypertension • Angina • Hyperthyroidism • Migraine prophylaxis
Timolol (Blocadren)		PO	4–5		• Migraine prophylaxis • Hypertension • Decrease mortality following MI • Angina
Sotalol (Betapace, sorine)		PO, IV	3–6		• Ventricular arrhythmias • Atrial fibrillation flutter
Labetalol (Trandate)	No (affinity for β_1, β_2, and α_1 sites)	PO, IV	3–6		• Hypertension • Hypertensive emergency
Carvedilol (Coreg)		PO	5		• CHF • Hypertension • Post MI LV dysfunction

III. Pharmacology of the Eye

CHOLINERGIC AND ADRENERGIC DRUGS FOR TREATING CONDITIONS OF THE EYE

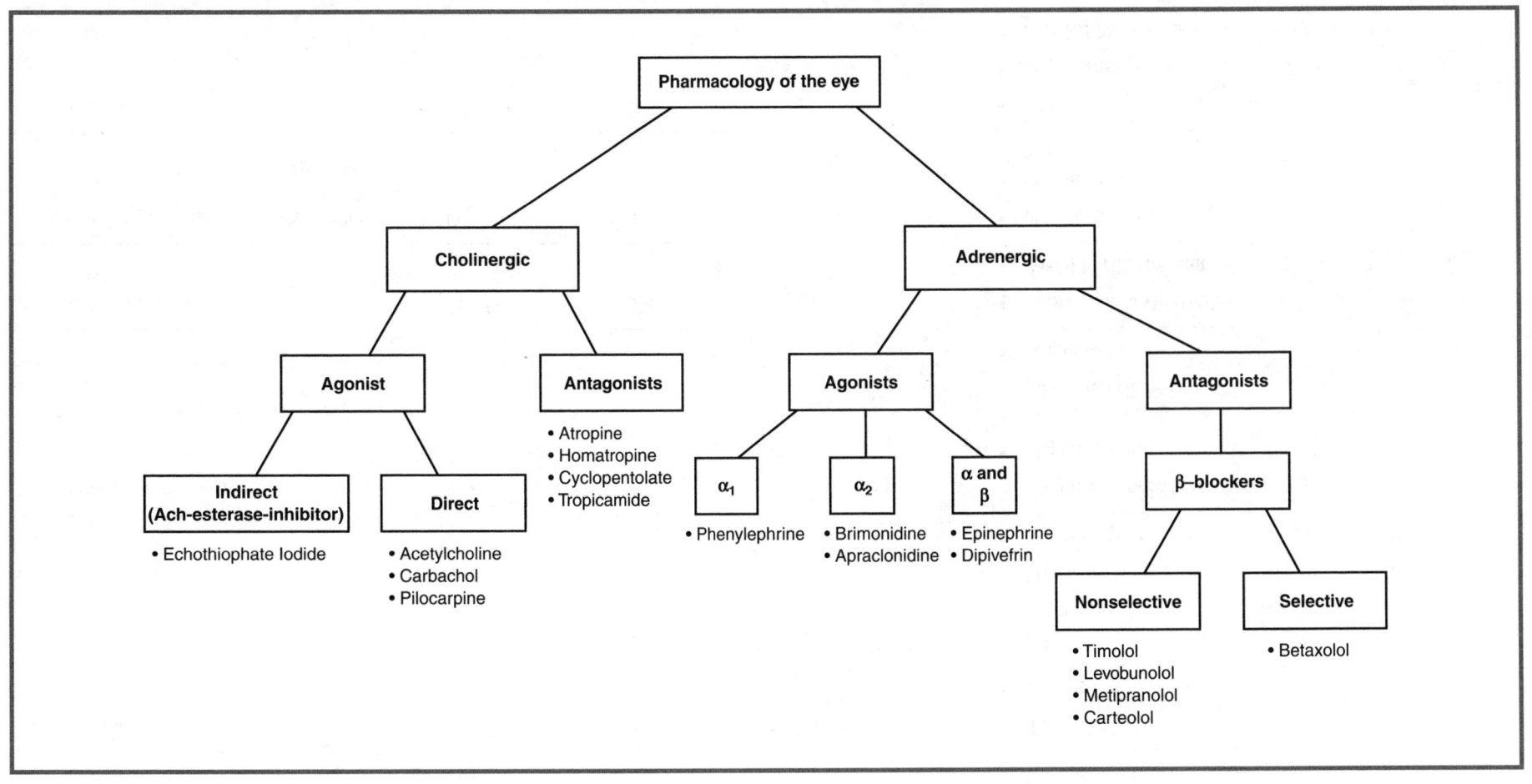

EYE RECEPTOR MECHANISMS

Area	Mechanism
Dilator muscle	• Adrenergic stimulation of α_1-receptors on muscle causes pupil to dilate.
Pupillary sphincter muscles	• Cholinergic stimulation of muscarinic receptors on these muscles cause the pupils to constrict.
Ciliary body	• Cholinergic stimulation of muscarinic receptors causes a contraction of the ciliary body leading to increased accommodation. • Adrenergic stimulation causes ciliary muscle to relax, allowing for far vision; produces aqueous humor.

CHOLINERGIC AGENTS, MIOTIC AGENTS

Drug	Mechanism of Action	Clinical Uses	Drawbacks and Side Effects*
Acetylcholine (Miochol-E)	• Stimulates cholinergic receptors causing miosis via constriction of the pupillary muscle	• Miosis for opthalmic surgery	• Blurry vision • Symptoms of toxicity consistent with cholinergic overdrive
Carbachol (Isopto Carbachol, Miostat)	• Potentiation of accommodation via constriction of the ciliary muscle • Reduces intraocular pressure by widening trabecular spaces to increase outflow of aqueous humor	• Treatment of glaucoma • Miosis for opthalmic surgery • Treatment of glaucoma	• Diarrhea • Urination • Miosis
Pilocarpine (Isopto Carpine, Pilopine HS)			• Bradycardia, Bronchospasm
Echothiophate Iodide (Phospholine Iodide)	• Inhibitor of cholinesterase causing increased activity of acetylcholine • Stimulates cholinergic receptors causing miosis via constriction of the pupillary muscle • Potentiation of accommodation via constriction of the ciliary muscle • Reduces intraocular pressure by widening trabecular spaces to increase outflow of aqueous humor		• Emesis • Lacrimation • Salivation

*Eye drops must be used with care because they can cause lethal complications, such as hypertensive crisis and ventricular arrhythmias.

Continued

CHOLINERGIC AGENTS, MIOTIC AGENTS (Continued)

Drug	Mechanism of Action	Clinical Uses	Drawbacks and Side Effects*
Mydriatics and Cycloplegics			
Atropine (Isopto Atropine) Homatropine (Isopto Homatropine)	• Cholinergic antagonist at muscarinic receptors on the iris and ciliary body causes cycloplegia and mydriasis	• Decrease post surgical inflammation (prevents iris from adhering to the cornea and relaxes the ciliary muscle and reduces vascular permeability) • Prevent adhesion formation in inflammatory conditions such as uveitis and procedures • Dilation for eye examinations	• May precipitate acute glaucoma in patients with a narrow anterior chamber angle • Blurry vision • Toxicity manifests as muscarinic toxicity (copy from page 87)
Cyclopentolate (Cyclogyl)		• Good for corneal abrasions (decreases pain from ciliary muscle spasm) or mild conditions where cycloplegia and mydriasis are desired	
Tropicamide (Mydriacyl)		• Produces dilation of pupil; useful for funduscopic examinations	
Adrenergic Agents			
Phenylephrine (Neosynephrine)	• α_1-Agonist at radial muscle of the iris	• Often added in small concentration to OTC drops to whiten the sclera via vasoconstriction	• Causes rebound dilation and redder eyes
Brimonidine (Alphagan)	• Reduces production of aqueous humor • Increases outflow of aqueous humor	• Treatment of glaucoma	• Burning, stinging of the eye • Blurred vision
Epinephrine (Epifrin, Glaucon)	• Causes conjunctival constriction • Causes slight mydriasis • Reduces intraocular pressure (mainly by increasing outflow and slight decrease in aqueous humor production)	• Treatment of glaucoma by reducing intraocular pressure via increased outflow and decreased production of aqueous humor	• Localized burning and irritation • Localized allergic reaction • Accumulation of melanin granules • Can cause lethal hypertensive crisis or ventricular arrhythmias by entering systemic vasculature via nasal cavity from tear duct

Dipivefrin (Propine)	• Transformed into epinephrine once in the eye and has same beneficial effects	• Treatment of glaucoma • Lipophilic version of epinephrine (leads to better absorption through the cornea)	• Absorption into the eye reduces therapeutic dose so systemic side effects of epinephrine are decreased
Apraclonidine (Iopidine)		• Treatment and prevention of perioperative intraocular pressure elevation	
Ocular β-blockers			
Timolol (Timoptic)	• Theoretically decreases aqueous humor formation via receptors on the ciliary body	• Treatment of open angle glaucoma • Treatment of ocular hypertension	• Localized irritation and burning • CNS effects include lethargy, light-headedness, fatigue, memory loss • CV effects include bradycardia, hypotension, syncope, arrhythmias, wheezing, pulmonary edema, CHF, and death
Levobunolol (Betagan)			
Betaxolol (Betoptic)			
Metipranolol (Optipranolol)			
Carteolol (Ocupress)			

*Eye drops must be used with care because they can cause lethal complications, such as hypertensive crisis and ventricular arrhythmias.

CLINICALLY IMPORTANT STRUCTURES OF THE EYE AND THEIR RECEPTORS

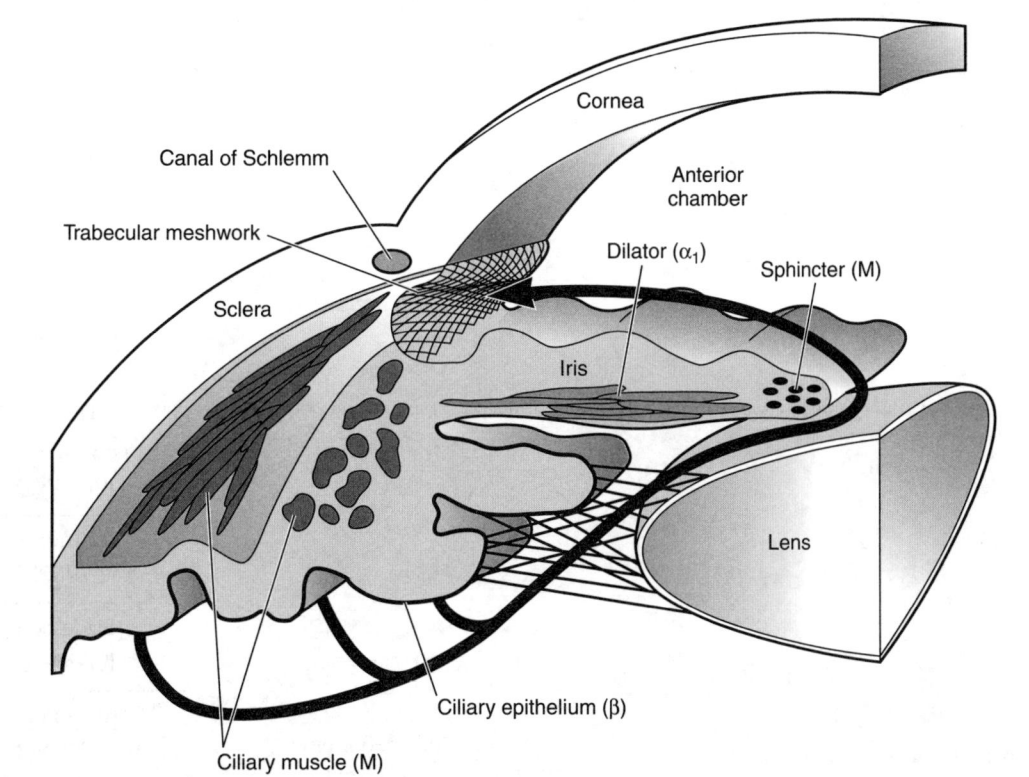

The heavy arrow shows the flow of aqueous humor from its secretion by the ciliary epithelium to its drainage through the canal of Schlemm (M, muscarinic; α_1, alpha receptor; β, beta receptor).

Cornea

Canal of Schlemm

Anterior chamber

Trabecular meshwork

Dilator (α_1)

Sphincter (M)

Sclera

Iris

Lens

Ciliary epithelium (β)

Ciliary muscle (M)

Modified from Trevor AJ, Katzung BG, Masters SB: *Katzung & Trevor's Pharmacology Examination & Board Review*, 6th ed, p 54. Originally published by Appleton & Lange. © 2002 by the McGraw-Hill Companies, Inc.

CHAPTER 4
PSYCHIATRIC MEDICATIONS

I. ANTIPSYCHOTICS

Classification of Antipsychotics

Typical Antipsychotics

Atypical Antipsychotics

II. ANTIDEPRESSANTS

Classification of
Antidepressants

Acute Actions
of Antidepressants

Tricyclic Antidepressants

Heterocyclics Antidepressants

Selective Serotonin
Reuptake Inhibitors

Serotonin Norepinephrine
Reuptake Inhibitors

Monoamine Oxidase
Inhibitors

**III. MOOD STABILIZING
AGENTS**

Mood Stabilizing Agents

IV. ANXIOLYTICS

Classification of
Anxiolytics

Anxiolytic Medications

**V. MEDICATIONS FOR
DISORDERS
DIAGNOSED IN
CHILDHOOD**

ADHD

VI. DRUGS OF ABUSE

Drugs of Abuse: The Facts

TERMS TO LEARN

Akathisia	An inner sense of restlessness.
Delirium Tremens (DTs)	Autonomic instability, hallucinations, tremor, hypertension, tachycardia, and risk of seizures associated with cessation of alcohol ingestion.
Dyskinesias	Abnormal involuntary movement.
Dystonia	Muscle spasm, stiffness.
Extrapyramidal Syndrome (EPS)	Parkinson-like syndrome, akathisias, and dystonias. Evolution appears as follows: • Acute dystonia develops over hours • Akinesia develops over days • Akathisia develops over weeks • Tardive dyskinesia develops over months
Neuroleptic Malignant Syndrome (NMS)	Characterized by muscular rigidity, fever, and autonomic instability; associated with the use of neuroleptic medications (eg, haloperidol).
Obsessive Compulsive Disorder (OCD)	Anxiety disorder that is characterized by recurrent, unwanted, intrusive thoughts and/or behaviors.
Posttraumatic Stress Disorder (PTSD)	Anxiety disorder that develops after exposure to one or more traumatic events. Symptoms include flashbacks, nightmares, hypervigilence.
Premenstrual Dysphoric Disorder (PMDD)	Severe form of premenstrual syndrome characterized by depression symptoms, irritability, and tension before menstruation. Occurs in 3–8% of women.
Seasonal Affective Disorder (SAD)	Type of depression that seems to affect a person at a certain time of the year. It is more common in the late fall and winter months but can be at other times of the year.
Serotonin Syndrome	Caused by overactivation of central 5-HT receptors; symptoms include abdominal pain, diarrhea, sweating, fever, tachycardia, hypertension, delirium, myoclonus; can induce cardiovascular shock and death.

Tardive Dyskinesia (TD)	Irreversible syndrome of involuntary choreoathetoid movements associated with chronic use of neuroleptic medications; typically involves mouth, face, limbs, and trunk.
Toxic Epidermal Necrolysis (TENS)	Potentially life threatening rare dermatologic reaction, widespread erythema, necrosis, and bullous detachment of the epidermis and mucous membranes. Usually a drug reaction however, can have other etiologies such as infection or malignancy.
Trigeminal Neuralgia	Sharp, stabbing pain that occurs in one or more divisions of the trigeminal nerve.
Wernicke-Korsakoff Syndrome	Neurologic disorder caused by thiamine deficiency; often seen in chronic alcoholic patients; symptoms include confusion, ataxia, and memory impairment.

I. Antipsychotics

CLASSIFICATION OF ANTIPSYCHOTICS

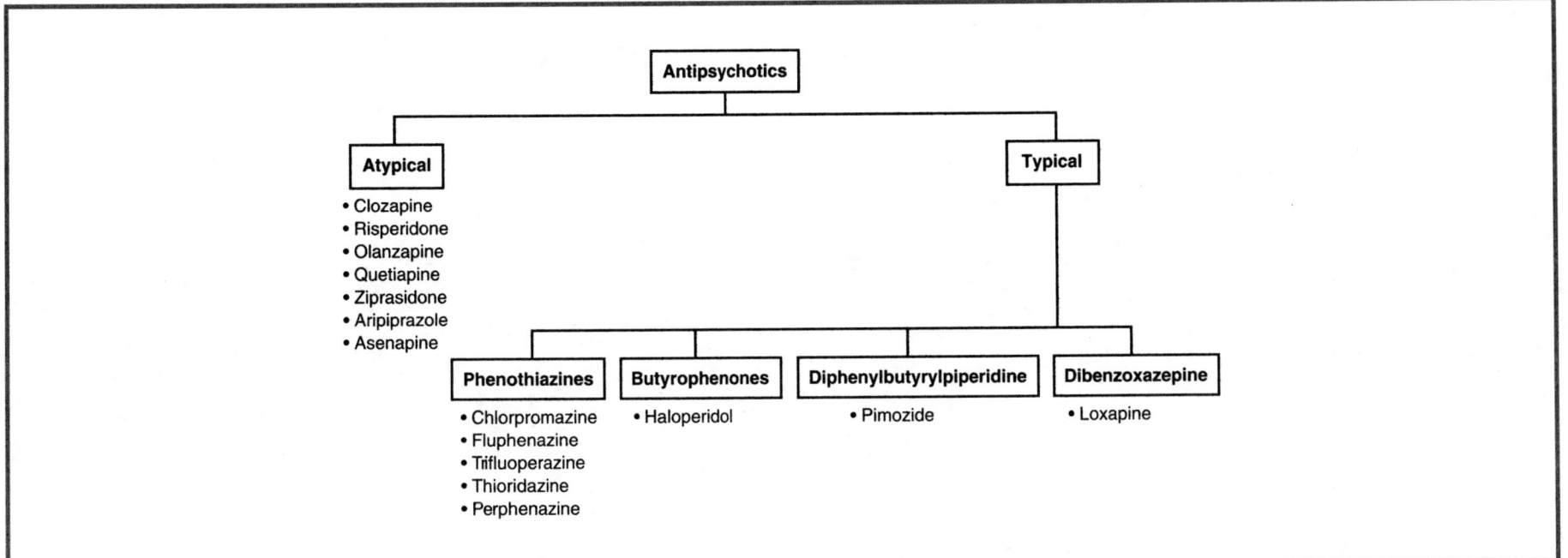

TYPICAL ANTIPSYCHOTICS

Drug	Pharmacokinetics	Mechanism of Action		Clinical Uses	Drawbacks and Side Effects
Phenothiazines					
Chlorpromazine (Thorazine)	A: IM, IV, PO	D: Widely distributed, crosses BBB M: Hepatic (P450) E: Parent drugs and metabolites excreted in urine > feces	• Blocks dopamine D2 post synaptic receptor	Low • Intractable hiccups • Nausea and vomiting • Schizophrenia/psychotic features associated with mental illnesses	• QT prolongation (esp Thioridazine) • NMS • TD • EPS • Increased risk of death in elderly patients with dementia-related psychosis with all typical antipsychotics • Inhibits P450 enzymes (except Trifluoperazine and Loxapine)
Thioridazine (Mellaril)	A: PO			Low • Schizophrenia/psychotic features associated with mental illnesses	
Fluphenazine (Prolixin, Permitil)	A: IM, PO, SC			High • Schizophrenia/psychotic features associated with mental illnesses	
Trifluoperazine (Stelazine)	A: PO			High • Schizophrenia/psychotic features associated with mental illnesses • Nonpsychotic anxiety	
Perphenazine	A: PO			High • Schizophrenia • Nausea and vomiting	
Butyrophenones					
Haloperidol (Haldol)	A: IM, IV, PO			High • Schizophrenia/psychotic features associated with mental illnesses	
Diphenylbutylpiperidinesd					
Pimozide (Orap)	A: PO			High • Tourette syndrome	
Dibenzoxazepine					
Loxapine (Loxitane)	A: IM, PO			High • Psychotic features associated with mental illnesses	

Continued

TYPICAL ANTIPSYCHOTICS (Continued)

- Potency refers to the D2 binding
- High potency typical antipsychotics are more likely to produce EPS
- Low potency typical antipsychotics are more likely to have nonneurologic side effects associated with anticholinergic, antihistamine, and a blockade effect and include increased risk of weight gain and metabolic disturbances
- Generally better at treating the positive symptoms of schizophrenia (ie, hallucinations, delusions)

ATYPICAL ANTIPSYCHOTICS

Drug	Pharmacokinetics	Mechanism of Action	Clinical Uses and General Information	Drawbacks and Side Effects
Clozapine (Clozaril, FazaClo)	**A:** PO, IM (clozapine, quetiapine, and asenapine are PO only) **B:** Highly protein bound **D:** Widely distributed, crossed BBB **M:** Hepatic (P450) **E:** Metabolites excreted in feces and urine	• Antagonism at $5\text{-}HT_2$ and D_2 receptors	• Treatment of refractory schizophrenia due to significant adverse effects	• Agranulocytosis • Myocarditis • Orthostatic hypotension • Sedation • Seizures • Excessive salivation • Inhibits P450 enzymes
Risperidone (Risperdal)			• Bipolar mania • Bipolar I maintenance • Schizophrenia • Autism in children	• Sedation • Weight gain • Hyperprolactinemia (highest risk with Risperdal) • Increased risk of suicidal thoughts and behaviors in children, adolescents, and young adults (with Seroquel and aripiprazole) • Increased risk of death in elderly patients with dementia-related psychosis with all atypical antipsychotics • Inhibits P450 enzymes (except Quetapine, Zisprasidone, Asenapine and Iloperidone)

Olanzapine (Zyprexa)	• Bipolar mania
	• Bipolar I maintenance
	• Schizophrenia
	• Agitation with bipolar disorder or schizophrenia
Quetiapine (Seroquel)	• Adjunctive therapy in depression
	• Bipolar maintenance
	• Schizophrenia
Ziprasidone (Geodon)	• Bipolar mania
	• Bipolar maintenance
	• Schizophrenia
	• Acute agitation in schizophrenia
Aripiprazole (Abilify)	• Adjunctive therapy in depression
	• Schizophrenia
	• Bipolar mania
Asenapine (Saphris)	• Schizophrenia
	• Bipolar mania
Paliperidone (Invega)	• Schizophrenia (adults and children)
	• Schizoaffective disorder
Iloperidone (Fanapt)	• Schizophrenia

- Greater risk of weight gain and metabolic disturbances than even low potency typical antipsychotics
- Less risk of EPS
- Generally better at treating the negative symptoms of schizophrenia (ie, flat affect, anhedonia)

II. Antidepressants

CLASSIFICATION OF ANTIDEPRESSANTS

Antidepressants

TCAs	**Heterocyclics**	**SNRIs**	**SSRIs**	**Irreversible MAO A and B inhibitors**	**Reversible MAO A inhibitor**	**Irreversible MAO B inhibitor**
• Imipramine • Amitriptyline • Clomipramine • Nortriptyline • Doxepine • Amoxapine • Desipramine	• Bupropion • Trazodone • Mirtazapine	• Venlafaxine • Desvenlafaxine • Duloxetine	• Fluoxetine • Citalopram • Fluvoxamine • Paroxetine • Sertraline • Escitalopram • Vilazodone	• Phenelzine • Isocarboxazid • Tranylcypromine	• Moclobemide	• Selegiline • Rasagiline

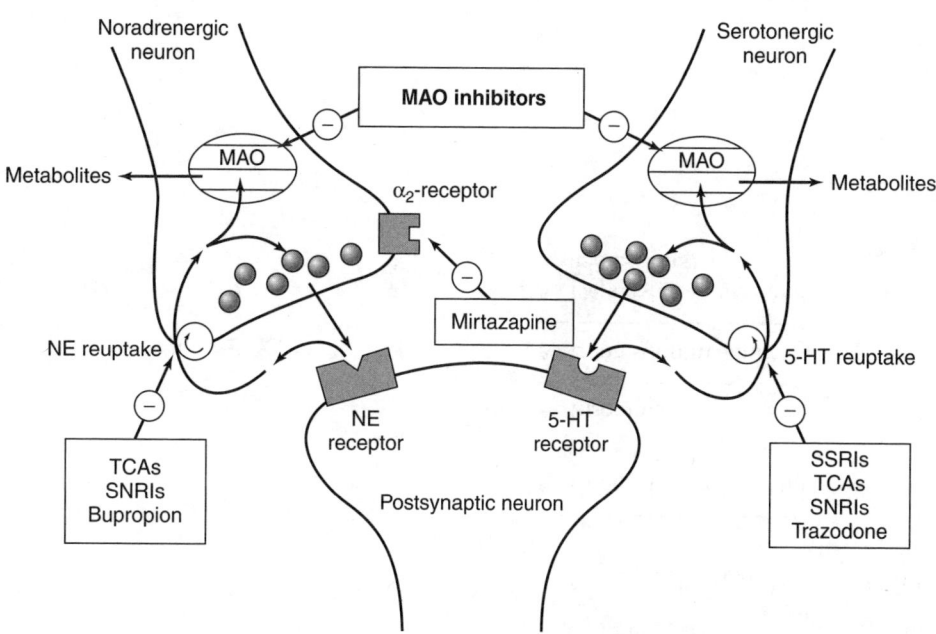

Many antidepressants may require administration for a number of weeks before achieving clinical efficacy.

Modified from Trevor AJ, Katzung BG, Masters SB: *Katzung & Trevor's Pharmacology Examination & Board Review*, 6th ed, p 270. Originally published by Appleton & Lange. © 2002 by the McGraw-Hill Companies, Inc.

TRICYCLIC ANTIDEPRESSANTS

Drug	Pharmacokinetics	Mechanism of Action	Clinical Uses	Drawbacks and Side Effects
Imipramine (Tofranil)	**A:** PO (Imipramine and Amitriptyline are also IM)	Inhibit NE and 5-HT reuptake increasing their levels in the synapse	• Nocturnal enuresis in children • Depression	• Increased risk of suicidal thoughts and behaviors in children, adolescents, and young adults
Amitriptyline (Elavil)	**D:** Widely distributed, crossed BBB		• Depression (adults and adolescents)	• Sexual dysfunction
Clomipramine (Anafranil)	**B:** Highly protein bound **M:** Hepatic (P450)		• OCD (adults and children)	• Sedation • Overdose associated with coma, cardiac toxicity (PR and QT prolongation); treat with NaHCO$_3$
Nortriptyline (Pamelor)	**E:** Metabolites excreted in urine > feces		• Depression in adults	• Inhibit P450 enzymes (except Doxepin and Amoxapine)
Doxepin (Silenor)			• Depression (adults and adolescents) • Insomnia	
Amoxapine			• Depression in adults	
Desipramine (Norpramin)			• Depression (adults and adolescents)	

HETEROCYCLICS ANTIDEPRESSANTS

Drug	Pharmacokinetics	Mechanism of Action	Clinical Uses and General Information	Drawbacks and Side Effects
Bupropion (Wellbutrin, Zyban, Budeprion, Forfivo, Aplenzin)	**A:** PO **M:** Hepatic (P450) **E:** Metabolites excreted in urine > feces	• Weakly inhibits NE and DA reuptake • Metabolite inhibits reuptake of NE	• Depression • SAD • Smoking cessation	• Neuropsychiatric events including depression, suicidal thoughts, and suicide • Increased risk of suicidal thoughts and behaviors in children, adolescents, and young adults • Headache • Xerostomia • Seizure • Less likely to cause sexual dysfunction • Inhibits P450 enzymes
Trazadone (Oleptro)		• Inhibits 5-HT reuptake • Blocks α_1 and H_1	• Depression	• Sedation (often exploited for insomnia) • Orthostatic hypotension • Increased risk of suicidal thoughts and behaviors in children, adolescents, and young adults • Inhibits P450 enzymes
Mirtazapine (Remeron)		• α_2 presynaptic antagonist leading to increased NE and 5-HT release into the synapse • Antagonist at 5-HT_2, 5-HT_3, H_1, α_1, and M	• Depression	• Sedation (often exploited for insomnia) • Weight gain • Xerostomia • Increased risk of suicidal thoughts and behaviors in children, adolescents, and young adults • Less likely to cause sexual dysfunction • Inhibits P450 enzymes

SELECTIVE SEROTONIN REUPTAKE INHIBITORS

Drug	Pharmacokinetics	Mechanism of Action	Clinical Uses and General Information	Drawbacks and Side Effects
Fluoxetine (Prozac)	A: PO, well absorbed M: Hepatic (P450) E: Majority of metabolites excreted in urine	Inhibits 5-HT reuptake increasing synaptic levels of 5-HT	• Depression (adults and pediatrics) • PMDD • Bulimia • Panic disorder • OCD (adults and pediatrics)	• Withdrawal syndrome including nausea, vomiting, diarrhea (most notable with Paroxetine, least risk with Fluoxetine due to its long $t_{1/2}$ of 4–6 days) • Sexual dysfunction • Serotonin syndrome • Increased risk of suicidal thoughts and behaviors in children, adolescents, and young adults • Inhibit P450 enzymes
Citalopram (Celexa)			• Depression (adults)	
Escitalopram (Lexapro)			• Depression (adults and pediatrics) • Generalized anxiety disorder	
Fluvoxamine (Luvox)			• OCD (adults and pediatrics)	
Paroxetine (Paxil)			• Depression • Panic disorder • PMDD • PTSD • SAD • OCD	
Sertraline (Zoloft)			• OCD • Panic disorder • PMDD • PTSD • SAD	
Vilazodone (Viibryd)			• Depression	

SEROTONIN NOREPINEPHRINE REUPTAKE INHIBITORS

Venlafaxine (Effexor)

A: PO
M: Hepatic
E: Metabolites excreted in urine > feces

Inhibit 5-HT and NE reuptake with greater effect on NE

- Depression
- Panic disorder
- Generalized anxiety disorder
- Social anxiety disorder

Desvenlafaxine (Pristiq, Khedezla)

- Depression

Duloxetine (Cymbalta)

- MDD
- Diabetic neuropathy
- Generalized anxiety disorder
- Fibromyalgia
- Chronic musculoskeletal pain

- Increased risk of suicidal thoughts and behaviors in children, adolescents, and young adults
- Hypertension
- Withdrawal symptoms include dizziness, nausea, and irritability
- Inhibit P450 enzymes
- Induces P450 enzymes (Desvenlafaxine only)

MONOAMINE OXIDASE INHIBITORS

Drug	Pharmacokinetics	Mechanism of Action	Clinical Uses and General Information	Drawbacks and Side Effects
Irreversible Monoamine Oxidase A and B Inhibitors				
Phenelzine (Nardil)	**A:** PO (Selegiline is also TD) **M:** Hepatic (P450) **E:** Metabolites excreted primarily in urine	• Inhibits MAO A and B • Increases presynaptic NE, DA, and 5-HT	• Depression • Side effects profile including dietary restrictions limit usefulness	• Contraindicated with drugs rich in amines or those that elevate synaptic amines (ie, amphetamines, SSRIs, TCAs, and λ dopa) or with foods that are rich in tyramine and other sympathomimetic amines as congestion causes hypertensive crisis • Orthostatic hypotension • Weight gain • Increased risk of suicidal thoughts and behaviors in children, adolescents, and young adults
Isocarboxazid (Marplan)				
Tranylcypromine (Parnate)				• Inhibits P450 enzymes (Tranylcypromine only)
Reversible Selective Monoamine Oxidase A Inhibitor				
Moclobemide (Manerix)		• Inhibits MAO A • Increases presynaptic NE, DA, and 5-HT	• Depression	• Insomnia • Tremor • Inhibits P450 enzymes
Irreversible Selective Monoamine Oxidase B Inhibitors				
Selegiline (Eldepryl, Emsam, Zelapar)		• Irreversible MAO B inhibitor • Also inhibits MAO A at higher levels	• Parkinson's disease • Depression	• Dyskinesia • Nausea • Orthostatic hypotension • Increased risk of suicidal thoughts and behaviors in children, adolescents, and young adults
Rasagiline (Azilect)		• Irreversible MAO B inhibitor	• Parkinson's disease	• Inhibit P450 enzymes

III. Mood Stabilizing Agents

MOOD STABILIZING AGENTS

Drug	Pharmacokinetics	Mechanism of Action	Clinical Uses	Drawbacks and Side Effects
Lithium (Lithobid)	• **A:** PO; completely absorbed from GI tract in about 8 hours; peak plasma concentration ~2–4 hours after an oral dose • **D:** In ECF with gradual accumulation; slow passage through BBB (CSF concentration 40% of plasma concentration) • **E:** ~95% eliminated in unchanged urine	• Not well defined • May decrease availability of IP$_3$ and DAG second messengers	• Bipolar disorder	• Narrow therapeutic window • Tremor • Sedation • Ataxia • Polydipsia/polyuria • Nephrogenic diabetes insipidus • Leukocytosis • Thyroid dysfunction • Prenatal use associated with congenital cardiac anomalies (ie, Ebstein's anomaly) • Cardiac arrhythmia • Flattened or inverted T waves

Continued

MOOD STABILIZING AGENTS (Continued)

Drug	Pharmacokinetics	Mechanism of Action	Clinical Uses	Drawbacks and Side Effects
Carbamazepine (Tegretol, Carbatrol, Epitol, Equetro)	**A:** PO; variable rate of absorption; peak blood levels 6–8 hours after administration **B:** 75–90% binding to plasma proteins **M:** Hepatic (P450) **E:** Parent drug and metabolites excreted in urine	• Blocks Na$^+$ channels	• Anticonvulsant • Trigeminal neuralgia • Bipolar mania	• Contraindicated in pregnancy (neural tube defects) • Nausea/vomiting • Dizziness • Drowsiness • Induces P450 enzymes • Dermatologic reactions (including TENS and SJS) • Patients of Asian descent should be screened for HLA-B*1502 variant (due to increased risk for SJS)
Valproate (Depakene, Depacon, Depakote, Stavzor)	**A:** PO, IV; absorbed well; peak blood levels ~1–6 hours (enteric coated preparation is absorbed in basic pH of small intestine, decreasing nausea and stomach cramps) **B:** 80% serum protein binding **M:** Hepatic (P450) **E:** Majority excreted as metabolites in urine	• Increased availability of GABA • Enhances or mimics the action of GABA at postsynaptic receptors	• Anticonvulsant • Migraine prophylaxis • Bipolar mania	• Contraindicated in pregnancy (neural tube defects) • Headache • Tremor • Somnolence • Nausea/vomiting • Hair loss • Thrombocytopenia • Hepatic failure resulting in fatalities • Pancreatitis • Inhibits P450 enzymes • Induces P450 enzymes

IV. Anxiolytics

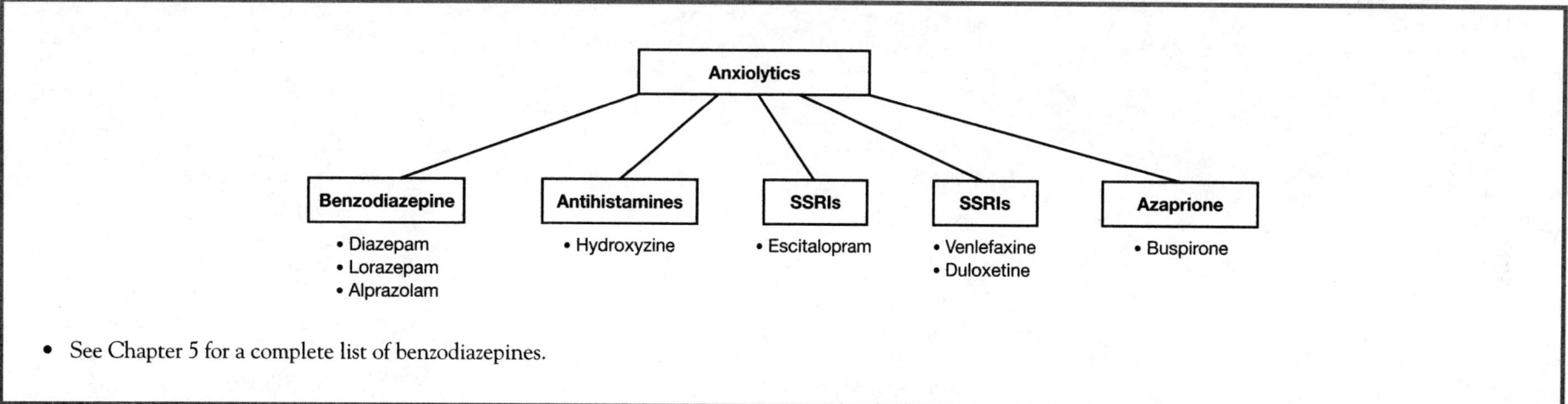

- See Chapter 5 for a complete list of benzodiazepines.

ANXIOLYTIC MEDICATIONS

Benzodiazepines

Alprazolam (Xanax, Niravam)	**A:** PO, IV, IM **B:** Highly bound to plasma proteins **M:** Hepatic (P450) **E:** Metabolites excreted in urine	• Enhances the inhibitory effect of GABA at the postsynaptic GABA receptor by increasing the frequency of chloride channel openings	• Anxiety disorder • Panic attacks	• Somnolence • Xerostomia • Appetite changes • Inhibits P450 enzymes (Diazepam only)
Diazepam (Valium, Diastat)	**A:** PO, IV, IM **B:** Highly bound to plasma proteins **M:** Hepatic (P450) **E:** Metabolites excreted in urine		• Anxiety disorder • Alcohol withdrawal • Muscle spasm • Status epilepticus	
Lorazepam (Ativan)	**A:** PO, IV, IM, PR **B:** Highly bound to plasma proteins **M:** Hepatic **E:** Metabolites excreted in urine		• Anxiety disorder • Insomnia due to anxiety • Status epilepticus • Anticonvulsant • Acute agitation	

Azapirone

Buspirone (Buspar)	**A:** PO **B:** Highly bound to plasma proteins **M:** Hepatic (P450) **E:** Metabolites excreted in urine	• Exact MOA unknown • High affinity at 5-HT$_{1A}$ and 5-HT$_2$ receptors	• Anxiety disorder	• Sedation • Dizziness

Antihistamine

Hydroxyzine (Vistaril)	**A:** PO, IM **M:** Hepatic **E:** Metabolites excreted in urine	• Competitive antagonist of histamine at H_1 receptors	• Anxiety • Antiemetic • Preop sedation • Pruritus	• Xerostomia • Dizziness • Inhibits P450 enzymes

Selective Serotonin Reuptake Inhibitors

Escitalopram (Lexapro)	**A:** PO, well absorbed **M:** Hepatic (P450) **E:** Majority of metabolites excreted in urine	• Inhibits 5-HT reuptake increasing synaptic levels of 5-HT	• Depression (adults and pediatrics) • Anxiety	• Sexual dysfunction • Serotonin syndrome • Increased risk of suicidal thoughts and behaviors in children, adolescents, and young adults • Inhibits P450 enzymes

Serotonin Norepinephrine Reuptake Inhibitors

Venlafaxine (Effexor)	**A:** PO **M:** Hepatic (P450) **E:** metabolites excreted in urine > feces	• Inhibit 5-HT and NE reuptake with greater effect on NE	• Depression • Panic disorder • Generalized anxiety disorder • Social anxiety disorder	• Increased risk of suicidal thoughts and behaviors in children, adolescents, and young adults • Hypertension • Withdrawal symptoms include dizziness, nausea, and irritability • Inhibits P450 enzymes
Duloxetine (Cymbalta)			• MDD • Diabetic neuropathy • Generalized anxiety disorder • Fibromyalgia • Chronic musculoskeletal pain	

Listed above are the FDA approved medications for anxiety, however, other medications from the above classes are also often clinically utilized.

V. Medications for Disorders Diagnosed in Childhood

Pervasive Developmental Disorder

- Autism
  - Risperdal (see Atypical Antipsychotics)
  - Abilify (see Typical Antipsychotics)

Tic Disorders

- Tourette
  - Pimozide (see Typical Antipsychotics)

Anxiety Disorders

- OCD
  - Clomipramine (see Tricyclic Antidepressants)
  - Fluoxetine (see Selective Serotonin Reuptake Inhibitors)
  - Fluvoxamine (see Selective Serotonin Reuptake Inhibitors)

Elimination Disorders

- Nocturnal Enuresis
  - Imipramine (see Tricyclic Antidepressants)

Mood Disorder

- Depression
  - Fluoxetine (see Selective Serotonin Reuptake Inhibitors)
  - Escitalopram (see Selective Serotonin Reuptake Inhibitors)

Psychotic Disorder

- Schizophrenia
  - Paliperidone (see Typical Antipsychotics)

ADHD

Stimulants

Drug	Pharmacokinetics	Mechanism	Indications	Adverse Effects
Dexmethylphenidate (Focalin)	**A:** PO **M:** Hepatic **E:** Metabolites excreted in urine	• Blocks reuptake of DA and NE into the presynaptic neurons	• ADHD	• Headache • Potential for drug dependency • Decreased appetite • Inhibits P450 enzymes (Methylphenidate only)
Methylphenidate (Concerta, Ritalin, Daytrana, Metadate, Methylin, Quillivant)	**A:** PO, TD **M:** Hepatic **E:** Metabolites excreted in urine		• ADHD • Narcolepsy	
Methamphetamine (Desoxyn)	**A:** PO **M:** Hepatic (P450) **E:** Metabolites excreted in urine	• Cause release of DA and NE from presynaptic nerve terminals		• Potential for drug dependency • Weight reduction plans are ineffective
Dextroamphetamine (Dexedrine, ProCentra, Zenzedi)	**A:** PO, TD **M:** Hepatic (P450) **E:** Parent drug and metabolites excreted in urine			• Potential for drug dependency • Serious cardiovascular events including sudden death in patients with structural cardiac abnormalities or other serious heart problems
Lisdexamfetamine (Vyvanse)	**A:** PO, TD **M:** Hydrolyzed in plasma to dextroamphetamine and L-lysine **E:** Metabolites excreted in urine		• ADHD in adults and children	• Potential for drug dependency

Norepinephrine Receptor Inhibitor

Drug	Pharmacokinetics	Mechanism	Indications	Adverse Effects
Atomoxetine (Strattera)	**A:** PO **M:** Hepatic (P450) **E:** Metabolites excreted in urine	• Inhibits the reuptake of NE	• ADHD	• Headache • Insomnia • Xerostomia • Increased risk of suicidal thoughts and behaviors in children, adolescents, and young adults • Inhibits P450 enzymes

Continued

ADHD (Continued)

Alpha Adrenergic Agonist

Guanfacine (Intuniv, Tenex)	**A:** PO **M:** Hepatic (P450) **E:** Parent drug and metabolites excreted in urine	• α_2 adrenergic agonist • Acts on chloride channels to increase NE in prefrontal cortex	• ADHD • PDD • Hypertension	• Arrhythmias • Chest pain • Dizziness
Clonidine (Kapvay)	• **A:** PO • **M:** Hepatic • **E:** Parent drug and metabolites excreted in urine	• α_2 adrenergic agonist • Increases NE in the prefrontal cortex	• ADD • Hypertension	• Hypotension

VI. Drugs of Abuse

DRUGS OF ABUSE: THE FACTS

Drug	Mechanism of Action	Intoxication Signs and Symptoms	Withdrawal Symptoms
Cannabinoid			
Marijuana (Mary Jane, Weed, Pot)	• THC is one of >80 psychoactive chemicals in marijuana • Bind to G-protein–coupled receptor that acts via cAMP • Highest concentration of binding sites located in basal ganglia, substantia nigra, globus pallidus, hippocampus, and brain stem	• Heightened mood • Increased appetite • Relaxation • Paranoia • Conjunctivitis	• Irritability • Depression • Nausea • Anorexia • Symptoms seem to peak 48 hours following cessation of use and can persist up to 7 days

Continued

DRUGS OF ABUSE: THE FACTS (Continued)

Drug	Mechanism of Action	Intoxication Signs and Symptoms	Withdrawal Symptoms
Hallucinogens			
Lysergic acid diethylamide (LSD)	• Exact MOA unknown • Chemically resembles NE, DA, and 5-HT • Appears to alter 5-HT turnover	• Synesthesia • Altered thinking • Anxiety • Paranoia • Delusions	• Panic attacks • Psychosis
Phencyclidine (PCP, wet)	• Noncompetitive antagonist at NMDA receptors • D_2 receptor agonist • DA reuptake inhibitor	• Euphoria • Anesthesia • Psychomotor agitation • Psychosis • Hyperthermia • Rotatory nystagmus	• Headache • Confusion • Paranoia
Opiates			
Heroin	• Acts at μ and δ opiate receptors in the CNS	• Euphoria • Analgesia • Respiratory depression • Constipation	• Chills • Piloerection • Nausea/vomiting • Diarrhea • Lacrimation

Sedatives			
Alcohol	• Exact MOA unknown • Seems to facilitate the action of GABA at the GABA$_A$ receptors • Inhibits the ability of glutamate to activate the NMDA receptor	• Loss of inhibition • Impaired judgment • Slurred speech • Ataxia	• Withdrawl: tremor, seizure • Delirium tremens: autonomic dysfunction, hallucinogens, delusions; associated with significant mortality • DTs treated with supportive care and benzodiazepines
Stimulants			
Caffeine	• Seems to work by blockade of presynaptic adenosine receptors	• Increased vigilance • Restlessness • Increased urination	• Fatigue • Headache • Irritability
Nicotine	• Activates presynaptic and postsynaptic cholinergic nicotinic receptors • Triggers release of NE, EPI, and DA	• Increased vigilance • Restlessness	• Irritability • Anxiety • Craving
Cocaine (crack, coke)	• Blocks reuptake of NE, 5-HT, and DA	• Euphoria • Restlessness	• Somnolence • Persistence of psychosis with LTU
Methamphetamine (crystal meth)	• Increases release on NE, 5-HT, and DA • Weak inhibitor of block MAO • Possibly active as direct catecholamine agonist	• Increased libido	• Post withdrawal syndrome following chronic use (mood swings, anhedonia, insomnia, suicidality) can persist for months
3,4-methylenedioxy-N-methylamphetamine (MDMA, Ecstasy)	• Indirect 5-HT agonist	• Mania • Hallucinations • Extroversion • Dry mouth • Bruxism	• Anxiety • Depression

CHAPTER 5
DRUGS AFFECTING NEUROLOGIC FUNCTION

I. DRUGS AFFECTING MOVEMENT DISORDERS

Classification of Drugs Used to Treat Parkinson's Disease

Drugs for the Treatment of Parkinson's Disease

Second-line Drugs for Parkinson's Disease

Third-line Drugs for Parkinson's Disease

Treatment of Other Movement Disorders

II. DRUGS FOR ALZHEIMER'S DISEASE

Classification of Drugs Used for Treatment of Alzheimer's Disease

Drugs for the Treatment of Alzheimer's Disease

III. SEDATIVES AND HYPNOTICS

Sedatives and Hypnotics: Benzodiazepines

Sedatives and Hypnotics: Barbiturates

Other Sedatives and Hypnotics

IV. ANTIEPILEPTIC DRUGS

Classification of Drugs for the Treatment of Epilepsy

Drugs for the Treatment of Epilepsy

Seizure Classifications

V. OPIOIDS

Opioids: Summary Table

Classification of Opioids

Opioid Agonists

VI. DRUGS FOR THE TREATMENT OF MIGRAINES

Classification of Drugs Used for Treatment of Migraines

Abortive Antimigraine Drugs

Prophylactic Migraine Drugs

VII. ANTISPASTIC DRUGS

Classification of Antispastic Drugs

Antispastic Drug Facts

VIII. LOCAL ANESTHETICS AND ADJUNCTIVE DRUGS

Local Anesthetics and Adjunctive Drugs: Summary Table

Classification of Local Anesthetics and Adjunctive Drugs

Local Anesthetics: Esters

Local Anesthetics and Adjunctive Agents: Amides and Other Nonesters

IX. GENERAL ANESTHETIC DRUGS

Classification of General Anesthetic Drugs

General Anesthetic Drugs: Inhaled

General Anesthetic Drugs: Intravenous Nonopioids

General Anesthetic Drugs: Intravenous Opioids

Four Components, Four Stages, and Four Keys to Anesthesia

Nonanesthetic Drugs Used During General Anesthesia

X. NEUROMUSCULAR BLOCKERS

Neuromuscular Blockers: Summary Table

Depolarizing Neuromuscular Blockers

Nondepolarizing Neuromuscular Blockers

Blepharospasm	Eyelid spasm.
Blood-to-Gas Partition Coefficient (B/G Coefficient)	An expression of solubility or the tendency of dissolved gas to come out of solution (ie, blood); low values indicate a fast-acting anesthetic.
Dysphagia	Difficulty swallowing.
Ergotism	Vasoconstriction leading to limb ischemia, gangrene, hypertension, and CNS disturbances; associated with the ingestion of ergots.
Lennox–Gastaut Syndrome	Childhood epileptic encephalopathy; syndrome of severe seizures, mental retardation, and characteristic EEG pattern.
Minimum Alveolar Concentration (MAC)	An expression of the concentration of inhaled anesthetic needed to keep 50% of patients from moving in response to surgical stimulus. Because it is a statistical measurement, all anesthetics are titrated until they produce the desired effect.
Pneumothorax	Air in the intrapleural space.
Strabismus	Nonparallel visual axis of the eyes.
West's Syndrome	Infantile spasms; age-specific form of generalized epilepsy.
Propofol-Related Infusion Syndrome	Syndrome characterized dysrhythmias, metabolic acidosis, hyperkalemia and rhabdomyolysis (with renal failure) associated with propofol use. Mortality rate of 33%.

I. Drugs Affecting Movement Disorders

CLASSIFICATION OF DRUGS USED TO TREAT PARKINSON'S DISEASE

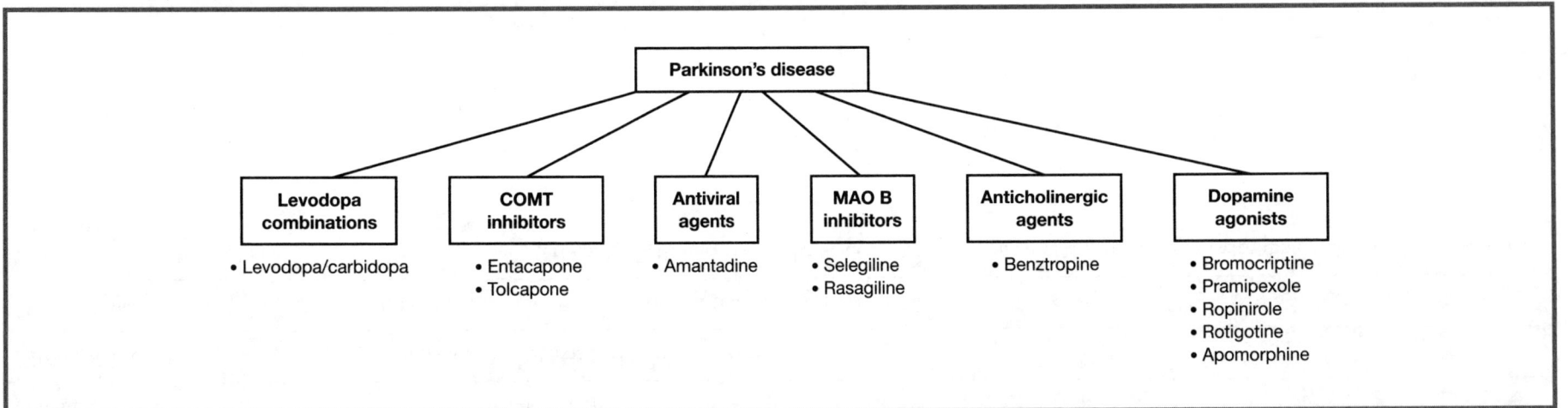

DRUGS FOR THE TREATMENT OF PARKINSON'S DISEASE

Drug	Pharmacokinetics	Mechanism of Action	Clinical Uses	Cautions	Side Effects
Antiviral					
Amantadine	• **A:** PO • **E:** Excreted unchanged in urine	• Antiviral drug used to treat influenza by inhibiting viral uncoating • Blocks or increases DA release in presynaptic fibers • DA release in the striatum	• Parkinson's disease • Drug-induced EPS • Treatment and prophylaxis for influenza A	• CHF • Patients prone to seizures • Renal impairment • Hepatic impairment • Narrow-angle glaucoma	• CNS disturbances (restlessness, depression, irritability, hallucinations, confusion) • GI disturbances (nausea, constipation, xerostomia)
Anticholinergics					
Benztropine (Cogentin)	• **A:** PO, IM, and IV • **M:** Hepatic (however, remaining pharmacokinetics are not well understood)	• Anticholinergic (muscarinic) • May inhibit reuptake and storage of DA	• Parkinson's disease • Dystonia • Drug-induced EPS	• BPH • Obstructive GI disease • Renal impairment • Hepatic impairment • Narrow-angle glaucoma	• Anticholinergic side effects
MAO B Inhibitors					
Selegiline (Emsam, Eldepryl, Zelapar)	• **A:** PO, TD • **D:** Crosses BBB • **M:** Hepatic (P450) metabolism to active metabolites • **E:** Metabolites excreted in urine	• MAO B irreversible inhibitor • Prolongs action of DA by preventing its breakdown • Interferes with DA reuptake • DA action in striatal region decreasing the symptomatic motor deficits of Parkinson's disease • May have neuroprotective effects	• Enhances effect of L-dopa thus may reduce on/off effects • Depression • ADHD in children • Parkinson's disease • Parkinson's disease	• Avoid concomitant use of TCAs, SSRIs, and SNRIs • Block MAO A as well at high doses • May increase adverse effects of L-dopa (psychosis, dyskinesia)	• Nausea • Headache • Insomnia • Inhibits P450 enzymes
Rasagiline (Azilect)	• **A:** PO • **M:** Hepatic (P450) • **E:** Metabolites excreted in urine				• Nausea • Headache • Dyskinesia • Orthostatic hypotension

SECOND-LINE DRUGS FOR PARKINSON'S DISEASE

Drug	Pharmacokinetics	Mechanism of Action	Clinical Uses	Cautions	Side Effects
Levodopa (Larodopa)	• **A:** PO; rapidly absorbed from the small intestine • **D:** Crosses the BBB and is then converted to DA; only 1–3% of oral dose reaches the CNS • **M:** Metabolized in lumen of intestine, liver, kidney, and stomach • **E:** Majority excreted as metabolites in urine	• DA precursor • Increases concentration of available DA	• Treatment of DA-deficient state found in Parkinson's disease	• Pyridoxine (B$_6$) (a cofactor of DA β-hydroxylase) can exacerbate some side effects • Nonselective MAO inhibitors can cause hypertensive crisis • Coadministration with phenothiazines, which block DA receptors • Psychotic patients (exacerbates symptoms) • Patients with open-angle glaucoma or cardiac disease	• On-off phenomenon (fluctuations in clinical effects) **Early:** • Anorexia, nausea, and vomiting due to activation of chemoreceptor zones in the brain (decreased if doses are divided or if taken with meals—tolerance develops to this side effect) • Orthostatic hypotension • Arrhythmias (increased DA is converted to NE) • These side effects are less prominent when the drug is coadministered with a decarboxylase inhibitor **Late:** • Dyskinesia: facial grimacing, restless feet syndrome (increased incidence when combined with decarboxylase inhibitor; managed with drug holidays, dose reduction, or pallidotomy) • Psychiatric and behavioral side effects (confusion, hallucinations, delusions) • Nightmares or anxiety

Drug	Pharmacokinetics	Mechanism	Use	Contraindications/Precautions	Adverse Effects
Carbidopa (Lodosyn)	• **A:** PO • **D:** Does not cross BBB • **E:** Excreted in urine	• Peripheral dopa decarboxylase inhibitor	• Prevents peripheral metabolism of L-dopa thus increasing the level in the CNS in Parkinson's disease	• Narrow-angle glaucoma • Psychotic disorders • Renal impairment • Hepatic impairment	• Agitation • Arrhythmia • Abdominal pain
Levodopa/ Carbidopa (Sinemet, Parcopa)	• **A:** PO • **E:** Both components excreted in urine	• Combination of L-dopa and carbidopa	• Maintains a more constant level of L-dopa in the CNS of Parkinson's patients thus reducing some of the side effects noted above		• Orthostatic hypotension • Impulse control disorder • Somnolence

COMT Inhibitors

Drug	Pharmacokinetics	Mechanism	Use	Contraindications/Precautions	Adverse Effects
Entacapone (Comtan)	• **A:** PO • **D:** Does not cross BBB • **M:** Hepatic • **E:** Primarily excreted as metabolites in feces	• Reversible, selective inhibitor of COMT • Decreases peripheral breakdown of L-dopa thus increasing its availability in the brain	• Reduces clinical fluctuations in Parkinson's patients receiving L-dopa therapy	• Glaucoma • Psychotic disorders • Renal impairment • Hepatic impairment	• Nausea • Dyskinesia • Inhibits P450 enzymes
Tolcapone (Tasmar)	• **A:** PO • **D:** Does not cross BBB • **M:** Hepatic • **E:** Primarily excreted as metabolites in feces				• Fatal hepatotoxicity • Rhabdomyolysis

THIRD-LINE DRUGS FOR PARKINSON'S DISEASE

Drug	Pharmacokinetics	Mechanism of Action	Clinical Uses and General Information	Contraindications	Side Effects
Dopamine Agonists					
Bromocriptine (Parlodel, Cycloset)	• A: PO • M: Hepatic (P450) • E: Metabolites excreted primarily in feces	• Activates postsynaptic DA receptors • Nigrostriatal region activation (enhanced motor control) • Tuberoinfundibular region activation (inhibits pituitary prolactin secretion)	• Parkinson's disease • Acromegaly • Hyperprolactinemia • Diabetes	• Cardiovascular disease • Psychotic disorder	• Risk of fibrotic valve thickening with LTU • Dizziness • Nausea • Headache • Inhibits P450 enzymes
Pramipexole (Mirapex)	• A: PO • E: Excreted unchanged in urine	• Preferential D$_2$ activity • Activates postsynaptic DA receptors	• Parkinson's disease • Restless legs syndrome	• CHF • Renal impairment	• Orthostatic hypotension • Somnolence
Ropinirole (Requip)	• A: PO • M: Hepatic (P450) • E: Primarily excreted as metabolites in feces	• D$_3$ > D$_2$ activity • Activates postsynaptic DA receptors		• Psychotic disorder • Renal impairment • Hepatic impairment	• Dizziness • Headache • Nausea • Dyskinesias
Rotigotine (Neupro)	• A: TD • M: Hepatic (P450) • E: Primarily excreted as metabolites in feces	• D$_1$, D$_2$, and D$_3$ activity • Believed to activate postsynaptic DA receptors		• Psychotic disorder • Cardiovascular disease	• Inhibits P450 enzymes (Ropinirole and Apomorphine only)
Apomorphine (Apokyn)	• A: SC • M: Hepatic (P450) • E: Primarily excreted as metabolites in feces	• Stimulates D$_2$ receptors in the caudate putamen	• Treatment of hypomobility episodes in Parkinson's disease	• Psychotic disorder • Renal impairment • Hepatic impairment	

TREATMENT OF OTHER MOVEMENT DISORDERS

Condition	Possible Medications
Enhances physiological tremor	• Propranolol
Essential tremor	• Propranolol • Primidone
Tourette's syndrome	• Haloperidol
Huntington's disease	• Fluphenazine • Pimozide • Haloperidol • Tetrabenazine • Ropinirole • Chlorpromazine • Risperidone • Olanzapine • Clozapine • Aripiprazole
Orthostatic tremor	• Clonazepam • Gabapentin

II. Drugs for Alzheimer's Disease

Acetylcholinesterase inhibitors are used to treat only the early stages of Alzheimer's disease. As the clinical efficacy of acetylcholinesterase inhibitors decreases, treatment shifts to a symptomatic approach, including standard psychiatric drugs such as antidepressants and antipsychotics (haloperidol, risperidone, and benzodiazepines).

CLASSIFICATION OF DRUGS USED FOR TREATMENT OF ALZHEIMER'S DISEASE

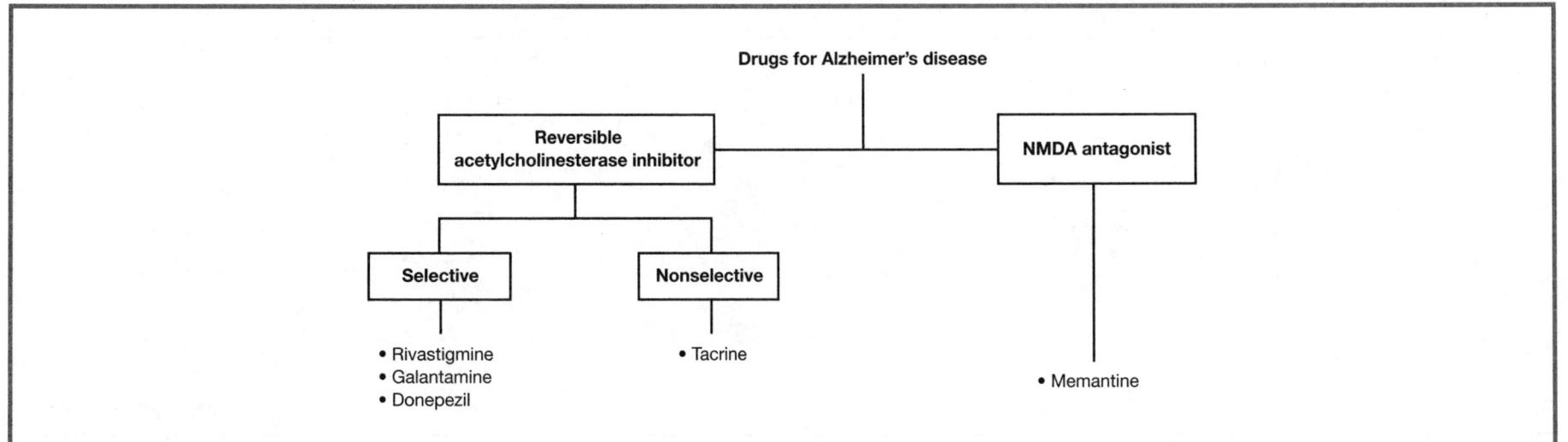

DRUGS FOR THE TREATMENT OF ALZHEIMER'S DISEASE

Drug	Pharmacokinetics	Mechanism of Action	Clinical Uses	Side Effects
Tacrine (Cognex)	• **A:** PO • **D:** Crosses BBB • **M:** Hepatic (P450) • **E:** Majority excreted as metabolites in urine	• Reversible acetylcholinesterase inhibitor • Increase the concentration of Ach in CNS synapses	• Alzheimer's disease however, clinical use limited by hepatotoxicity	• Nausea/vomiting • Abdominal pain • Diarrhea • Hepatotoxicity
Donepezil (Aricept)	• **A:** PO • **D:** Crosses BBB • **M:** Hepatic (P450) • **E:** Majority excreted as metabolites in urine		• Mild to severe Alzheimer's disease	• Nausea/vomiting • Anorexia • Diarrhea • Dizziness • Insomnia • Headache
Rivastigmine (Exelon)	• **A:** PO, TD • **D:** Crosses BBB • **M:** Hydrolysis in the brain and hepatic • **E:** Majority excreted as metabolites in urine		• Alzheimer's dementia • Parkinson's related dementia	
Galantamine (Razadyne)	• **A:** PO • **D:** Crosses BBB • **M:** Hepatic (P450)		• Mild to moderate Alzheimer's disease	
Memantine (Namenda)	• **A:** PO • **D:** Crosses BBB • **M:** Hepatic (P450) • **E:** Parent drug and metabolites excreted in urine	• NMDA receptor antagonist • Helps prevent Ca^{2+}-mediated excitotoxicity	• Moderate to severe Alzheimer's disease	• Dizziness • Headache • Vomiting • Confusion • Constipation

III. Sedatives and Hypnotics

As dosages increase, clinical results move from sedation to hypnosis to coma to death. ☞ SHoCkeD, where S stands for sedation, H for hypnotics and hypnosis, C for coma, and D for death.

SEDATIVES AND HYPNOTICS: BENZODIAZEPINES

Drug	Duration of Action	Pharmacokinetics	Mechanism of Action	Clinical Uses and General Information	Side Effects
Alprazolam (Xanax)	• Short ($t_{1/2}$ <12 hours)	• A: PO • M: Hepatic (P450) metabolism to active metabolites • E: Renal excretion of parent drug and metabolites	• Increase frequency of opening of Cl⁻ channel by GABA at the GABAₐ receptor	• Panic disorder • Anxiety	• Drowsiness • Irritability • Appetite changes
Midazolam (Versed)		• A: PO, PR, IM, IV • M: Hepatic (P450) metabolism to active metabolites • E: Renal excretion of metabolites		• Sedation	• Respiratory depression (caution especially in elderly pts) • Inhibits P450 enzymes
Oxazepam (Serax)		• A: PO • M: Hepatic metabolism • E: Renal excretion of metabolites		• Anxiety • Ethanol withdrawal	• Dizziness • Nausea
Triazolam (Halcion)		• A: PO • M: Hepatic (P450) metabolism to active metabolites • E: Renal excretion of metabolites		• Insomnia	• Drowsiness • Dizziness • Headache • Inhibits P450 enzymes

Estazolam (ProSom)	• Intermediate ($t_{1/2}$ 10–15 hours)	• **A:** PO • **M:** Hepatic (P450) metabolism to inactive metabolites • **E:** Renal excretion of metabolites	• Insomnia	• Drowsiness • Hypokinesia
Lorazepam (Ativan)		• **A:** PO, IM, IV • **M:** Hepatic metabolism to inactive metabolites • **E:** Renal excretion of metabolites	• Anxiety • Insomnia • Status epilepticus • Anesthesia premedication	• Respiratory depression • Sedation
Temazepam (Restoril)		• **A:** PO • **M:** Hepatic (P450) metabolism to inactive metabolites • **E:** Renal excretion of metabolites	• Insomnia	• Drowsiness • Dizziness
Chlordiazepoxide (Librium)	• Long ($t_{1/2}$ 25–100 hours)	• **A:** PO • **M:** Hepatic (P450) metabolism to active metabolites • **E:** Renal excretion of metabolites	• Anxiety • Ethanol withdrawal	• Syncope • Change in libido
Clonazepam (Klonopin)		• **A:** PO • **M:** Hepatic (P450) metabolism • **E:** Renal excretion of metabolites	• Panic disorder • Seizure disorder	• Drowsiness • Dizziness • Change in libido • Inhibits P450 enzymes (Diazepam only)

Continued

| 5. Drugs Affecting Neurologic Function

SEDATIVES AND HYPNOTICS: BENZODIAZEPINES (Continued)

Drug	Duration of Action	Pharmacokinetics	Mechanism of Action	Clinical Uses and General Information	Side Effects
Clorazepate (Tranxene)		• A: PO • M: Metabolism in the GI tract to active metabolite and hepatic (P450) to active metabolites • E: Renal excretion of metabolites		• Anxiety • Ethanol withdrawal	
Diazepam (Valium, Diastat)		• A: PO, PR, IM, IV • M: Hepatic (P450) metabolism to active metabolites • E: Renal excretion of metabolites		• Anxiety • Muscle spasm • Status epilepticus • Ethanol withdrawal	
Flurazepam (Dalmane)		• A: PO • M: Hepatic (P450) metabolism to active metabolites • E: Renal excretion of metabolites		• Insomnia	• Drowsiness • Dizziness • Inhibits P450 enzymes
Quazepam (Doral)		• A: PO • M: Hepatic (P450) metabolism to active metabolites • E: Renal excretion of metabolites			• Drowsiness • Dizziness • Headache • Inhibits P450 enzymes

- Good hypnotic drugs have a fast onset of action.

- Good sedative drugs have a slow onset of action.

- Sedatives and hypnotics have an antiepileptic effect when a methyl group is attached to a N within the ring (eg, phenobarbital).

Drug	Pharmacokinetics	Mechanism of Action	Clinical Uses	Side Effects
Amobarbital (Amytal)	• A: IM, IV • OOA: 1–5 minutes • DOA: 6–8 hours • M: Hepatic (P450) • E: Primarily excreted as metabolites in urine	• Increase duration of Cl^- channel opening by GABA at GABA$_A$ receptor thereby depressing the reticular activating system • At high doses, can perform same action without GABA	• Sedation • Insomnia	• Death • CNS depression (additive effects with alcohol and other CNS depressants) • Rash, dermatitis • Acute toxicity with overdose (respiratory, CV, and CNS depression, renal failure)
Butabarbital (Butisol)	• A: PO • OOA: 45–60 minutes • DOA: 6–8 hours • M: Hepatic (P450) • E: Primarily excreted as metabolites in urine		• Sedation • Insomnia • Preop sedation	• Chronic toxicity (abuse and addiction, tolerance and dependency can lead to status epilepticus during withdrawal) • P450 induction (LTU causes induction of these enzymes, which leads to tolerance and decreased efficacy of other drugs as well) • Decreased REM time (causes rebound REM with anxiety following drug removal)
Mephobarbital (Mebaral)	• A: PO • OOA: 30–60 minutes • DOA: 10–16 hours • M: Hepatic (P450) (metabolized to phenobarbital) • E: Primarily excreted as metabolites in urine		• Sedation • Anticonvulsant	• May precipitate acute intermittent porphyria in susceptible patients • Treat overdose with diuresis and by making urine basic (NaHCO$_3$) to keep the molecules charged and increase urinary excretion • Methohexital has a black box warning for sedation

Continued

SEDATIVES AND HYPNOTICS: BARBITURATES (Continued)

Drug	Pharmacokinetics	Mechanism of Action	Clinical Uses	Side Effects
Secobarbital (Seconal)	• A: PO • OOA: 10–15 minutes • DOA: 3–4 hours • M: Hepatic (P450) • E: Primarily excreted as metabolites in urine		• Sedation • Insomnia • Preop sedation	
Phenobarbital (Luminal)	• A: PO, IM, IV • OOA: 5–50 minutes • DOA: 4–10 hours • M: Hepatic (P450) • E: Primarily excreted as metabolites in urine		• Sedation • Preop sedation • Anticonvulsant	
Thiopental	• A: IV • OOA: 60 seconds • DOA: 5–30 minutes • M: Hepatic (P450) • E: Primarily excreted as metabolites in urine		• Reduction of elevated ICP • Anticonvulsant • Anesthesia	

Methohexital (Brevital)	• **A:** IM, IV, PR	• Anesthesia
	• **OOA:** 2–15 minutes	
	• **DOA:** 10–45 minutes	
	• **M:** Hepatic (P450)	
	• **E:** Primarily excreted as metabolites in urine	
Pentobarbital (Nembutal)	• **A:** PO, IM, IV, PR	• Preop/procedural sedation
	• **OOA:** Immediate–1 hour	• Hypnotic
	• **DOA:** 15 minutes–4 hours	• Refractory status epilepticus
	• **M:** Hepatic (P450)	• Sedation for intubated patients
	• **E:** Primarily excreted as metabolites in urine	• Reduction of elevated ICP

OTHER SEDATIVES AND HYPNOTICS

Drug	Pharmacokinetics	Mechanism of Action	Clinical Uses	Side Effects
Buspirone (Buspar)	• A: PO; well absorbed • M: Hepatic (P450) metabolism to active metabolites • E: Primarily excreted as metabolites in urine	• Exact mechanism of action unknown • 5-HT$_{1A}$, 5-HT$_2$, and DA agonist	• Generalized anxiety disorder • Nonsedating • Limited abuse potential • Does not potentiate CNS depressive effects of ethanol	• Drowsiness • Nervousness • Nausea • Paresthesias
Chloral hydrate	• A: PO, PR • M: Prodrug, metabolized to trichloroethanol (active metabolite) by alcohol dehydrogenase • E: Primarily excreted as metabolites in urine	• Exact mechanism of action unclear • CNS depressant	• Sedative/hypnotic	• Displaces coumarins from plasma binding proteins increasing its anticoagulant properties • Metabolite (TCE) with questionable carcinogenicity
Zolpidem (Ambien, Edluar, Intermezzo, Zolpimist)	• A: PO • M: Rapid hepatic (P450) metabolism • E: Primarily excreted as metabolites in urine	• Nonbenzodiazepine that selectively binds to the benzodiazepine-1 (BZ$_1$) receptor on GABA$_A$ receptor	• Insomnia • Actions similar to benzodiazepines without the tolerance or dependency problems • Safer than benzodiazepines • Overdose can be treated with flumazenil	• Respiratory depression when large doses are combined with other sedative/hypnotics or alcohol • Headache • Drowsiness • Dizziness • Ataxia

Zaleplon (Sonata)	• **A:** PO • **M:** Hepatic (P450) • **E:** Primarily excreted as metabolites in urine	• Binds to omega 1 receptor on the α subunit of the $GABA_A$ receptor complex	• Insomnia	• Headache • Dizziness • Eye pain
Eszopiclone (Lunesta)		• Exact MOA unknown • Agonist at benzodiazepine receptor on $GABA_A$ receptor complexes		• Headache • Unpleasant taste • Dry mouth • Somnolence
Ramelteon (Rozerem)		• Selective agonist of melatonin receptors MT_1 and MT_2 within the suprachiasmatic nucleus of the hypothalamus		• Dizziness • Nausea

IV. Antiepileptic Drugs

CLASSIFICATION OF DRUGS FOR THE TREATMENT OF EPILEPSY

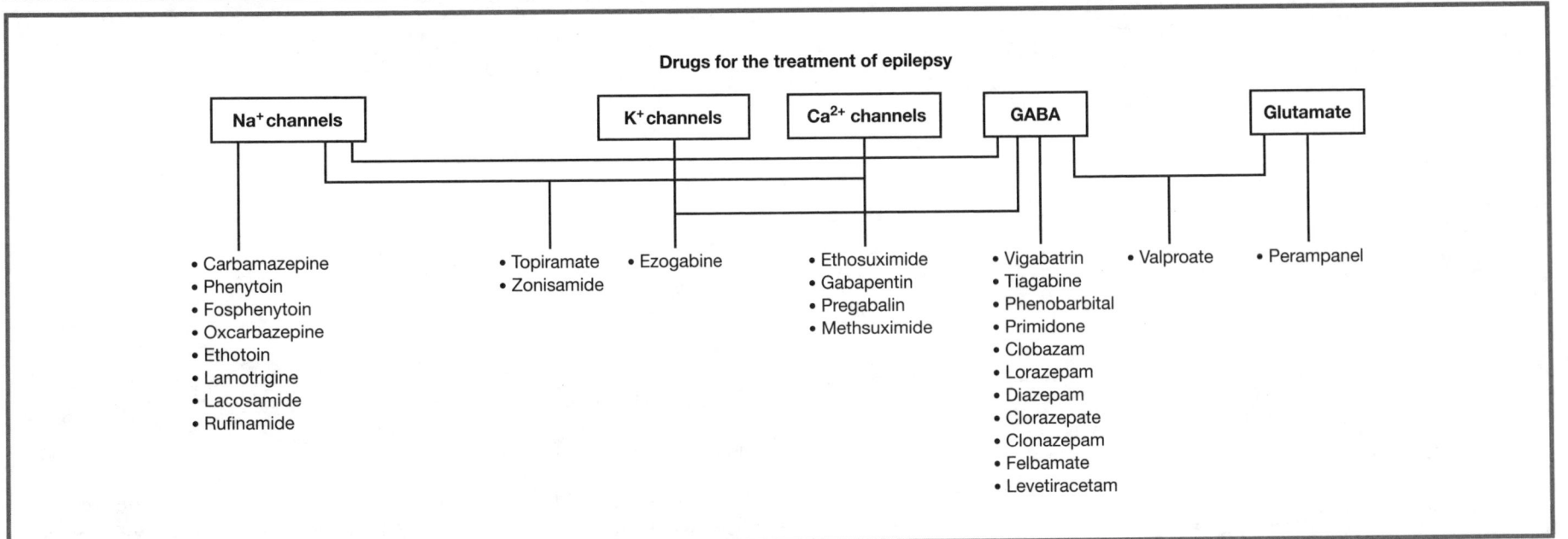

Drugs for the treatment of epilepsy

| Na⁺ channels | K⁺ channels | Ca²⁺ channels | GABA | Glutamate |

- Carbamazepine
- Phenytoin
- Fosphenytoin
- Oxcarbazepine
- Ethotoin
- Lamotrigine
- Lacosamide
- Rufinamide

- Topiramate
- Zonisamide

- Ezogabine

- Ethosuximide
- Gabapentin
- Pregabalin
- Methsuximide

- Vigabatrin
- Tiagabine
- Phenobarbital
- Primidone
- Clobazam
- Lorazepam
- Diazepam
- Clorazepate
- Clonazepam
- Felbamate
- Levetiracetam

- Valproate

- Perampanel

DRUGS FOR THE TREATMENT OF EPILEPSY

Drug	Pharmacokinetics	Mechanism of Action	Clinical Uses	Side Effects
Vigabatrin (Sabril)	• **A:** PO • $t_{1/2}$: 6–8 hours • **E:** Primarily excreted unchanged in urine	• Irreversible GABA-T inhibitor • Prolongs the action of GABA by inhibition of its degradation by GABA-T	• Infantile spasms • Refractory complex partial seizures in children and adults	• Vision loss • Somnolence • Headache • Fatigue
Tiagabine (Gabitril)	• **A:** PO • $t_{1/2}$: 2–9 hours • **M:** Hepatic (P450) • **E:** Primarily excreted as metabolites in feces	• Blocks reuptake of GABA	• Partial seizures	• Somnolence • Dizziness • Nausea
Phenobarbital (Luminal)	• **A:** PO, IM, IV • $t_{1/2}$: 20–90 hours (depending on patient profile) • **M:** Hepatic (P450) • **E:** Primarily excreted as metabolites in urine	• Increase duration of Cl^- channel opening by GABA at $GABA_A$ receptor	• Sedation • Preop sedation • Anticonvulsant • Status epilepticus	• Sedation • Tolerance • Dependence • Induces P450 enzymes
Primidone (Mysoline)	• **A:** PO • $t_{1/2}$: 5–16 hours • **M:** Hepatic (P450) metabolism to two active agents (phenobarbital and phenylethylmalonamide [PEMA]) • **E:** Primarily excreted as metabolites in urine		• Seizures (grand mal, psychomotor, and focal)	• Ataxia • Impotence • Nausea/vomiting • Drowsiness • Induces P450 enzymes

Continued

DRUGS FOR THE TREATMENT OF EPILEPSY (Continued)

Drug	Pharmacokinetics	Mechanism of Action	Clinical Uses	Side Effects
Clobazam (Onfi)	• A: PO • $t_{1/2}$: 36–82 hours • M: Hepatic (P450) • E: Primarily excreted as metabolites in urine	• Increase frequency of opening of Cl⁻ channel by GABA at the GABA$_A$ receptor	• Adjunctive therapy of seizures associated with Lennox–Gastaut syndrome	• Somnolence • Aggression • Hypersalivation • Inhibits P450 enzymes • Induces P450 enzymes
Lorazepam (Ativan)	• A: PO, IM, IV • $t_{1/2}$: 14–42 hours • M: Hepatic metabolism to inactive metabolites • E: Renal excretion of metabolites		• Acute anticonvulsant • Status epilepticus • Anxiety • Insomnia • Anesthesia premedication	• Somnolence • Decreased libido • SIADH
Diazepam (Valium, Diastat)	• A: PO, PR, IM, IV • $t_{1/2}$: 20–100 hours • M: Hepatic (P450) metabolism to active metabolites • E: Renal excretion of metabolites		• Acute anticonvulsant • Status epilepticus • Muscle spasm • Alcohol withdrawal • Sedative • Febrile seizure prophylaxis	• Hypotension • Decreased libido • Drowsiness • Inhibits P450 enzymes
Clorazepate (Tranxene)	• A: PO • $t_{1/2}$: 6–50 hours • M: Metabolism in the GI tract to active metabolite and hepatic (P450) to active metabolites • E: Renal excretion of metabolites		• Anxiety • Alcohol withdrawal • Seizures	• Hypotension • Somnolence • Xerostomia • Decreased libido

Clonazepam (Klonopin)	• **A:** PO • $t_{1/2}$: 17–60 hours • **M:** Hepatic (P450) • **E:** Renal excretion of metabolites		• Panic disorder • Seizures	• Somnolence • Decreased libido • Ataxia
Levetiracetam (Keppra)	• **A:** IV, PO • $t_{1/2}$: 6–8 hours • **M:** Some enzymatic hydrolysis • **E:** Excreted primarily unchanged in urine	• Exact MOA unknown • Seems to work on voltage-dependent N type and facilitation of GABAergic inhibitory activity	• Myoclonic seizures • Tonic–clonic seizures • Partial-onset seizures	• CNS (drowsiness, dizziness) • Behavioral changes in children and adults • Weakness • Anorexia • Pharyngitis • Vomiting
Felbamate (Felbatol)	• **A:** PO • $t_{1/2}$: 20–38 hours • **M:** Hepatic (P450) • **E:** Parent drug and metabolites excreted in urine	• Exact MOA unknown • Weak inhibitory effects at GABA receptor binding	• Adjunctive and monotherapy for partial seizures and seizures associated with Lennox–Gastaut syndrome	• CNS (dizziness, somnolence, headache) • GI (nausea, vomiting) • Purpura in children • Inhibits P450 enzymes • Induces P450 enzymes
Topiramate (Topamax, Topiragen, Trokendi)	• **A:** PO • $t_{1/2}$: 21 hours • **M:** Hepatic (minor) • **E:** Primarily excreted unchanged in urine	• Multiple mechanisms of action • Blocks neuronal voltage-dependent Na^+ channels • Enhances GABA action • Antagonizes glutamate receptors	• Adjunctive and monotherapy for partial and generalized seizures • Adjunctive therapy for seizures associated with Lennox–Gastaut syndrome • Migraine prophylaxis	• CNS (cognitive slowing, confusion, dizziness, somnolence) • Anorexia/weight loss • Renal stone formation • Inhibits P450 enzymes • Induces P450 enzymes

Continued

DRUGS FOR THE TREATMENT OF EPILEPSY (Continued)

Drug	Pharmacokinetics	Mechanism of Action	Clinical Uses	Side Effects
Valproate (Depacon, Depakene, Stavzor)	• A: IV, PO • $t_{1/2}$: 7–19 hours • M: Hepatic (P450) • E: Primarily excreted as metabolites in urine	• Increased availability of GABA and enhances/mimics GABA at postsynaptic sites	• Seizures • Mania • Migraine prophylaxis	• CNS (dizziness, tremor, headache, somnolence) • GI (pancreatitis, nausea, vomiting) • Alopecia • Hepatic failure • Neural tube defects in pregnant women • Inhibits P450 enzymes • Induces P450 enzymes
Pregabalin (Lyrica)	• A: PO • $t_{1/2}$: 6 hours • E: Excreted primarily unchanged in urine	• Binds to voltage gated Ca^{2+} channels to influence the release of excitatory neurotransmitters	• Adjunctive therapy in partial seizures • Fibromyalgia • Postherpetic neuralgia • Neuropathic pain in diabetes and spinal cord injury	• CNS (headache, somnolence, dizziness) • Weight gain • Peripheral edema
Gabapentin (Neurontin, Gralise)	• A: PO • $t_{1/2}$: 5–7 hours • E: Excreted unchanged in urine	• Exact MOA unknown • Seems to work on voltage-gated Ca^{2+} channels to influence the release of excitatory neurotransmitters	• Epilepsy • Postherpetic neuralgia	• CNS (drowsiness, dizziness) • Behavioral changes in children

Drug	Pharmacokinetics	Mechanism of Action	Indications	Adverse Effects
Ethosuximide (Zarontin)	• **A:** PO • $t_{1/2}$: 50 hours • **M:** Hepatic (P450) • **E:** Primarily excreted as metabolites in urine	• Reduces Ca^{2+} current through T channels	• Absence (petit mal) seizures	• Rashes (urticaria, SJS, DRESS) • GI (abdominal pain, diarrhea, anorexia) • CNS (headaches, dizziness, lethargy)
Methsuximide (Celontin)	• **A:** PO • $t_{1/2}$: 2–4 hours • **M:** Hepatic (P450) • **E:** Metabolites excreted in urine	• Increases seizure threshold through action on type T voltage sensitive Ca^{2+} channels • Depresses conduction in the motor cortex	• Treatment of refractory absence seizures	• Inhibits P450 enzymes
Zonisamide (Zonegran)	• **A:** PO • $t_{1/2}$: 63 hours • **M:** Hepatic (P450) • **E:** Metabolites and parent drug excreted in urine	• Exact MOA unknown • Seems to work through action at Na^+ and Ca^{2+} channels to stabilize neuronal membranes	• Adjunctive therapy for partial seizures	• CNS (dizziness, somnolence) • Anorexia/weight loss • Renal stone formation
Perampanel (Fycompa)	• **A:** PO • $t_{1/2}$: 105 hours • **M:** Hepatic (P450) • **E:** Primarily excreted as metabolites in feces	• Noncompetitive glutamate receptor antagonist	• Adjunctive therapy for the treatment of partial-onset seizures with or without secondarily generalized seizures	• Severe neuropsychiatric disturbances (anger, homicidal ideations) • Induces P450 enzymes
Ezogabine (Potiga)	• **A:** PO • $t_{1/2}$: 6 hours • **M:** Hepatic • **E:** Excreted primarily as metabolites in urine	• Binds to voltage-gated K^+ channels to regulate neuronal excitability • May also act on GABA-mediated pathways	• Adjunctive therapy in partial-onset seizures	• Retinal abnormalities with possible vision loss • CNS (drowsiness, dizziness)

Continued

DRUGS FOR THE TREATMENT OF EPILEPSY (Continued)

Drug	Pharmacokinetics	Mechanism of Action	Clinical Uses	Side Effects
Carbamazepine (Tegretol, Carbatrol, Epitol, Equetro)	• A: PO • M: Hepatic (P450) (causes induction) • t$_{1/2}$: 25–45 hours • E: Primarily excreted as metabolites in urine	• Inhibits voltage-gated Na$^+$ channels stabilizing neuronal membranes in hyperactive neurons	• Partial seizures • Mixed pattern seizures • Generalized seizures • Trigeminal neuralgia • Bipolar disorder	• Hematologic (anemia, agranulocytosis) • Dermatologic (SJS, TENS) (screen Asian patients for HLA-B*1502 allele) • CNS (dizziness, drowsiness, headache) • GI (nausea, vomiting) • Induces P450 enzymes
Phenytoin (Dilantin, Phenytek)	• A: PO, IV • M: Hepatic (P450) (causes induction) • t$_{1/2}$: 7–42 hours • E: Primarily excreted as metabolites in urine		• Partial seizures • Complex partial seizures • Generalized seizures • Seizure prophylaxis • Status epilepticus	• Gingival hyperplasia • Purple glove syndrome • Induces P450 enzymes • Folic acid and vit D deficiencies • Drug-induced SLE • GU (Peyronie's disease) • CNS (dizziness, drowsiness, headache)
Fosphenytoin (Cerebyx)	• A: IM, IV • t$_{1/2}$: 7–42 hours • M: Hepatic • E: Primarily excreted as metabolites in urine			• Fosphenytoin is a product of phenytoin with improved aqueous solubility
Oxcarbazepine (Trileptal, Oxtellar)	• A: PO • t$_{1/2}$: 7–11 hours • M: Hepatic metabolism to active metabolite (MHD) • E: Primarily excreted as metabolites in urine		• Adjunctive therapy and monotherapy for the treatment of partial seizures	• GI (nausea, vomiting) • CNS (dizziness, drowsiness, headache, diplopia) • Induces P450 enzymes

Ethotoin (Peganone)	• **A:** PO • $t_{1/2}$: 3–9 hours • **M:** Hepatic • **E:** Primarily excreted as metabolites in urine and feces	• Stabilizes seizure threshold and decreases spread in mechanism likely similar to phenytoin	• Generalized tonic–clonic or complex partial seizures	• CNS (dizziness, tremor, headache, somnolence) • GI (nausea, vomiting, gingival hyperplasia) • SJS • SLE-like syndrome • Inhibits P450 enzymes
Lamotrigine (Lamictal)	• **A:** PO • $t_{1/2}$: 25–42 hours • **M:** Hepatic and renal • **E:** Primarily excreted as metabolites in urine	• Inhibits voltage-gated Na^+ channels and glutamate stabilizing neuronal membranes in hyperactive neurons	• Adjunctive therapy for the treatment of partial seizures, primary generalized seizures, and Lennox–Gastaut syndrome • Bipolar disorder	• Dermatologic (SJS, TENS, angioedema) • Increased half-life with coadministration with valproate • GI (nausea, vomiting) • CNS (insomnia, somnolence, ataxia)
Lacosamide (Vimpat)	• **A:** IV, PO • $t_{1/2}$: 13 hours • **M:** Hepatic (P450) • **E:** Metabolites and parent drug excreted in urine	• Seems to work through action at Na^+ channels to stabilize neuronal membranes and prevent repetitive firing	• Partial-onset seizures	• CNS (dizziness, fatigue, tremor, diplopia) • GI (nausea, vomiting) • Inhibits P450 enzymes
Rufinamide (Banzel)	• **A:** PO • $t_{1/2}$: 6–10 hours • **E:** Primarily excreted as metabolites in urine	• Exact MOA unknown • Prolongs inactive state of Na^+ channels	• Adjunctive therapy for the treatment of seizures associated with Lennox–Gastaut syndrome	• CNS (dizziness, fatigue, headache, somnolence) • GI (nausea, vomiting) • Shortens QT interval • Inhibits P450 enzymes • Induces P450 enzymes

SEIZURE CLASSIFICATIONS

Seizure Type	Description	Protocol
Partial seizures	• Simple: seizure in a discrete region of the brain without altered consciousness • Complex: simple seizure with altered consciousness • Partial with secondary generalization: begins as a simple seizure and then spreads throughout the cortex	• Carbamazepine • Ethotoin • Felbamate • Fosphenytoin • Lacosamide • Levetiracetam • Oxcarbazepine • Phenytoin • Primidone • Tiagabine • Topiramate • Valproate • Vigabatrin • Adjunctive therapies (lamotrigine, ezogabine, pregabalin, zonisamide, perampanel)
Generalized (grand mal) seizures	• Seizures that arise from bilateral brain hemispheres without focal onset • Accompanied by loss of consciousness	• Carbamazepine • Ethotoin • Fosphenytoin • Lamotrigine • Levetiracetam • Phenytoin • Primidone • Topiramate • Valproate

Absence (petite mal) seizures	• Brief lapses in consciousness without loss of postural control	• Ethosuximide • Methsuximide
Myoclonic seizures	• Sudden, brief muscle contraction involving one part of the body	• Levetiracetam
Infantile spasms	• Seizure disorder of early childhood or infancy • Usually occurs in the first year of life • Characterized by myoclonic seizures and mental retardation	• Vigabatrin
Status epilepticus	• Prolonged seizure activity without recovery of consciousness or discrete seizures without regaining consciousness in the interim	• Diazepam • Fosphenytoin • Lorazepam • Phenobarbital • Phenytoin
Lennox–Gastaut syndrome	• Syndrome associated with severe seizures of various types and mental retardation in the first 7 years of life. Several different etiologies include genetic, traumatic, infectious, or even ischemic episodes	• Felbamate • Lamotrigine • Rufinamide • Adjunctive therapies (topiramate, clonazepam)

V. Opioids

Endogenous opioids include dynorphins, enkephalins, and endorphins.

OPIOIDS: SUMMARY TABLE

General Pharmacokinetics	Mechanism of Action	Clinical Uses of Opioid Agonists	Adverse Effects			
			Acute Side Effects	Chronic Side Effects	Toxicities	Abstinence Syndrome
• Well absorbed via intramuscular, subcutaneous, and mucosal sites; PO administration often accompanied by extensive first-pass metabolism • Distribution depends on chemical properties of each opioid; some readily cross the BBB, all readily cross the placenta • Most undergo hepatic metabolism to polar metabolites • Renal excretion of polar metabolites	• MOA relies on endogenous receptors: • μ_1—analgesic receptors found supraspinally • μ_2—analgesic receptors found in the spinal cord, also mediate respiratory depression and GI transit depression • δ—unknown function in humans • κ_1—analgesic receptors found in the spinal cord • κ_3—analgesic receptors found supraspinally	• Analgesia: mild to moderate pain • Acute pulmonary edema: calms patient and slows respiration • MI: analgesic and sedative effects • Preanesthetic medication: sedative, analgesic • Anesthetic • Antitussive • Antidiarrheal	• Nausea and vomiting • Constipation • Mental clouding • Muscular rigidity • Euphoria • Dysphoria • Respiratory center depression • Miosis	• Tolerance • Cross tolerance throughout the class • Physiologic dependence	• Overdose leading to coma with respiratory depression and hypotension can be fatal • Additive CNS depression when combined with EtOH, sedative/hypnotics, anesthetics, antipsychotics, TCAs, or antihistamines	• Rhinorrhea and lacrimation • Yawning • Anxiety and hostility • Chills and gooseflesh • Muscle aches • Diarrhea

CLASSIFICATION OF OPIOIDS

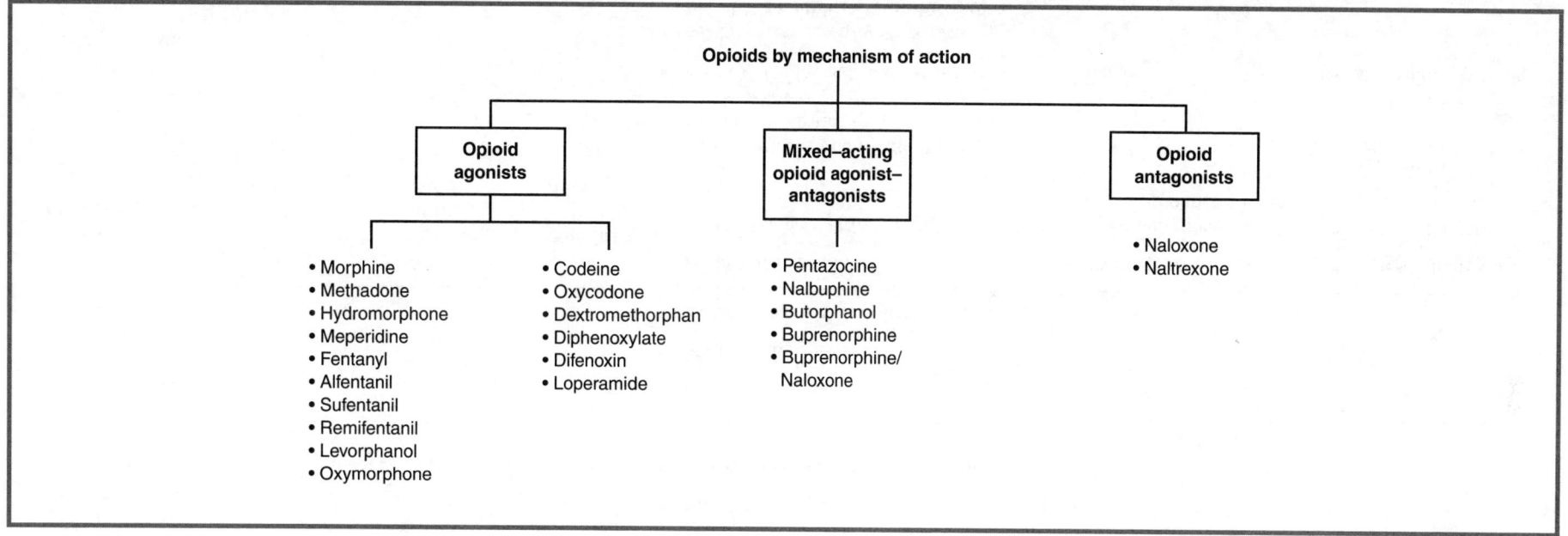

Opioids by mechanism of action

Opioid agonists
- Morphine
- Methadone
- Hydromorphone
- Meperidine
- Fentanyl
- Alfentanil
- Sufentanil
- Remifentanil
- Levorphanol
- Oxymorphone
- Codeine
- Oxycodone
- Dextromethorphan
- Diphenoxylate
- Difenoxin
- Loperamide

Mixed-acting opioid agonist-antagonists
- Pentazocine
- Nalbuphine
- Butorphanol
- Buprenorphine
- Buprenorphine/ Naloxone

Opioid antagonists
- Naloxone
- Naltrexone

OPIOID AGONISTS

Drug	Receptor Effects			Pharmacokinetics	Clinical Uses	Side Effects
	μ	δ	κ			
Morphine (MS Contin, Duramorph, Kadian, Avinza, Infumorph, Astramorph)	• Agonist	• Agonist	• Agonist	• **A:** IV, IM, SC, PO, PR; epidural, intrathecal • **M:** Hepatic (P450); extensive first-pass metabolism after PO administration • **E:** Excreted as parent drug and metabolites in urine	• Analgesia	• See summary table • Itching from histamine release
Levorphanol				• **A:** PO • **M:** Hepatic • **E:** Excreted as metabolites in urine	• Analgesic • Acts as NE/5-HT reuptake inhibitor • NMDA antagonism	• See summary table
Oxymorphone (Opana)				• **A:** PO • **M:** Hepatic • **E:** Excreted as metabolites in urine	• Analgesic	• See summary table
Methadone (Dolophine, Methadose)	• Agonist	• Agonist at high doses	• Agonist at high doses	• **A:** PO, IM, SC, IV • **DOA:** Longest acting opioid • **M:** Hepatic (P450) • **E:** Parent drug and metabolites excreted in urine	• Chronic pain • Heroin detoxification and maintenance therapy	• See summary table • QT prolongation • Induces P450 enzymes
Hydromorphone (Dilaudid, Exalgo)				• **A:** PO, IM, IV, SC, and rectal • **M:** Hepatic: extensive first-pass metabolism after PO administration • **E:** Excreted primarily in urine as metabolites	• Analgesic	• See summary table

Meperidine (Demerol, Meperitab)	• **A:** PO, IM, IV, and SC • **M:** Hepatic metabolism to normeperidine; stimulates the hepatic microsomal system to regulate its own metabolism • **E:** Excreted as metabolites in urine	• Analgesic	• Potential for causing seizures (avoid in epileptics)
Fentanyl (Actiq, Abstral Lazanda, Subsys Onsolis, Fentora, Duragesic)	• **A:** IV, IM, SL, nasal spray, buccal, TD • **M:** Hepatic (P450) • **E:** Excreted primarily as metabolites in urine	• Analgesic	• See summary table • Inhibits P450 enzymes (Fentanyl only)
Alfentanil (Alfenta)	• **A:** IV • **M:** Hepatic (P450) • **E:** Primarily excreted as metabolites in urine	• Analgesic	
Sufentanil (Sufenta)	• **A:** IM, IV, and epidural • **M:** Hepatic (P450) and small intestine metabolism • **E:** Excreted primarily as metabolites in urine	• Analgesic • Adjunct for anesthesia	
Remifentanil (Ultiva)	• **A:** IV • **M:** Plasma and tissue esterases • **E:** Excreted as metabolites in urine	• Induction and maintenance of anesthesia	• See summary table

Continued

OPIOID AGONISTS (Continued)

Drug	Receptor Effects μ	δ	κ	Pharmacokinetics	Clinical Uses	Side Effects
Moderate to Weak Opioid Agonists						
Codeine	μ Agonist	δ Agonist at high doses	κ Agonist at high doses	• A: PO, IM, and SC • D: Readily crosses BBB • M: Hepatic (P450); produg converted to morphine • E: Primarily excreted in urine as metabolites	• Analgesic	• See summary table • Respiratory depression and death in children after T&A with rapid metabolism due to CYP206 rapid metabolism
Oxycodone (Oxycontin, Oxecta, Roxicodone)				• A: PO • M: Hepatic (P450) • E: Primarily excreted in urine as metabolites	• Analgesic	• See summary table
Dextromethorphan (Delsym, Robitussin DM)				• A: PO • M: Hepatic (P450) • E: Primarily excreted as metabolites in urine	• Antitussive	• See summary table less risk of side effects due to lower agonist qualities • Inhibits P450 enzymes (Dextromethorphan only)
Diphenoxylate (Lomotil)				• A: PO • M: Hepatic • E: Primarily excreted in feces as metabolites and parent drug	• Antidiarrheal	• Small amount of atropine added to prevent abuse
Difenoxin (Motofen)				• A: PO • M: Hydrolysis in blood • E: Primarily excreted as metabolites in feces and urine		

Loperamide (Imodium)				• **A:** PO • **M:** Hepatic • **E:** Metabolites and parent drug excreted in feces	• Treatment of diarrhea		
Mixed Agonist/Antagonists							
Nalbuphine (Nubain)	μ Antagonist	No significant δ activity	κ Agonist	• **A:** IM, IV, and SC • **M:** Hepatic (P450) • **E:** Primarily excreted as metabolites in feces	• Analgesic • Adjunct to anesthesia		• Sedation • Dizziness • Sweating • Nausea
Pentazocine (Talwin)	Partial μ agonist			• **A:** PO, IM, IV • **M:** Hepatic • **E:** Primarily excreted as metabolites in urine	• Analgesic • Obstetrical pain		• Anxiety • Hallucinations • Cause less respiratory depression than full agonist
Butorphanol (Stadol)				• **A:** IM, IV, or nasal spray • **M:** Hepatic • **E:** Primarily excreted as metabolites in urine	• Analgesic • Migraine • Obstetrical pain • Adjunct to anesthesia		• Physical dependence • Milder withdrawal symptoms
Buprenorphine (Buprenex, Butrans Subutex)			κ Antagonist	• **A:** IM, IV, SL, TD • **M:** Hepatic (P450) • **E:** Primarily excreted as metabolites in feces	• Analgesic • Opioid dependence		
Buprenorphine and Naloxone* (Suboxone, Zubsolv)				• **A:** SL • **M:** Hepatic (P450) • **E:** Excreted as metabolites in urine and feces	• Maintenance therapy of opioid dependence		

Continued

OPIOID AGONISTS (Continued)

Drug	Receptor Effects			Pharmacokinetics	Clinical Uses	Side Effects
	μ	δ	κ			
Opioid Antagonist						
Naloxone (Narcan)	μ Antagonist	δ Antagonist	κ Antagonist	• **A:** IM, IV, and SC; poor oral efficacy • **DOA:** 1–2 hours • Short-acting so repeated administration is required • **M:** Hepatic • **E:** Primarily excreted as metabolites in urine	• Treatment of acute opioid overdose	• Can precipitate an intense abstinence syndrome in opioid-dependent patients
Naltrexone (ReVia, Vivitrol)				• **A:** PO, IM • **DOA:** 24–48 hours • **M:** Hepatic • **E:** Primarily excreted as metabolites in urine	• Treatment of acute opioid overdose • Adjunctive therapy in alcohol dependency programs	

*There are numerous combination formulations that combine opioids with other medications such as NSAIDs and acetaminophen.

VI. Drugs for the Treatment of Migraines

CLASSIFICATION OF DRUGS USED FOR TREATMENT OF MIGRAINES

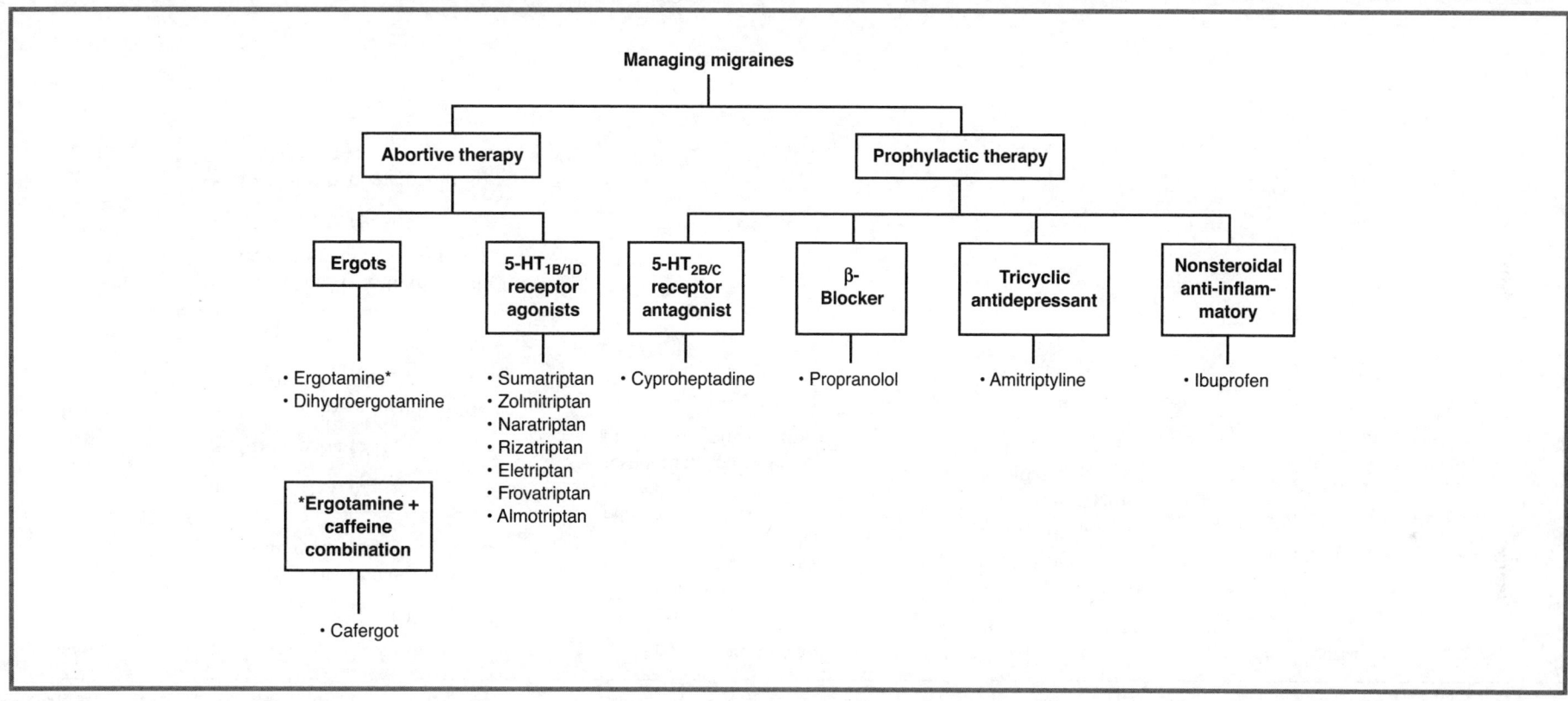

Drug	Pharmacokinetics	Mechanism of Action	Clinical Uses	Drawbacks and Side Effects
Ergots				
Ergotamine (Ergomar)	• A: SL • M: Hepatic (P450) • E: Majority of metabolites excreted in feces	• 5-HT$_{1B/1D}$ receptor agonists • Thought that stimulation of these receptors causes vasoconstriction of intracranial vessels and inhibits release of peptides involved in sterile neurogenic inflammatory response from the sensory processes of the trigeminal nerve	• Abortive antimigraine medications • Best used at the onset of the headache • Almost always administered with caffeine	• Ergotism • GI problems (nausea, vomiting, diarrhea) • Uterine contractions • Contraindicated with potent inhibitors of CYP3A4 which can precipitate ergotism • Use with cautions in patients with cardiovascular disease • Inhibit P450 enzymes
Dihydro-ergotamine (DHE-45, Migranal)	• A: SC, IM, IV, or intranasal • M: Hepatic (P450) • E: Majority of metabolites excreted in feces			
Caffeine and Ergotamine				
Ergotamine and caffeine (Cafergot, Migergot)	• A: PO or PR; caffeine seems to help ergotamine absorption • M: Hepatic (P450) • E: Majority of metabolites excreted in feces			

5-HT$_{1B/1D}$ Receptor Agonists

Drug	Pharmacokinetics	Indications/Mechanism	Adverse Effects/Cautions
Sumatriptan (Imitrex, Alsuma, Sumavel)	• **A:** SC, PO, TD or intranasal; poorly absorbed • **M:** Hepatic • **E:** Metabolites excreted in urine	• Abortive antimigraine therapy • Very high and selective affinity for 1D$_\alpha$, 1D$_\beta$, and 1F receptors with little affinity for other 5-HT or monoamine receptors • Do not produce ergotism • No GI upset (as seen with ergots)	• Limit dose of agents metabolized by MAO A in patients taking MAO inhibitors • Paresthesias • Warm/cold sensations • Neck/throat/jaw/chest pain/tightness/pressure • Nausea • Dizziness • Sleepiness • Arrhythmias • Caution in patients with pre-existing vascular disease (angina, CVA, MI) • Caution in patients with HTN
Zolmitriptan (Zomig)	• **A:** PO; intranasal; well absorbed • **M:** Hepatic (P450) • **E:** Primarily excreted as metabolites in urine		
Naratriptan (Amerge)	• **A:** PO; well absorbed • **M:** Hepatic (P450) • **E:** Parent drug and metabolites excreted in urine		
Rizatriptan (Maxalt)	• **A:** PO; complete absorption • **M:** Metabolized by MAO A to inactive metabolite (minor amount of active metabolite formed) • **E:** Primarily excreted as metabolites in urine		

Continued

ABORTIVE ANTIMIGRAINE DRUGS (Continued)

Drug	Pharmacokinetics	Mechanism of Action	Clinical Uses	Drawbacks and Side Effects
Eletriptan (Relpax)	• **A:** PO; well absorbed • **M:** Hepatic (P450) • **E:** Metabolites excreted in feces			
Frovatriptan (Frova)	• **A:** PO; well absorbed • **M:** Hepatic (P450) • **E:** Metabolites excreted in urine and feces			
Almotriptan (Axert)	• **A:** PO; well absorbed • **M:** Hepatic (P450) • **E:** Metabolites and parent drug excreted in urine			

PROPHYLACTIC MIGRAINE DRUGS

Drug	Class	Pharmacokinetics	Mechanism of Action	Clinical Uses	Side Effects
Cyproheptadine (Periactin)	• 5-HT$_{2B/C}$ receptor antagonists • Histamine I$_A$ antagonist	• **A:** PO • **M:** Hepatic • **E:** Primarily excreted as metabolites in urine	• Unknown • 5-HT$_{2B/C}$ and histamine antagonism	• Prophylactic antimigraine therapy • Allergic conditions	• Nausea • Drowsiness • Weight gain • Weakness
Propranolol (Inderal)	• β-Blocker	• **A:** PO and IV; well absorbed • **M:** Hepatic (P450) • **E:** Metabolites excreted in urine	• 5-HT$_{2B/C}$ receptor antagonist in doses employed	• Prophylactic antimigraine therapy • HTN • Angina • IHSS • Pheochromocytoma • Tachydysrhythmias	• Bronchoconstriction • Hypotension • Bradycardia • Sexual dysfunction • Cannot be abruptly discontinue • Inhibits P450 enzymes
Amitriptyline (Elavil)	• TCA	• **A:** PO • **M:** Hepatic (N-demehtylation and P450) • **E:** Metabolites excreted in urine	• Possesses some 5-HT$_2$ blocking properties • As methysergide and cyproheptadine	• Prophylactic antimigraine therapy • Antidepressant	• Cardiotoxicity including quinidine-like cardiac conduction block • Anticholinergic side effects • Hypotension due to α_1-blockade • Sexual dysfunction • Sedation • Increased risk for SI/suicidal behavior in children–young adults • Inhibits P450 enzymes
Ibuprofen (Advil, Motrin numerous other brand names)	• Nonsteroidal anti-inflammatory	• **A:** PO; well absorbed • **M:** Hepatic (Oxidation and P450) • **E:** Metabolites excreted in urine	• Appears to act by inhibiting synthesis of prostaglandins including prostacyclin	• Prophylactic antimigraine therapy • Also effective in treating mild to moderate migraines	• Gastritis with risk of ulceration, perforation, and bleeding • Increased risk of cardiovascular thrombotic events • Contraindicated in pain control for perioperative CABG patients • Inhibits P450 enzymes

VII. Antispastic Drugs

CLASSIFICATION OF ANTISPASTIC DRUGS

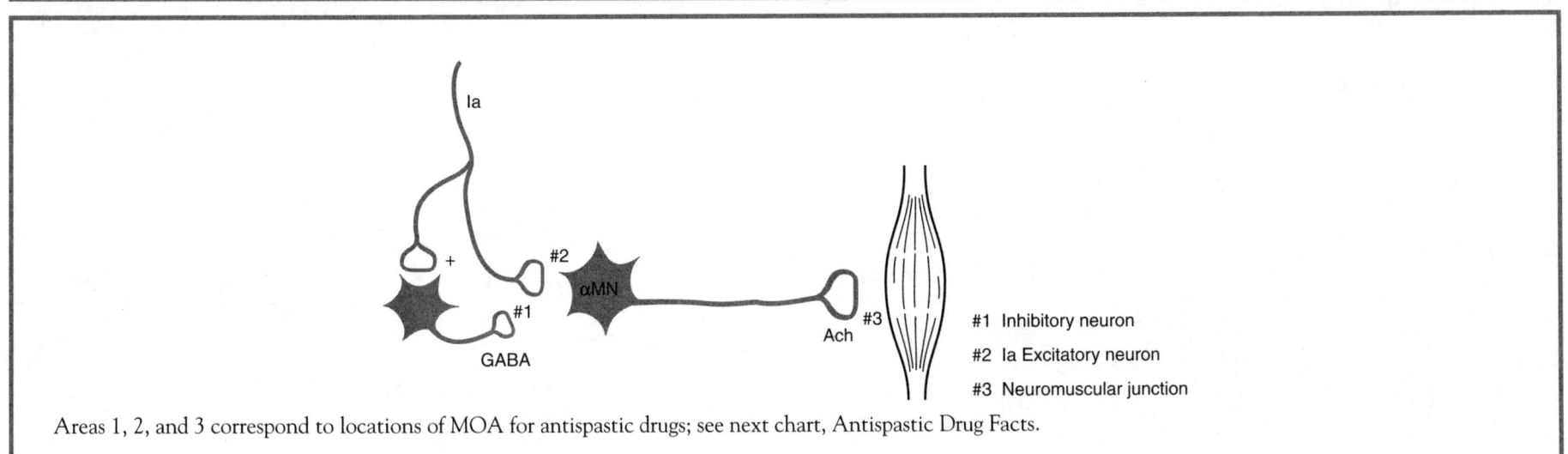

Areas 1, 2, and 3 correspond to locations of MOA for antispastic drugs; see next chart, Antispastic Drug Facts.

#1 Inhibitory neuron

#2 Ia Excitatory neuron

#3 Neuromuscular junction

ANTISPASTIC DRUG FACTS

Drug	Pharmacokinetics	Mechanism of Action	Clinical Uses	Side Effects
Baclofen (Lioresal, Gablofen)	• **A:** Intrathecal and PO; rapidly absorbed from GI tract • **M:** Hepatic (minor) • $t_{1/2}$: 3–4 hours • **E:** Primarily excreted unchanged in urine and feces	• Structural analog of GABA • $GABA_B$ agonist at terminal of 1a afferent neuron • Decreases release of excitatory amino acid neurotransmitter • May also decrease pain via inhibition of substance P release • Acts at site #2 (see preceding chart Mechanism of Action of Antispastic Drugs)	• Spasticity associated with multiple sclerosis • Clonus and muscular rigidity in patients with spinal cord injuries	• Sedation • Dizziness • Hypotension • Headache • Seizures • Weakness • Hyperpyrexia and reflex spasficity associated with abrupt cessation of intrathecal administration
Botulinum toxin (BoTox)	• **A:** IM • **D:** Does not enter systemic circulation in measurable quantities	• Enters motor neuron nerve terminal and inhibits release of Ach release from presynaptic membrane by interfering with SNAP/SNARE proteins on vesicles • Acts at site #3 (see preceding chart Mechanism of Action of Antispastic Drugs)	• Local antispastic in disorders such as cerebral palsy, cervical dystonia, blepharospasm, strabismus, bladder dysfunction • Cosmetic treatment of wrinkles • Primary axillary hyperhidrosis • Chronic migraine	• Spread beyond injection site that can lead to generalized muscle weakness, diplopia, dysarthria, breathing difficulties
Carisoprodol (Soma)	• **A:** PO • **M:** Hepatic (P450) • **E:** Metabolites excreted in urine	• Unknown • May decrease postsynaptic neural transmission in the spinal cord	• Treatment of musculoskeletal pain/spasm	• Drowsiness • Dizziness

Continued

ANTISPASTIC DRUG FACTS (Continued)

Drug	Pharmacokinetics	Mechanism of Action	Clinical Uses	Side Effects
Chlorzoxazone (Parafon Forte, Lorzone)	• **A:** PO • **M:** Hepatic (Glucuronidation and P450) • **E:** Metabolites excreted in urine	• Decrease postsynaptic neural transmission in the spinal cord and subcortical regions of the brain	• Muscular spasm	• Drowsiness • Dizziness • Inhibits P450 enzymes
Cyclobenzaprine (Flexeril, Fexmid, Amrix)	• **A:** PO • **M:** Hepatic (P450) • **E:** Metabolites excreted in urine	• Acts on α and γ motor neurons to reduce somatic motor activity	• Muscular spasm	• Drowsiness • Dizziness • Xerostomia
Dantrolene (Dantrium, Revonto)	• **A:** IV and PO; poorly absorbed from GI tract • $t_{1/2}$: 4–8 hours • **M:** Hepatic (P450) • **E:** Parent drug and metabolites excreted in feces and urine	• Interferes with release of calcium from sarcoplasmic reticulum • Acts at site #3 (see preceding chart Mechanism of Action of Antispastic Drugs)	• Spasticity • Malignant hyperthermia	• General muscle weakness • Hepatotoxicity
Diazepam (Valium)	• **A:** IV and PO; good absorption • $t_{1/2}$: 20–80 hours • **M:** Hepatic (P450) • **E:** Active metabolites excreted in urine	• Positive allosteric modulation of $GABA_A$ • Acts at $GABA_A$ receptors on the terminal portion of the 1a axon • Acts at site #1 (see preceding chart Mechanism of Action of Antispastic Drugs)	• Spasticity associated with multiple sclerosis • Clonus and muscular rigidity in patients with spinal cord injuries	• Sedation • Respiratory depression • Physiologic dependence • Inhibits P450 enzymes

Drug	Pharmacokinetics	Mechanism of Action	Indications	Adverse Effects
Metaxalone (Skelaxin)	• **A:** PO • **M:** Hepatic (P450) • **E:** Metabolites excreted in urine	• Exact MOA unknown • May act in the CNS as a depressant to interrupt the pain/spasm cycle	• Muscular spasm	• Drowsiness • Dizziness • Nausea and vomiting
Methocarbamol (Robaxin)	• **A:** IM, IV, PO • **M:** Hepatic • **E:** Metabolites excreted in urine	• CNS depressant	• Muscular spasm	• Drowsiness • Dizziness • Angioedema
Orphenadrine (Norflex)	• **A:** IM, IV, PO • **M:** Hepatic (P450) • **E:** Metabolites excreted in urine	• Seems to work via a central atropine-like action	• Muscular spasm	• Drowsiness • Dizziness • Hallucinations, euphoria • Inhibits P450 enzymes
Tizanidine (Zanaflex)	• **A:** PO; absorbed rapidly and completely • **M:** Hepatic (P450) • **E:** Metabolites excreted in urine and feces	• Short acting α_2 and imidazoline agonist • Acts centrally to increase presynaptic inhibition of motor neurons • Decreases release of excitatory amino acid neurotransmitter at site #2 (see preceding chart Mechanism of Action of Antispastic Drugs)	• Spasticity associated with multiple sclerosis • Clonus and muscular rigidity in patients with spinal cord injuries	• Dry mouth • Sedation • Dizziness • Hypotension • Bradycardia

VIII. Local Anesthetics and Adjunctive Drugs

LOCAL ANESTHETICS AND ADJUNCTIVE DRUGS: SUMMARY TABLE

Pharmacokinetics		Mechanism of Action	Adverse Effects
Potency	**Dosing**		
• Measure of lipid solubility (ability to penetrate a hydrophobic environment) • Decreased pH decreases potency due to the inability of the cation to reach the site of action	• Maximum tolerated dose increased with slow administration or coadministration with vasoconstrictors (decrease drug removal by blood) or sedative/hypnotic drugs (increase seizure threshold) • Maximum tolerated dose decreased with hepatic disease • Maximum tolerated dose varies with drug	• Smaller, unmyelinated neurons are preferentially blocked by local anesthetics (ie, pain fibers) • As neuronal size and myelination increase, the effect decreases • Pain fibers > temperature > touch > proprioception > skeletal muscle tone	• CNS: Drowsiness, dizziness, tinnitus, diplopia, sedation, seizures (avoid IV injection) • CV: Arrhythmias, hypotension • Immunologic: Allergic reaction to PABA metabolite of choline esters • Pulm: Respiratory arrest

CLASSIFICATION OF LOCAL ANESTHETICS AND ADJUNCTIVE DRUGS

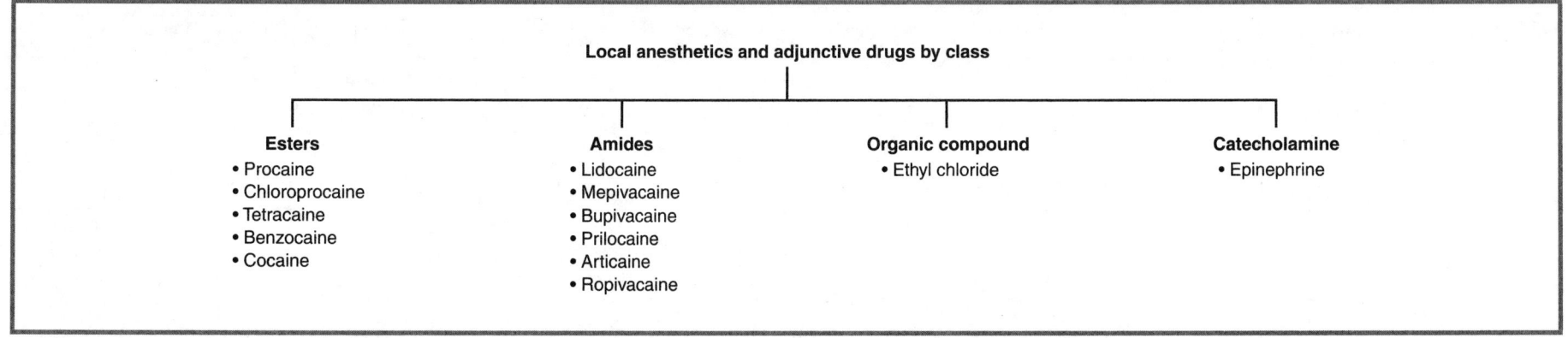

Local anesthetics and adjunctive drugs by class

Esters
• Procaine
• Chloroprocaine
• Tetracaine
• Benzocaine
• Cocaine

Amides
• Lidocaine
• Mepivacaine
• Bupivacaine
• Prilocaine
• Articaine
• Ropivacaine

Organic compound
• Ethyl chloride

Catecholamine
• Epinephrine

LOCAL ANESTHETICS: ESTERS

Drug	Pharmacokinetics	Mechanism of Action	Clinical Uses	Side Effects
Procaine (Novacain)	• **DOA:** Short • **OOA:** Slow • **M:** Rapid hydrolysis in plasma by plasma esterases; metabolites include PABA • **E:** Water soluble metabolites excreted in urine	• Blocks nerve conduction by decreasing the membrane permeability of the neuron to Na^+ • Inhibits neuronal depolarization	• Spinal anesthesia (mixed with tetracaine in obstetrics) • Local infiltration • Peripheral nerve block	• Low toxicity • Vasodilation
Chloroprocaine (Nesacaine)	• **DOA:** Short • **OOA:** Rapid • **M:** Rapid hydrolysis in plasma by plasma esterases; metabolites include PABA • **E:** Water soluble metabolites excreted in urine		• Local infiltration • Epidural anesthesia • Peripheral nerve block	
Tetracaine (Pontocaine)	• **DOA:** Long • **OOA:** Slow • **M:** Rapid hydrolysis in plasma by plasma esterases and hepatic metabolism, metabolites include PABA • **E:** Water soluble metabolites excreted in urine		• Topical anesthesia • Spinal anesthesia • Peripheral nerve block	• Vasodilation

Continued

LOCAL ANESTHETICS: ESTERS (Continued)

Drug	Pharmacokinetics	Mechanism of Action	Clinical Uses	Side Effects
Cocaine	• **DOA:** Short • **OOA:** Slow • **M:** Hydrolyzed in numerous tissues • **E:** Parent drug and metabolites excreted in urine	• Cocaine also blocks reuptake of NE, DA, and 5-HT at nerve synapse	• Topical	• Vasoconstriction • CNS stimulation • Hypertension • Tachycardia • Arrhythmias
Benzocaine (numerous brand name preparations)	• **DOA:** Short • **OOA:** Slow • **M:** Metabolized by plasma esterases and hepatic • **E:** Metabolities excreted in urine	• Accumulates within phospholipid cell membrane and deforms Na^+ channel resulting in decreased Na^+ conductance	• Topical sprays, creams, otic drops, sunburn and teething preparations	• Methemoglobinemia

LOCAL ANESTHETICS AND ADJUNCTIVE AGENTS: AMIDES AND OTHER NONESTERS

Drug	Pharmacokinetics	Mechanism of Action	Clinical Uses	Side Effects
Amide				
Lidocaine (Xylocaine)	• **DOA:** Intermediate • **OOA:** Rapid • **M:** Hepatic (P450)	• Blocks nerve conduction by decreasing the membrane permeability of the neuron to Na⁺ • Inhibits neuronal depolarization	• Topical creams and sprays • Local infiltration • Epidural anesthesia • Spinal • Peripheral nerve block	• In general, local anesthetics are low in toxicity • Methemoglobinemia is seen with lidocaine, articaine, and prilocaine • Bupivacaine is most often associated with cardiovascular collapse
Mepivacaine (Carbocaine)	• **DOA:** Intermediate • **OOA:** Rapid • **M:** Hepatic		• Local infiltration • Peripheral nerve block	
Bupivacaine (Marcaine, Sensorcaine)	• **DOA:** Long • **OOA:** Slow • **M:** Hepatic (minor P450) • **E:** Metabolites excreted in urine		• Local infiltration • Epidural (intense analgesia with minimal motor block) • Spinal anesthesia • Peripheral nerve block • Sympathetic nerve block • Retrobulbaronesthesia	

Continued

LOCAL ANESTHETICS AND ADJUNCTIVE AGENTS: AMIDES AND OTHER NONESTERS (Continued)

Drug	Pharmacokinetics	Mechanism of Action	Clinical Uses	Side Effects
Prilocaine (Citanest)	• **DOA:** Intermediate • **OOA:** Rapid • **M:** Hepatic and renal metabolism		• Local infiltration primarily for dental procedures • Peripheral nerve block	
Articaine/ epinephrine (Articadent, Orabloc, Septocaine, Zorcaine)	• **DOA:** Long • **OOA:** Rapid • **M:** Plasma hydrolysis and hepatic • **E:** Metabolites excreted in urine		• Local anesthesia particularly for dental procedures	
Ropivacaine (Naropin)	• **DOA:** Long • **OOA:** Rapid • **M:** Hepatic (P450) • **E:** Metabolites excreted in urine		• Epidural anesthesia (block or infusion) • Local anesthesia • Obstetrical anesthesia	

Organic Compound

Ethyl chloride	• **DOA:** Short • **OOA:** Rapid	Volatile liquid anesthetizes via rapid cooling during evaporation	• Topical anesthesia for minor surgery, injections, and dermatologic procedures • Treatment of myofascial pain • Anesthesia in nonclinical setting (athletic events)	• Flammable • Alteration of skin pigmentation following application • Hypersensitivity • Renal and hepatic toxicity prevent LTU

Catecholamine (Adrenergic Agonist)

Epinephrine	• **DOA:** Intermediate • **OOA:** Rapid • **M:** Enzymatic degradation in liver and kidneys	• Vasoconstriction • Mixed with local anesthetics to prolong duration of action of drug	Reduces blood flow to anesthetized area to decrease removal of local anesthetic	• Toxicity from systemic absorption • Increased HR, BP, cardiac output • Decreased renal blood flow

IX. General Anesthetic Drugs

CLASSIFICATION OF GENERAL ANESTHETIC DRUGS

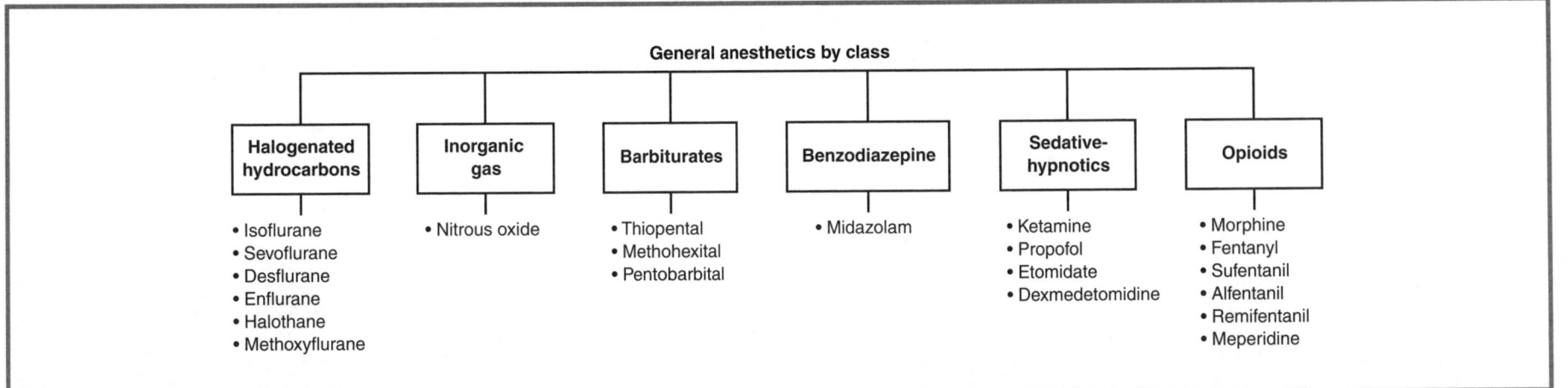

General anesthetics by class

Halogenated hydrocarbons	Inorganic gas	Barbiturates	Benzodiazepine	Sedative-hypnotics	Opioids
• Isoflurane • Sevoflurane • Desflurane • Enflurane • Halothane • Methoxyflurane	• Nitrous oxide	• Thiopental • Methohexital • Pentobarbital	• Midazolam	• Ketamine • Propofol • Etomidate • Dexmedetomidine	• Morphine • Fentanyl • Sufentanil • Alfentanil • Remifentanil • Meperidine

GENERAL ANESTHETIC DRUGS: INHALED

Drug	MAC	B/G	Pharmacokinetics*	Clinical Uses	Side Effects
Halogenated Hydrocarbons					
☞ "Halogenated Hydrocarbons are inHaled as a vapor and eliminated via exHalation" "All increase ICP and decrease BP"					
Isoflurane (Forane, Terrell)	1.15%	1.4	• **A:** Inhaled as a vapor • **M:** Minimal hepatic (P450) metabolism • **E:** Exhalation	• Bronchodilator • Depth of anesthesia can be rapidly adjusted • Cardiac output sustained • Arrhythmias uncommon • Potentiates action of skeletal muscle relaxants	• Increases ICP • Increases HR • Decreases BP • Hepatitis • Malignant hyperthermia • Inhibits P450 enzymes
Sevoflurane (Ultane, Sojourn)	1.7%	0.69	• **A:** Inhaled as a vapor • **M:** Minimal hepatic (P450) metabolism • **E:** Exhalation	• Bronchodilator • Low pungency, least irritating • Good for induction • Potentiates action of skeletal muscle relaxants	• Increases ICP • Decreases BP • Hepatitis • Malignant hyperthermia • QT prolongation
Desflurane (Suprane)	6%	0.42	• **A:** Inhaled; high vapor pressure requires special vaporizer • **M:** Minimal hepatic metabolism to fluoride • **E:** Exhalation	• Very rapid induction and recovery • Potentiates action of skeletal muscle relaxants	• Increases ICP • Hepatitis • Malignant hyperthermia

Continued

GENERAL ANESTHETIC DRUGS: INHALED (Continued)

Drug	MAC	B/G	Pharmacokinetics*	Clinical Uses	Side Effects
Enflurane (Ethrane)	1.68%	1.9	• **A:** Inhaled as a vapor • **M:** Minimal hepatic (P450) metabolism • **E:** Exhalation	• Smooth adjustments of depth of anesthesia are possible • Adequate skeletal muscle relaxant	• Increases ICP • Hepatitis • Decreases BP • Malignant hyperthermia
Halothane (Fluothane)	0.74%	2.4	• **A:** Inhaled as a vapor • **M:** 20–25% oxidized in liver and kidney to trifluoroacetic acid • **E:** Exhalation	• Low pungency • Bronchodilator • Minimal postoperative nausea and vomiting	• Increases ICP • Decreases ventilation • Decreases BP • Hepatotoxicity
Inorganic Gas					
Nitrous oxide	105%	0.47	• **A:** Inhaled as a gas at room temperature • **M:** Minimal metabolism • **E:** Exhalation	• Nonflammable, nonirritating • Little toxicity • Does not increase ICP • Rapid onset, short duration, and rapid recovery • Used in combination with intravenous and other inhalation agents to decrease their dosage requirements	• Insufficient to produce surgical anesthesia as a sole agent • No muscle relaxation

GENERAL ANESTHETIC DRUGS: INTRAVENOUS NONOPIOIDS

Drug	Pharmacokinetics	Clinical Uses	Side Effects
Barbiturates			
Thiopental	• **A:** IV • **OOA:** Rapid • **DOA:** Short • **M:** Hepatic • **E:** Metabolites excreted in urine	• Rapid recovery • Used during induction	• No analgesia • Possible hyperalgesia at subanesthetic doses • Peripheral vasodilation • Respiratory depression • Thiopental should be avoided in patients with abnormalities in porphyrin metabolism • Induces P450 enzymes (Pentobarbital)
Methohexital (Brevital)			
Pentobarbital (Nembutal)			
Benzodiazepines			
Midazolam (Versed)	• **A:** IV, IM, PO, PR • **OOA:** Rapid • **DOA:** Short • **M:** Hepatic (P450) • **E:** Metabolites excreted in urine	• 100% reversible with antagonist (flumazenil) • Anterograde amnesia • Preoperative anxiolysis; adjunct to local/regional/general anesthesia • ICU sedation	• Dose-related dependence • Drug interactions due to P450 metabolism • Possible CV depression • Does not reach complete surgical anesthesia as a sole agent • Inhibits P450 enzymes
Sedative/Hypnotics			
Ketamine (Ketalar)	• **A:** IV, IM, PO • **OOA:** Rapid • **DOA:** Short • **M:** Hepatic (P450) • **E:** Metabolites excreted in urine	• Produces dissociative anesthesia • No loss of consciousness • Rapid recovery • Low doses provide analgesia • Airway patency maintained • Used in short surgeries and painful procedures, especially in pediatrics	• CV stimulation • Increases ICP • Diplopia • Nystagmus • Emergence reactions (agitation)

Continued

GENERAL ANESTHETIC DRUGS: INTRAVENOUS NONOPIOIDS (Continued)

Drug	Pharmacokinetics	Clinical Uses	Side Effects
Propofol (Diprivan, Fresenius Propoven)	• **A:** IV • **OOA:** Rapid • **DOA:** Short • **M:** Hepatic (P450) • **E:** Primarily excreted as metabolites in urine	• Used for induction • Maintenance of anesthesia during short cases • ICU sedation • Antiemetic properties	• Contraindicated in patients with egg or soy allergies • Requires metabolism to end effect following long infusions or high doses • Decreases ventilation • Decreases BP • Decreases ICP • PRIS • Inhibits P450 enzymes
Etomidate (Amidate)	• **A:** IV • **OOA:** Rapid • **DOA:** Short • **M:** Hepatic and plasma metabolism • **E:** Renal	• Used for induction • Supplement during maintenance • Rapid recovery	• Transient adrenal suppression • Decreases ICP • Nausea and vomiting • Myoclonus
Dexmedetomidine (Precedex)	• **A:** IV • **OOA:** Rapid • **DOA:** Short • **M:** Hepatic (Glucuronidation, Methylation and P450) • **E:** Metabolites excreted in urine	• α_2 agonist in the brainstem that inhibits NE release and, thus, produces sedation	• Decreases BP • Decreases HR • Decrease ventilation • Inhibits P450 enzymes
Remifentanil (Ultiva)	• **A:** IV • **OOA:** Immediate • **DOA:** Short • **M:** Blood and tissue esterases • **E:** Metabolites excreted in urine	• Binds to μ receptors in the CNS to alter pain perception • Induction and maintenance of anesthesia	• Decreases BP • Decreases HR

Drug	Pharmacokinetics	Clinical Uses	Drawbacks and Side Effects
Morphine (Duramorph, Astramorph, Infumorph)	• **A:** IV, IM, SC, PO • **OOA:** Intermediate • **DOA:** Intermediate • **M:** Hepatic • **E:** Renal	• Reduce dysphoria associated with pain • Increase pain tolerance • Reduce amount of other anesthetic agent when administered simultaneously • Used in patient-controlled analgesia, preoperative anxiolysis/analgesia/sedation, adjuncts to other anesthetics, and regional anesthesia • Minimal cardiovascular depression	• Histamine release • Nausea and vomiting • Respiratory depression • Decreased cough reflex • Venodilation (decreased BP) • Constipation • Inhibits P450 enzymes (Fentanyl only)
Fentanyl	• **A:** IV, IM, transdermal, PO, nasal spray, buccal, SL • **OOA:** Rapid • **DOA:** Intermediate • **M:** Hepatic (P450) • **E:** Renal		
Sufentanil (Sufenta)	• **A:** IV • **OOA:** Immediate • **DOA:** Short • **M:** Small intestine and hepatic (P450) • **E:** Renal	• More potent than fentanyl • Adjunct or primary anesthetic • Mixed with bupivacaine in epidural • Rapid recovery	• Respiratory depression • Constipation
Alfentanil (Alfenta)	• **A:** IV • **OOA:** Immediate • **DOA:** Short • **M:** Small intestine and hepatic (P450) • **E:** Renal	• Adjunct or primary anesthetic • Rapid recovery	

Continued

GENERAL ANESTHETIC DRUGS: INTRAVENOUS OPIOIDS (Continued)

Drug	Pharmacokinetics	Clinical Uses	Drawbacks and Side Effects
Remifentanil (Ultiva)	• **A:** IV • **OOA:** Immediate • **DOA:** Short • **M:** Plasma/tissue esterases • **E:** Renal	• Adjunct or primary anesthetic • Rapid recovery	• Respiratory depression • Hypotension • Nausea and vomiting • Bradycardia • Headache
Meperidine (Demerol)	• **A:** IV, IM, PO, SC • **OOA:** Intermediate • **DOA:** Intermediate • **M:** Hepatic • **E:** Renal	• Adjunct to other anesthetic • Obstetric anesthesia • Preoperative and short-term IV pain control	• Lowers seizure threshold

Brand names are IV forms only.

FOUR COMPONENTS, FOUR STAGES, AND FOUR KEYS TO ANESTHESIA

Components of Good Anesthesia	1. Loss of consciousness and amnesia: patient does not respond to command and will have no recall of surgical procedures; produced by nitrous oxide, benzodiazepines, or very low doses of any general anesthetic 2. Analgesia: elimination of the sensation of pain; produced by IV narcotic analgesics 3. Blunting of protective reflexes: primarily blunting of protective airway reflexes; produced by general anesthetics 4. Muscle relaxation: reduction in the resting muscle tone; produced by paralytic agents
Stages of Anesthesia	1. Analgesia (buzz): produced by nitrous oxide or ketamine, patient remains conscious 2. Excitement (spazz): deeper level of analgesia during which the patient is unresponsive, but because the cortex is depressed, there is disinhibition of activity and the patient flails 3. Surgical anesthesia (out): blunts protective reflexes, provides amnesia, eliminates sensation of pain, creates a still and bloodless field for surgeon 4. Medullary depression (death): cardiovascular and respiratory centers cease to function leading to death
Keys to Anesthesia	1. Maintain homeostasis: oxygenation and ventilation 2. Protection of the patient from injury 3. Provide a bloodless field (via vasoconstriction provided by adjuncts such as epinephrine) 4. Optimize patient's medical condition before and after surgery

NONANESTHETIC DRUGS USED DURING GENERAL ANESTHESIA

Class	Example	Clinical Use	Side Effects
Sedatives	• Benzodiazepines (eg, midazolam)	• Sedation	• Decrease pain tolerance
Paralytic agents	• Depolarizing (eg, succinylcholine) and nondepolarizing (eg, pancuronium)	• Prevent movement during procedures • Causes muscular relaxation, easing surgical access	• No analgesia or amnesia

X. Neuromuscular Blockers

NEUROMUSCULAR BLOCKERS: SUMMARY TABLE

Class	Pharmacokinetics				Mechanism of Action	Clinical Uses
	Administration	Onset of Action	Distribution	Metabolism		
☞ NM blockers ending in "Onium" are all sterOid derivatives; those ending in "Urium", "Urine" or "Uranine" are all isoqUinoline derivatives	IV	Important for determining appropriate time for intubation	All are ionized, therefore limited distribution occurs	Steroid derivatives must undergo hepatic biotransformation to achieve their active form	All NM blockers are nondepolarizing EXCEPT succinylcholine, which causes depolarization	Used by anesthesiologists in the OR for surgical muscular relaxation

DEPOLARIZING NEUROMUSCULAR BLOCKERS

Drug	Class	Pharmacokinetics	Mechanism of Action	Side Effects
Succinylcholine (Anectine, Quelicin)	• Dimer of acetylcholine	• **DOA:** 4–6 minutes • **OOA:** 30–60 seconds • **M:** Via plasma pseudocholinesterase • **E:** Metabolites excreted in urine	• Acts like a nicotinic agonist at the NMJ causing initial depolarization followed by blockade of any further neuromuscular transmission • Causes fasciculations followed by paralysis due to persistent depolarization of the end plate	• Hyperkalemia (especially in patients with muscular dystrophy, peripheral nerve dysfunction, burn or spinal cord injury) • Increased intraocular pressure • Increased intragastric pressure (emesis) • Muscle pain/damage • Slight histamine release • Stimulates autonomic ganglia • Stimulates cardiac muscarinic receptors causing bradycardia • Interactions with other medications (eg, aminoglycosides)

NONDEPOLARIZING NEUROMUSCULAR BLOCKERS

Drug	Class	Pharmacokinetics	Mechanism of Action	Side Effects
Cisatracurium (Nimbex) Atracurium		• DOA: 20–35 minutes • OOA: 2–3 minutes • M: Ester hydrolysis and Hofmann elimination	• Act as competitive Ach antagonists at the neuromuscular junction	• 3× potency of atracurium thus lower toxicity due to decreased dosing requirements • Major metabolite (laudanosine) has long $t_{1/2}$, crosses BBB and may cause seizures • Histamine release • Hypotension (due to histamine release and ganglionic blockade)
Pancuronium	• Steroid derivatives	• DOA: 60–100 minutes • OOA: 2–3 minutes • M: Hepatic (minor) • E: Primarily excreted unchanged in urine		• Vagal blockade results in increased heart rate, blood pressure, and cardiac output
Vecuronium		• DOA: 45 minutes • OOA: 3 minutes • M: Hepatic (minor) • E: Parent drug and metabolites excreted in feces > urine		• Low incidence of toxicity
Rocuronium		• DOA: 30 minutes • OOA: 2 minutes • M: Hepatic (minor) • E: Parent drug and metabolites excreted in feces > urine		• Low incidence of toxicity

CHAPTER 6

MEDICATIONS AFFECTING CARDIAC AND RENAL FUNCTION

I. ANTIHYPERTENSIVE DRUGS

Classification of Antihypertensive Drugs

Antihypertensives: Classification of Antiadrenergic Agents

Antihypertensives: Antiadrenergic Agents

Antihypertensives: β-Blockers

Antihypertensives: Classification of Vasodilators

Antihypertensives: Vasodilators

Antihypertensives: Calcium Channel Blockers and Angiotensin Antagonists

Antihypertensives: Classification of Angiotensin/Renin Agents

Drugs that Affect Angiotensin Action

The Functions of Angiotensin

Antihypertensives: Classification of Diuretics

Thiazide, Loop, and Potassium-Sparing Diuretics

Carbonic Acid Inhibitor and Osmotic Diuretics

Serum Electrolyte Effects of Diuretics

II. ANTIANGINAL DRUGS

Classification of Antianginal Drugs

Antianginals: Organic Nitrates, Calcium Channel Blockers, and β-Blocker

Effects of Nitrates Combined with β-Blockers

Mechanisms of Action of Antianginal Drugs

III. ANTIARRHYTHMICS

Classification of Antiarrhythmic Drugs

Class I Antiarrhythmics

Classes II, III, and IV Antiarrhythmics

IV. MANAGING CONGESTIVE HEART FAILURE

Classification of CHF Drugs

CHF Therapy: Positive Inotropic Drugs

CHF Therapy: Diuretics and ACE Inhibitors

V. ANTIHYPER-LIPIDEMIC DRUGS

Classification of Antihyperlipidemic Drugs

Antihyperlipidemics: Bile Acid Sequestrants and Nicotinic Acid

Antihyperlipidemics

Antihyperlipidemic: Fibric Acid Derivatives

Effects of Antihyperlipidemics on Lipoproteins

VI. MANAGING COAGULOPATHY

Classification of Drugs to Reduce Clotting

Coagulation Cascade

Drugs Used to Reduce Clotting: Anticoagulants, Thrombolytics, and Antiplatelets

Classification of Drugs to Facilitate Clotting/Reverse

Anticoagulation

Drugs Used to Facilitate Clotting/Reverse Anticoagulation

Acanthosis Nigricans	Warty growths and hyperpigmentation characteristically found in the axilla and groin; associated with certain drugs, endocrine disorders, obesity, or malignancy.
Alopecia	Absence or loss of hair.
Angina	Chest discomfort caused by insufficient cardiac blood flow resulting in cardiac ischemia.
Conn's Syndrome	Primary hyperaldosteronism.
Hypertensive Emergnecy	Hypertensive urgency with end-organ damage.
Hypertensive Urgency	Severely elevated BP (systolic >220 or diastolic >120) with no evidence of end-organ damage.
Hypertrichosis	Excessive hair growth.
Lupus-Like Syndrome	Drug-induced syndrome resembling the symptoms associated with SLE; rarely demonstrates nephritic component.
Pheochromocytoma	Catecholamine-secreting tumor of the adrenal gland.
Quinidine Syncope	Recurrent light-headedness and fainting associated with use of quinidine.
Reye's Syndrome	A rare syndrome of encephalitis and hepatic dysfunction seen in children recovering from a viral illness linked to aspirin.
Rhabdomyolysis	Destruction of skeletal muscle cells.
Thrombotic Thrombocytopenic Purpura	Coagulopathy seen in adults; associated with central nervous system involvement.
Tinnitis	Ringing in the ears.
Tolerance	Repeated administration of medication leads to decreased effectiveness.
Torsade de Pointes	A ventricular arrhythmia often induced by antiarrhythmic drugs (especially those that prolong the QT interval). Its morphology is that of a polymorphic ventricular tachycardia often with an increasing then decreasing QRS amplitude.
Wolff-Parkinson-White Syndrome	Syndrome associated with ventricular arrhythmias due to the presence of an accessory conduction pathway between the SA and AV nodes.

I. Antihypertensive Drugs

CLASSIFICATION OF ANTIHYPERTENSIVE DRUGS

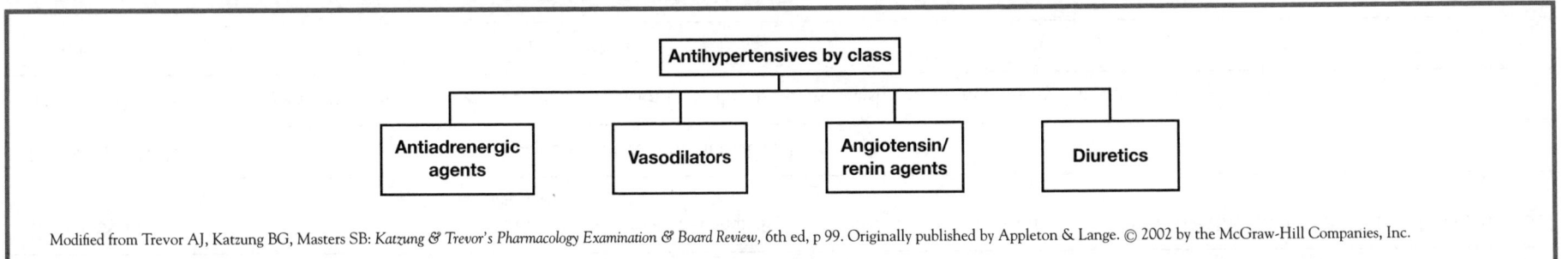

Modified from Trevor AJ, Katzung BG, Masters SB: *Katzung & Trevor's Pharmacology Examination & Board Review*, 6th ed, p 99. Originally published by Appleton & Lange. © 2002 by the McGraw-Hill Companies, Inc.

ANTIHYPERTENSIVES: CLASSIFICATION OF ANTIADRENERGIC AGENTS

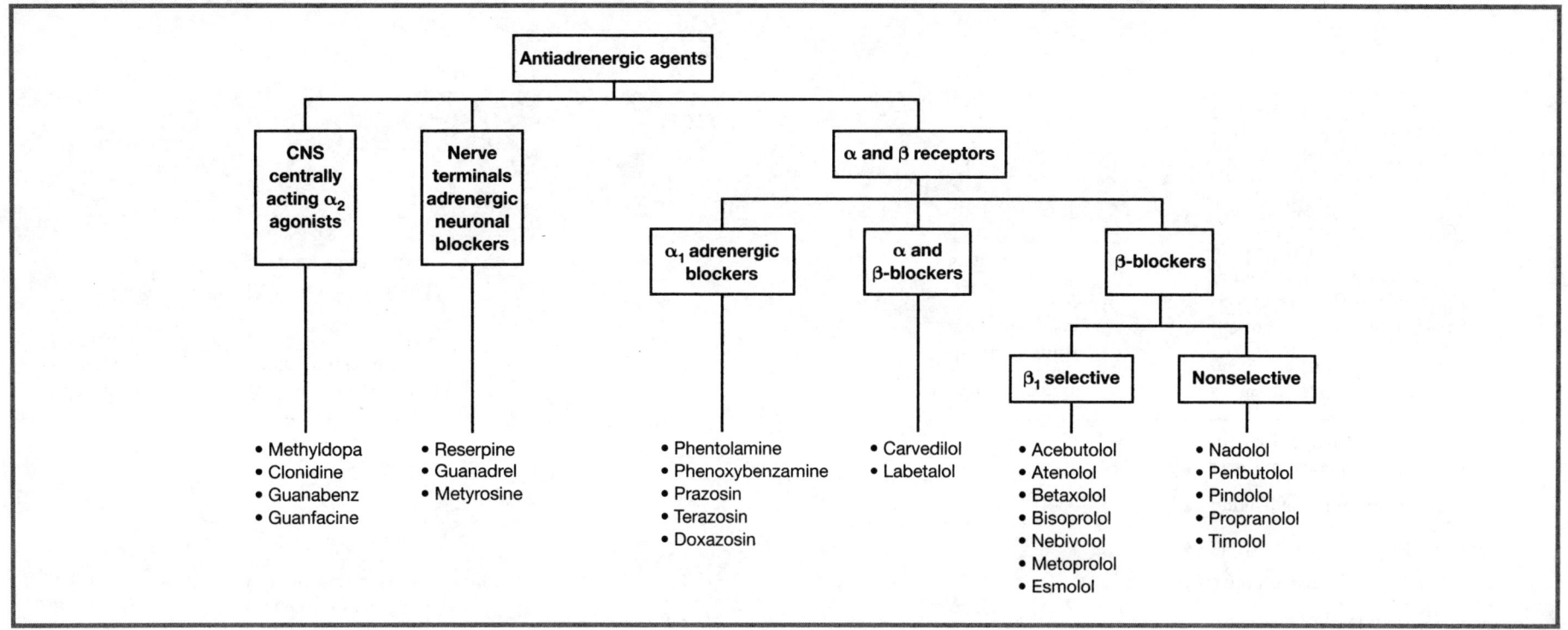

Drug	Pharmacokinetics	Mechanism of Action	Clinical Uses	Side Effects
Centrally Acting α_2 Agonists				
Methyldopa	• **A:** PO and IV • **M:** Hepatic and intestinal metabolism by COMT • **E:** Parent drug and metabolites excreted primarily in urine	• Believed to work in the relay area of the solitary nucleus • Act as α_2-receptor agonists to reduce sympathetic tone to peripheral structures (decrease peripheral resistance, HR, and plasma renin activity)	• Hypertension	• Plasma volume is increased (body's attempt to reestablish homeostasis) leading to mild edema • Sedation, dizziness, and headache (diminish as tolerance develops) • Mild bradycardia • Flu-like symptoms with fever • Lupus-like syndrome • Positive Coombs' test with no increase in hemolytic anemia
Clonidine (Catapres, Duraclon, Kapvay)	• **A:** PO, transdermal patch, and epidural • **M:** Hepatic • **E:** Majority excreted unchanged in urine		• Hypertension • Epidural infusion for pain management	• Drowsiness, dizziness, and headache (subside with tolerance) • Plasma volume is increased (body's attempt to reestablish homeostasis) leading to mild edema • Xerostomia • Constipation • Patch can cause itching, irritation, and redness

Guanabenz (Wytensin)	• **A:** PO • **M:** Site of metabolism unknown • **E:** Metabolites excreted in urine		• Hypertension	• Confusion/mental depression • Antimuscarinic side effects • Headache • Nausea
Guanfacine (Intuniv, Tenex)	• **A:** PO • **M:** Hepatic (P450) • **E:** Parent drug and metabolites excreted in urine			

Adrenergic Neuronal Blockers

Reserpine (Serpasil)	• **A:** PO • **M:** Hepatic • **E:** Parent drug and metabolites excreted in feces > urine	• Blocks reuptake of NE and DA into vesicle within the neuron by inhibiting Mg ATPase • Depletion of neurotransmitters leads to decreased activity in blood vessels and heart	• Hypertension • Used only rarely (due to CNS side effects) in small doses with other drugs like diuretics and β-blockers • Schizophrenia	• Severe depression • Sedation • Bradycardia • TTP

Continued

ANTIHYPERTENSIVES: ANTIADRENERGIC AGENTS (Continued)

Drug	Pharmacokinetics	Mechanism of Action	Clinical Uses	Side Effects
Guanadrel (Hylorel)	• A: PO • M: Hepatic • E: Parent drug and metabolites excreted in urine	• Replaces NE bound to ATP in vesicles • Results in decreased NE released with nerve stimulation • Leads to reduced arteriolar vasoconstriction	• Moderate to severe hypertension	• Angina • Edema (peripheral and pulmonary) • Fatigue • Severe diarrhea
Metyrosine (Demser)	• A: PO • M: Majority excreted unchanged in urine	• Competitive inhibitor of tyrosine hydroxylase • Reduces synthesis of NE and EPI causing decreased BP	• Prophylaxis and treatment of hypertension associated with pheochromocytomy • Chronic treatment for malignant pheochromocytoma	• Severe diarrhea • EPS (see section on Antipsychotics in Chapter 4 for more information) • Allergic reactions
Nonselective α-Adrenergic Blockers				
Phentolamine (Regitine, Rogitine)	• A: IM, IV • M: Hepatic • E: Primarily excreted as metabolites in urine	• α-Adrenergic blockade leads to decreased systemic vascular resistance • Results in decreased BP	• Diagnosis of pheochromocytoma • Prophylaxis and treatment of hypertension associated with pheochromocytomy	• Reflex tachycardia • Orthostatic hypotension • GI disturbances (nausea, diarrhea) • Weakness
Phenoxy-benzamine (Dibenzyline)	• A: PO • M: Hepatic metabolism; irreversible • E: Metabolites excreted in urine and feces			

Selective α-Adrenergic Blockers

Prazosin (Minipress)	• **A:** PO • **M:** Hepatic metabolism to active metabolites • **E:** Parent drug and metabolites excreted in bile and feces	• α_1 blockade causing decreased arterial tone	• Hypertension • BPH • Cause less reflex tachycardia than nonselective α-adrenergic blockers	• First dose orthostatic hypotension (can lead to syncope) requires careful dosing (usually before bed) • Dizziness • Drowsiness (will subside) • Headache • Peripheral edema • Palpitations
Terazosin (Hytrin)	• **A:** PO • **M:** Hepatic metabolism to active metabolites • **E:** Parent drug and metabolites excreted in urine and feces			
Doxazosin (Cardura)	• **A:** PO • **M:** Hepatic (P450) • **E:** Parent drug and metabolites excreted in bile and feces			

ANTIHYPERTENSIVES: β-BLOCKERS

Drug	Pharmacokinetics	Mechanism of Action	Clinical Uses	Side Effects
Acebutolol (Sectral)	• **A:** PO • **M:** Hepatic • **E:** Metabolites excreted in urine and feces	• Selective β_1 antagonist	• HTN • Ventricular arrhythmias	• Headache • Fatigue • Dizziness • Inhibits P450 enzymes (Acebutolol and Betaxolol only)
Atenolol (Tenormin)	• **A:** PO • **M:** Hepatic (minimal) • **E:** Parent drug excreted in urine, metabolites excreted in feces		• HTN • Angina • Post MI	
Betaxolol (Kerlone)	• **A:** PO • **M:** Hepatic (P450) • **E:** Metabolites excreted primarily in urine		• HTN	
Bisoprolol (Zebeta)	• **A:** PO • **M:** Hepatic (P450) • **E:** Parent drug and metabolites excreted in urine			
Nebivolol (Brevibloc)	• **A:** PO • **M:** Hepatic (P450) • **E:** Metabolites excreted in feces and urine			
Metoprolol (Lopressor, Toprol)	• **A:** PO, IV • **M:** Hepatic (P450) • **E:** Metabolites excreted primarily in urine		• HTN • Angina • Rate control in SVT and a fib/flutter • Myocardial infarction	• Hypotension • Diarrhea • Dizziness • Inhibits P450 enzymes

Drug	Pharmacokinetics	Mechanism of Action	Indications	Side Effects
Esmolol (Brevibloc)	• **A:** IV • **M:** Metabolized by esterases in blood • **E:** Primarily excreted as metabolites in urine		• Class II antiarrhythmic • SVT • Management of intra/postoperative HTN or tachycardia	• Hypotension • Nausea • Dizziness
Carvedilol (Coreg)	• **A:** PO • **M:** Hepatic (P450) • **E:** Metabolites excreted primarily in feces	• Nonselective β antagonist (decreases HR and plasma renin activity; increases plasma volume) • Nonselective α antagonist (decreases peripheral resistance)	• HTN • Heart failure • LV dysfunction following MI	• Hypotension • Fatigue • Dizziness • Weight gain
Labetalol (Trandate)	• **A:** PO, IV • **M:** Hepatic • **E:** Metabolites excreted primarily in urine		• HTN • Hypertensive emergency	• Orthostatic hypotension • Fatigue • Dizziness • Weight gain
Nadolol (Corgard)	• **A:** PO • **E:** Excreted unchanged in urine	• Nonselective β antagonist	• HTN • Angina	• Sleep disturbances (drowsiness, insomnia)
Penbutolol (Levatol)	• **A:** PO • **M:** Hepatic • **E:** Metabolites excreted primarily in urine		• HTN	• Bradycardia • Fatigue • Dizziness

Continued

ANTIHYPERTENSIVES: β-BLOCKERS (Continued)

Drug	Pharmacokinetics	Mechanism of Action	Clinical Uses	Side Effects
Pindolol	• A: PO • M: Hepatic (P450 minor) • E: Metabolites excreted in feces and urine		• HTN • Angina	• Edema • Sleep disturbances (drowsiness, insomnia) • Inhibits P450 enzymes
Propranolol (Hemangeol, Inderal, InnoPran)	• A: PO, IV • M: Hepatic (P450) • E: Metabolites excreted primarily in urine		• HTN • Essential tremor • Migraine prophylaxis • Angina • Tachyarrhythmias • IHSS pheochromocytoma • Post MI mortality reduction • Class II antiarrhythmic	• Bronchospasm • Hypotension • Inhibits P450 enzymes
Timolol	• A: PO • M: Hepatic (P450) • E: Parent drug and metabolites excreted in urine		• HTN • Migraine prophylaxis • Prevention of MI	• Bradycardia • Fatigue • Dizziness • Inhibits P450 enzymes

Avoid abrupt cessation of β-blockers to avoid increased HR, BP, and risk of angina.
Use nonselective β-blockers with caution in the setting of asthma, COPD, DM, and PVD.

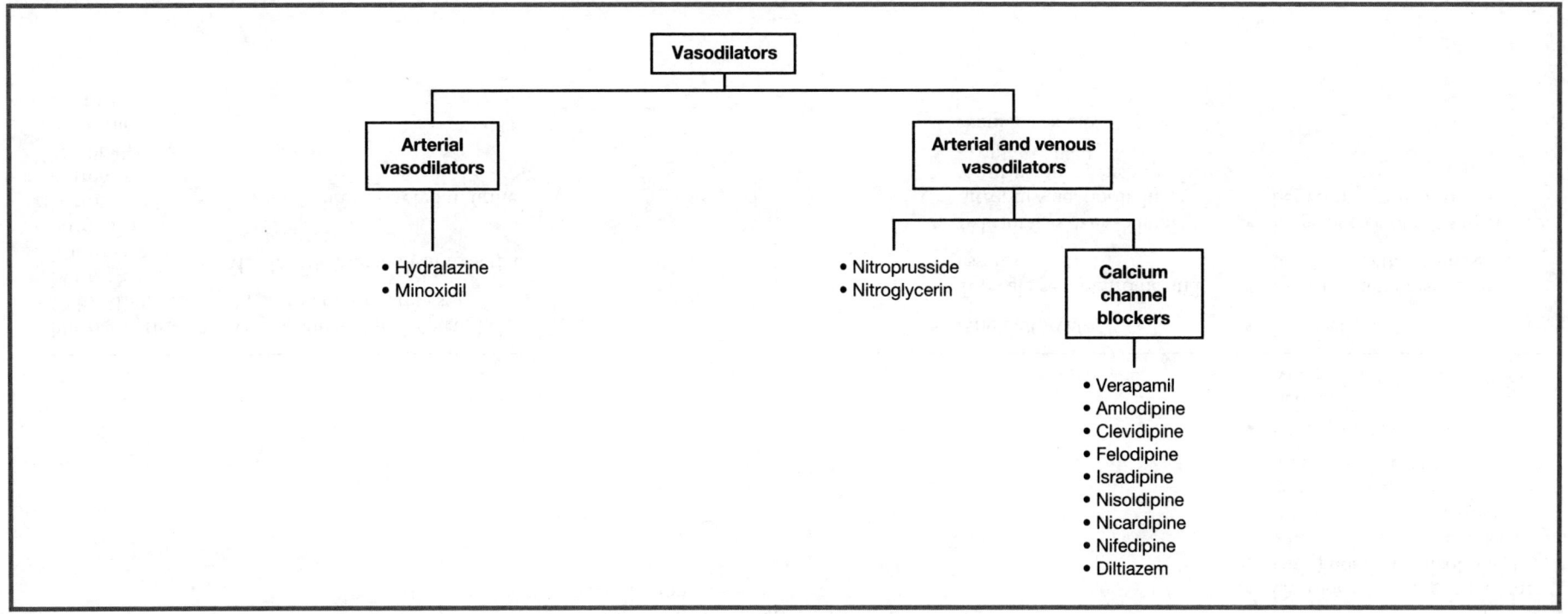

ANTIHYPERTENSIVES: VASODILATORS

Drug	Pharmacokinetics	Mechanism of Action	Clinical Uses	Side Effects
Arterial and Venous Vasodilator				
Nitroprusside (Nitropress)	• **A:** IV • **M:** Local metabolism by tissues and erythrocytes • **E:** Metabolites excreted in urine	• Converted to nitric oxide intracellularly, which activates guanylate cyclase, leading to an increase in cGMP causing dephosphorylation of myosin light chain resulting in relaxation of vascular smooth muscle resulting in vasodilation	• Acute hypertensive emergencies • Acute decompensated heart failure	• Hypotension • Byproduct of metabolism is cyanide, which is metabolized by the liver by rhodanase to thiocyanate (water soluble and excreted in urine) • Cyanide poisoning in patients with poor diets (alcoholics) where it leads to decreased sulfur availability or when administered in high doses for long period of time • Drug is broken down by UV light so IV bag must be wrapped in foil
Nitroglycerin (Nitro-Bid, Nitro-Dur, Minitran, Nitro-Time, Nitrolingual, NitroMist, Nitronal, Nitrostat, Rectiv)	• **A:** Translingual sublingual, PO, IV, ointment, or patches • **M:** Hepatic metabolism to active metabolites • **E:** Metabolites excreted in urine	• Topical use for chronic and fissures • Angina/CAD	• Advantages over sodium nitroprusside: not light sensitive, inexpensive, readily available, no cyanide toxicity	• Headache • Repeated administration leads to a loss of effectiveness • Large degree of cross tolerance between organic nitrates

Arterial Vasodilators

Hydralazine (Apresoline, NovoHylazin, Nu-Hydral)	• **A:** PO, IM, and IV • **M:** Extensive first-pass hepatic metabolism; hepatic acetylation (certain patient populations have varying rates of acetylation) • **E:** Parent drug and metabolites excreted in urine	• Arteriole smooth muscle relaxation and vasodilation (probably through action on cAMP and Ca^{2+})	• Hypertension • Hypertensive emergency in pregnancy • Hypertensive emergency	• Toxicity in slow acetylators • Tachycardia • Headache • Dizziness • Nausea • Sweating • Flushing • Lupus-like syndrome
Minoxidil	• **A:** PO and topical • **M:** Hepatic • **E:** Parent drug and metabolites excreted in urine	• Inhibits PDE leading to increased levels of cAMP, which through Ca^{2+} modulation leads to arterial smooth muscle relaxation and vasodilation	• Hypertension • Alopecia	• Exacerbation of angina • Massive fluid retention • Hypertrichosis (hair growth) • ECG changes • Pericarditis

Drug	Pharmacokinetics	Mechanism of Action	Clinical Uses	Side Effects
Calcium Channel Blockers				
Verapamil (Calan, Isoptin, Verelan)	• **A:** PO, IV • **M:** Extensive first pass hepatic (P450) metabolism to active metabolites • **E:** Primarily excreted as metabolites in urine	• Block voltage sensitive calcium channels located primarily in the cardiac muscle and in vascular smooth muscle causing decreased intracellular Ca²⁺	• HTN • SVT/PSVT • Angina • Rate control in a fib	• Gingival hyperplasia • Constipation • Headache • Peripheral edema • Inhibits P450 enzymes
		• Block cyclic nucleotide PDE which increases cGMP and decreases Ca^{2+} influx • Results in dilation of peripheral arterioles and venules		
Diltiazem (Cardizem)	• **A:** PO, IV • **M:** Hepatic (P450) • **E:** Metabolites excreted in urine and feces		• HTN • Atrial fib/flutter • PSVT • Angina	• Headache • Peripheral edema • Inhibits P450 enzymes
Amlodipine (Norvasc)	• **A:** PO • **M:** Hepatic (P450) • **E:** Parent drug and metabolites excreted in urine		• HTN • Angina	• Peripheral edema • Inhibits P450 enzymes
Clevidipine (Cleviprex)	• **A:** IV • **M:** Hydrolysis and blood and extravascular tissues • **E:** Metabolites excreted in urine and feces		• HTN	• Atrial fibrillation • Fever • Insomnia • Nausea

Felodipine (Plendil, Renedil)	• **A:** PO • **M:** Hepatic (P450) • **E:** Primarily excreted as metabolites in urine		• Headache • Peripheral edema • Inhibits P450 enzymes
Isradipine	• **A:** PO • **M:** Hepatic (P450) • **E:** Metabolites excreted in urine and feces		• Inhibits P450 enzymes
Nisoldipine (Sular)	• **A:** PO • **M:** Hepatic (P450) • **E:** Primarily excreted as metabolites in urine		• Inhibits P450 enzymes
Nicardipine (Cardene)	• **A:** PO, IV • **M:** Hepatic (P450) • **E:** Metabolites excreted in urine and feces	• HTN • Acute HTN • Angina	• Flushing • Peripheral edema • Inhibits P450 enzymes
Nifedipine (Adalat, Afeditab, Procardia, Nifediac, Nifedical)	• **A:** PO • **M:** Hepatic (P450) • **E:** Primarily excreted as metabolites in urine	• HTN • Angina • HTN in pregnancy	• Flushing • Peripheral edema • Nausea • Dizziness • Inhibits P450 enzymes

ANTIHYPERTENSIVES: CLASSIFICATION OF ANGIOTENSIN/RENIN AGENTS

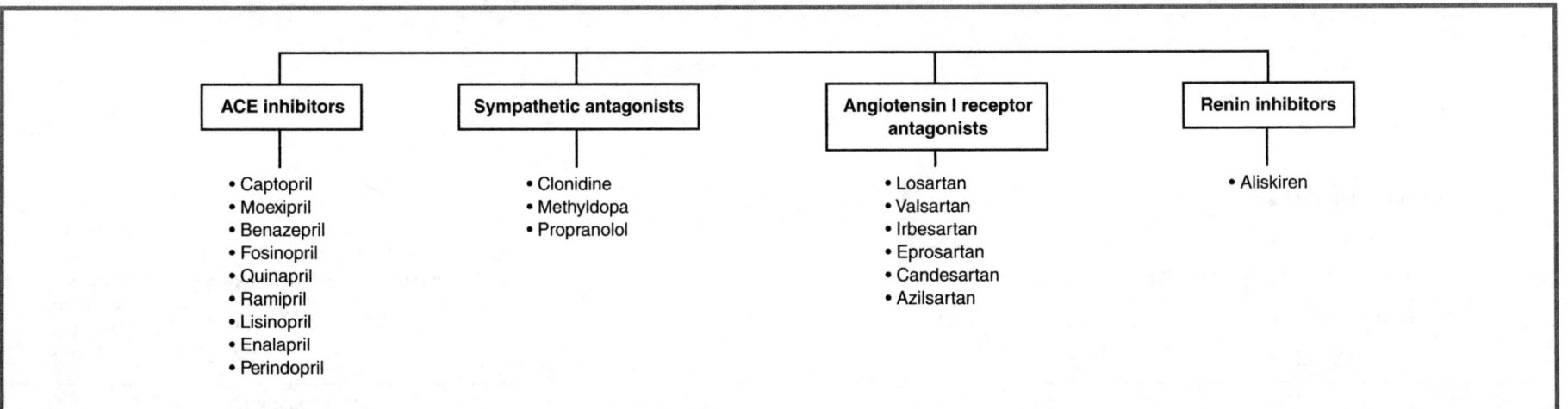

ACE inhibitors
- Captopril
- Moexipril
- Benazepril
- Fosinopril
- Quinapril
- Ramipril
- Lisinopril
- Enalapril
- Perindopril

Sympathetic antagonists
- Clonidine
- Methyldopa
- Propranolol

Angiotensin I receptor antagonists
- Losartan
- Valsartan
- Irbesartan
- Eprosartan
- Candesartan
- Azilsartan

Renin inhibitors
- Aliskiren

DRUGS THAT AFFECT ANGIOTENSIN ACTION

Drug	Pharmacokinetics	Mechanism of Action	Clinical Uses	Drawbacks and Side Effects
ACE Inhibitors				
Captopril (Capoten)	• **A:** PO • **M:** Prodrugs metabolized by intestinal wall and liver to active metabolite (Captopril P450) • **E:** Parent drug and metabolites excreted primarily in urine (Moexipril, Ramipril, and Fosinopril are also excreted in feces)	• Inhibit the formation of the potent vasoconstrictor angiotensin II from angiotensin by the inhibition of angiotensin-converting enzyme • Decrease peripheral resistance • Reduce the breakdown of bradykinin	• HTN • LV dysfunction following MI • Heart failure with reduced EF	• Angioedema • Cough (due to increased bradykinin) • Hyperkalemia • Renal failure • Contraindicated in pregnancy • Hypotension • Neutropenia
Moexipril (Univasc)			• HTN	
Benazepril (Lotensin)				
Perindopril (Aceon)			• HTN and stable CAD	
Ramipril (Altace)			• HTN • Heart failure post MI • Reduction in risk of CVA, MI, death	
Fosinopril (Monopril)			• HTN • Heart failure	
Quinapril (Accupril)				
Lisinopril (Prinivil, Zestril)	• **A:** PO • **E:** Excreted unchanged in urine			

Continued

DRUGS THAT AFFECT ANGIOTENSIN ACTION (Continued)

Drug	Pharmacokinetics	Mechanism of Action	Clinical Uses	Drawbacks and Side Effects
Trandolapril (Mavik)	• **A:** PO • **M:** Prodrugs metabolized by intestinal wall and liver to active metabolite • **E:** Parent drug and metabolites excreted primarily in urine and feces		• HTN • Asymptomatic LV dysfunction • Heart failure with reduced EF	
Enalapril (Vasotec, Epaned)	• **A:** IV, PO • **M:** Prodrugs metabolized by liver to active metabolite • **E:** Parent drug and metabolites excreted primarily in urine and feces		• HTN • Asymptomatic LV dysfunction • Heart failure with reduced EF	

Angiotensin Receptor Blockers

Drug	Pharmacokinetics	Mechanism of Action	Clinical Uses	Drawbacks and Side Effects
Losartan (Cozaar)	• **A:** PO • **M:** Hepatic (P450) metabolism to active metabolites • **E:** Parent drug and metabolites excreted in urine and feces	• Angiotensin II receptor blockade prevents the vasoconstriction caused by angiotensin II	• HTN • Neuropathy in patients with DM and HTN • Stroke reduction in patient with HTN and LVH	• Hyperkalemia • Fatigue • Contraindicated in pregnancy • Inhibits P450 enzymes (Losartan, Irbesartan, Eprosartan and Candesartan only)
Valsartan (Diovan)	• **A:** PO • **M:** Hepatic • **E:** Parent drug and metabolites excreted primarily in feces		• HTN • Heart failure • Neuropathy in patients with DM and HTN	

Irbesartan (Avapro)	• **A:** PO • **M:** Hepatic (P450 minor) • **E:** Parent drug and metabolites excreted in urine and feces		• HTN • Neuropathy in patients with DM and HTN
Eprosartan (Teveten)	• **A:** PO • **M:** Hepatic (minimal) • **E:** Parent drug and metabolites excreted primarily in feces		• HTN
Candesartan (Atacand)	• **A:** PO • **M:** Metabolized to active metabolite via hydrolysis within the intestinal wall and hepatic (P450 minor) • **E:** Primarily excreted unchanged in urine		• HTN • Heart failure
Azilsartan (Edarbi)	• **A:** PO • **M:** Metabolized to active metabolite via hydrolysis within the intestinal wall and hepatic (P450 minor) • **E:** Parent drug and metabolites excreted in urine and feces		• HTN
Renin Inhibitors			
Aliskiren (Tekturna)	• **A:** PO • **M:** Hepatic (P450 minor) • **E:** Parent drug excreted in feces and urine	• Renin inhibitor that results in the inhibition of angiotensinogen to angiotensin I	• HTN

Continued

DRUGS THAT AFFECT ANGIOTENSIN ACTION (Continued)

Drug	Pharmacokinetics	Mechanism of Action	Clinical Uses	Drawbacks and Side Effects
Sympathetic Antagonists				
Clonidine (Catapres)	• **A:** PO and transdermal • **M:** Hepatic • **E:** Majority excreted unchanged in urine	• Inhibit renin release by inhibiting the sympathetic nervous system • Renin release is the rate-limiting step in the renin-angiotensin system	• Hypertension • CHF	• Many adverse effects associated with the inhibition of the sympathetic nervous system due to nonselective nature of these medications • Bronchoconstriction • Hypotension • Bradycardia • Sexual dysfunction • Inhibits P450 enzymes (Propranolol only)
Methyldopa (Aldomet)	• **A:** PO and IV • **M:** Hepatic and intestinal metabolism by COMT • **E:** Parent drug and metabolites excreted in urine			
Propranolol (Inderal)	• **A:** PO and IV; well absorbed • **M:** Hepatic (P450) • **E:** Metabolites excreted in urine			

THE FUNCTIONS OF ANGIOTENSIN

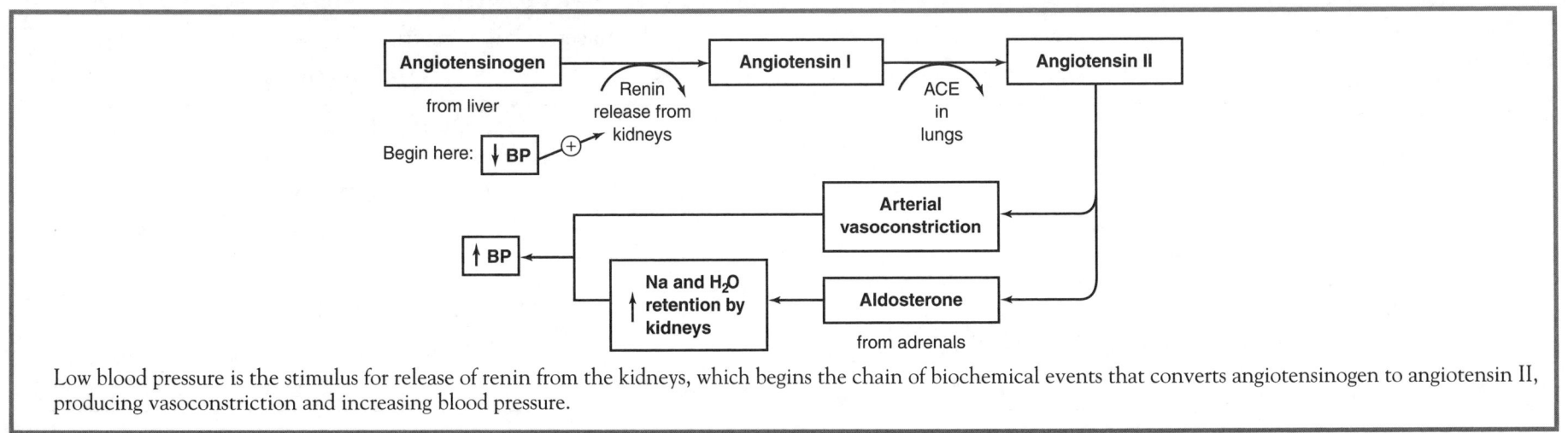

Low blood pressure is the stimulus for release of renin from the kidneys, which begins the chain of biochemical events that converts angiotensinogen to angiotensin II, producing vasoconstriction and increasing blood pressure.

ANTIHYPERTENSIVES: CLASSIFICATION OF DIURETICS

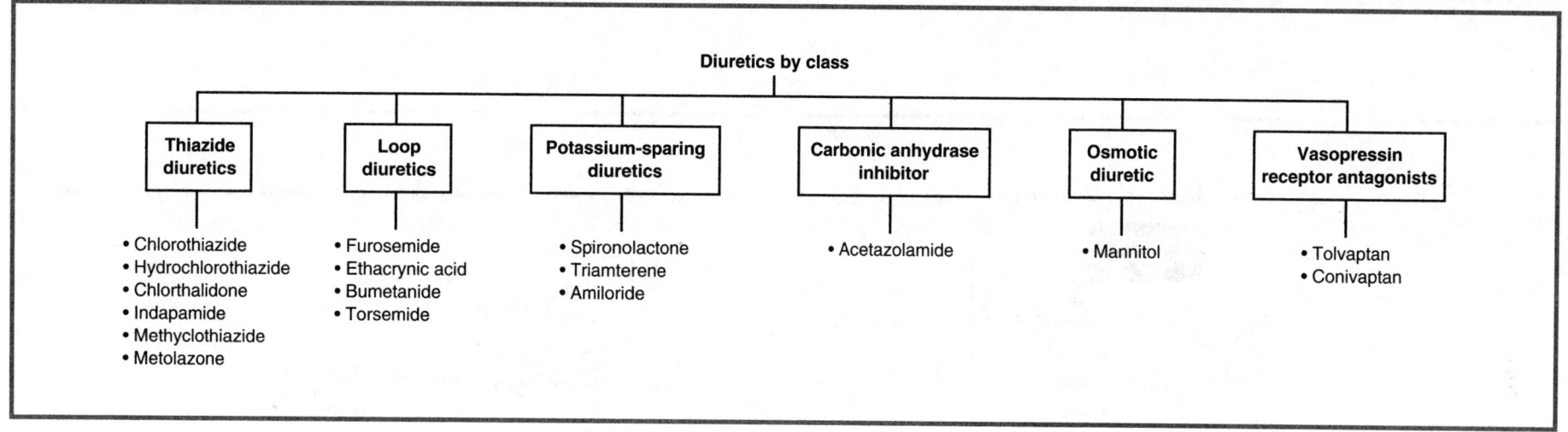

Diuretics by class

Thiazide diuretics	Loop diuretics	Potassium-sparing diuretics	Carbonic anhydrase inhibitor	Osmotic diuretic	Vasopressin receptor antagonists
• Chlorothiazide • Hydrochlorothiazide • Chlorthalidone • Indapamide • Methyclothiazide • Metolazone	• Furosemide • Ethacrynic acid • Bumetanide • Torsemide	• Spironolactone • Triamterene • Amiloride	• Acetazolamide	• Mannitol	• Tolvaptan • Conivaptan

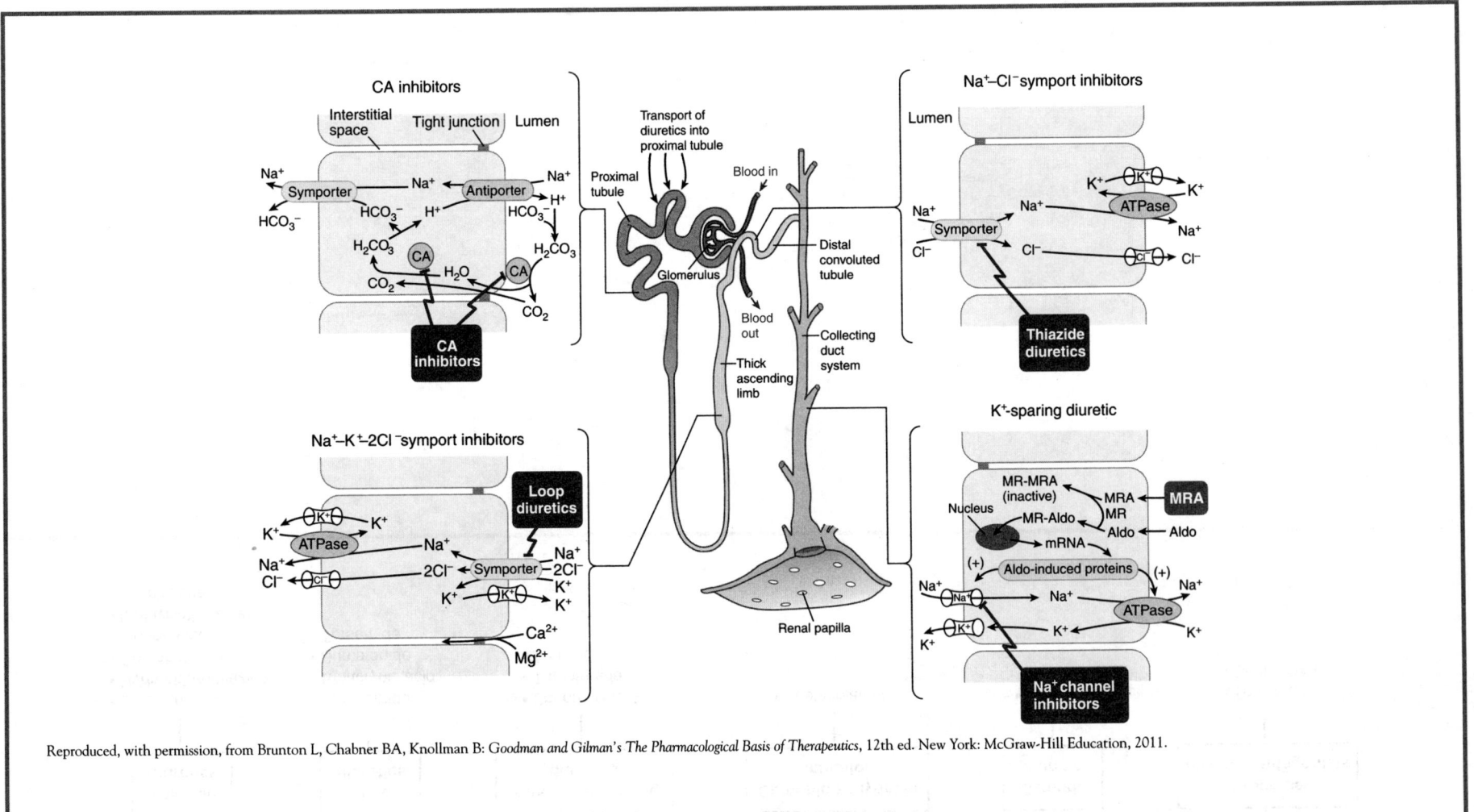

Reproduced, with permission, from Brunton L, Chabner BA, Knollman B: *Goodman and Gilman's The Pharmacological Basis of Therapeutics*, 12th ed. New York: McGraw-Hill Education, 2011.

THIAZIDE, LOOP, AND POTASSIUM-SPARING DIURETICS

Drug	Pharmacokinetics	Mechanism of Action	Clinical Uses and General Information	Side Effects
Thiazide Diuretics				
Chlorothiazide (Diuril)	• **A:** PO and IV • **E:** Unchanged in urine	• Increase urinary and salt output by inhibiting Na^+, Cl^- and water reabsorption in the distal tubule resulting in diuresis	• Hypertension • Edema	• Hypercalcemia • Hyperglycemia • Hyperlipidemia • Hypomagnesemia • Hyperuricemia (increased risk for gout) • Hypokalemia • Hyponatremia • Metabolic alkalosis • Muscle weakness • Pancreatitis
Hydrochlorothiazide (HCTZ)	• **A:** PO • **E:** Unchanged in urine			
Chlorthalidone	• **A:** PO • **E:** Unchanged in urine			
Indapamide	• **A:** PO • **M:** Hepatic • **E:** Metabolites excreted in urine			
Methyclothiazide	• **A:** PO • **E:** Excreted unchanged in urine			
Metolazone (Zaroxolyn)	• **A:** PO • **E:** Excreted unchanged in urine			

Continued

THIAZIDE, LOOP, AND POTASSIUM-SPARING DIURETICS (Continued)

Drug	Pharmacokinetics	Mechanism of Action	Clinical Uses and General Information	Side Effects
Loop Diuretics				
Furosemide (Lasix)	• **A:** IV, IM, and PO • **M:** Hepatic (minor) • **E:** Metabolites and parent drug excreted in urine	• Block reabsorption of Na^+ and Cl^- in the cortical and medullary regions of the ascending loop of Henle • Promote Ca^{2+} excretion	• Edema from CHF • Acute pulmonary edema • HTN	• Hyperglycemia (similar effect on pancreas as thiazides) • Hyperuricemia (increased risk for gout) • Hyponatremia • Hypokalemia • Excessive administration can lead to profound diuresis
Torsemide (Demadex)	• **A:** IV, PO • **M:** Hepatic (P450) • **E:** Metabolites and parent drug excreted in urine		• Edema from CHF • Hepatic cirrhosis • HTN	
Bumetanide (Bumex)	• **A:** IV, IM, and PO • **M:** Hepatic (minor) • **E:** Metabolites and parent drug excreted in urine and feces		• Edema from CHF	
Ethacrynic Acid (Edecrin)	• **A:** IV, PO • **M:** Hepatic (P450) • **E:** Metabolites and parent drug excreted in urine and feces		• Edema	

Potassium-Sparing Diuretics

Spironolactone (Aldactone)	• **A:** PO • **M:** Hepatic metabolism to active metabolites • **E:** Metabolites excreted in urine > feces	• Blocks the effects of aldosterone in the cortical collecting duct leading to Na^+ loss and K^+ retention	• CHF • HTN • Hypokalemia • Primary hyperaldosteronism • Edema	• Hepatotoxicity • DRESS syndrome • Hyperkalemia • CNS depression (drowsiness and lethargy) • Tumorigen • Antiandrogen effects (amenorrhea, gynecomastia) • GI (abdominal pain, GI hemorrhage)
Eplerenone (Inspra)	• **A:** PO • **M:** Hepatic (P450) • **E:** Metabolites excreted in urine > feces		• CHF • HTN	• Hyperkalemia • Hypertriglyceridemia
Triamterene (Dyrenium)	• **A:** PO • **M:** Hepatic • **E:** Parent drug and metabolites excreted in urine	• Blocks Na^+ reabsorption in the collecting duct and distal collecting tubule causing decreased intracellular Na^+ level causing dysfunction of the Na^+/K^+ ATPase leading to K^+ retention	• Edema	• Hyperkalemia (in patients with impaired renal function) • Nephrotoxicity • Nephrolithiasis • Metabolic acidosis
Amiloride (Midamor)	• **A:** PO • **E:** Parent drug excreted in urine and feces		• HTN	• Hyperkalemia (in patients with impaired renal function) • Metabolic acidosis

CARBONIC ACID INHIBITOR AND OSMOTIC DIURETICS

Drug	Pharmacokinetics	Mechanism of Action	Clinical Uses	Side Effects
Carbonic Anhydrase Inhibitor				
Acetazolamide (Acetazolam, Diamox)	• **A:** PO, IV • **E:** Parent drug excreted in urine	• Reversible inhibition of carbonic anhydrase resulting in decreased H^+ secretion at the renal tubule • Decreases production of aqueous humor	• Edema • Epilepsy • Glaucoma • Altitude sickness	• Paresthesias • Tinnitus • GI upset • Hypokalemia • Hyperchloremic metabolic acidosis (non gap)
Vasopressin Receptor Antagonists				
Tolvaptan (Samsca)	• **A:** PO • **M:** Hepatic (P450) • **E:** Metabolites excreted in feces	• Antagonism at the V_2 vasopressin receptor site causes excretion of free water	• Hyponatremia	• Nausea • Xerostomia • Initiation in inpatient settings where Na^+ can be closely monitored • Inhibits P450 enzymes
Conivaptan (Vaprisol)	• **A:** IV • **M:** Hepatic (P450) • **E:** Primarily excreted as metabolites in feces			• Fever • Orthostatic hypotension • Inhibits P450 enzymes
Osmotic Diuretic				
Mannitol (Osmitrol)	• **A:** IV • **M:** Minimal hepatic metabolism to glycogen • **E:** Primarily excreted unchanged in urine	• Increases osmotic pressure of glomerular filtrate thus increasing urine output by decreasing fluid and electrolyte resorption	• Reduction of intraocular pressure in glaucoma • Reduction of intracranial pressure with CNS edema	• Headache • Hypernatremia

SERUM ELECTROLYTE EFFECTS OF DIURETICS

In general, the opposite findings of serum electrolytes are seen in urine.

Type of Diuretic	Ca	Mg	Na	K	Uric Acid	Blood Sugar	Lipids	Metabolic Disturbance
Thiazide	↑	↓	↓	↓	↑	↑	↑	Hypokalemic metabolic alkalosis
Loop	↓	↓	↓	↓	↑	↑	—	
Potassium-sparing	—	↑	↓	↑	↑	—	—	Hyperchloremic metabolic acidosis
CAI	—	—	—	↓	↑	↑	—	
Osmotic	—	—	↑↓	↑	—	↑	—	Metabolic acidosis
Vasopressin Antagonists	—	↓	↓	↓	—	↑↓	—	

II. Antianginal Drugs

CLASSIFICATION OF ANTIANGINAL DRUGS

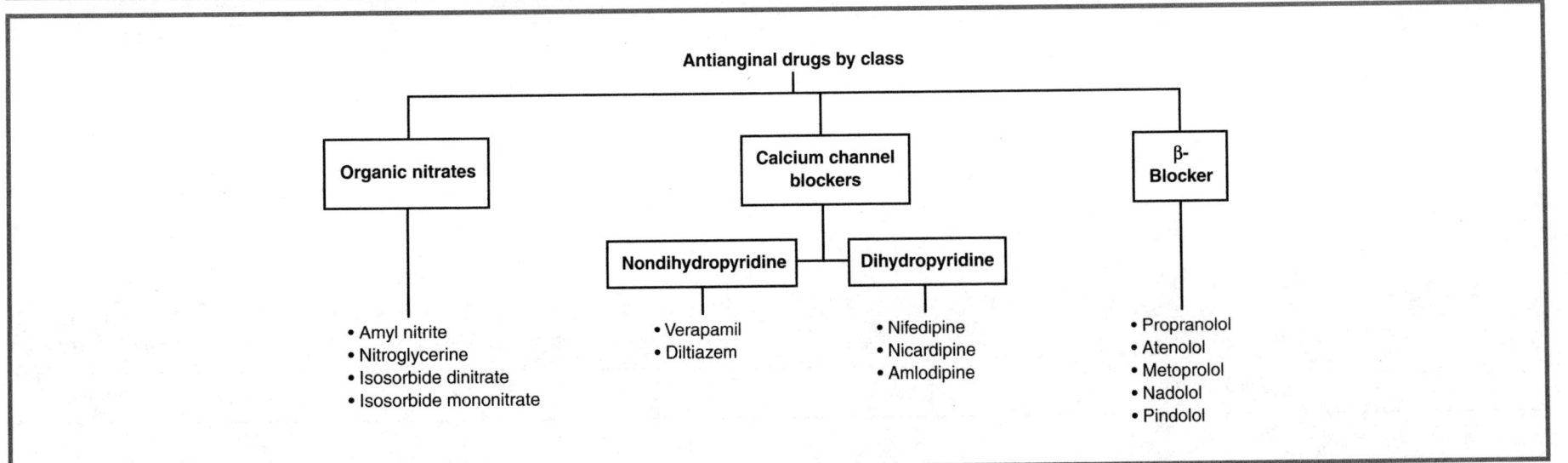

Drug	Pharmacokinetics	Mechanism of Action	Clinical Uses	Side Effects

Amyl nitrate	• **A:** Inhaled
	• **M:** Rapidly metabolized via hydrolytic denitration
	• **E:** Metabolites and parent drug excreted in urine
		• Converted to nitric oxide intracellularly which activates guanylate cyclase leading to the following cascade of events:
		
		  • Increase in cGMP
		  • Dephosphorylation of myosin light chain
		  • Relaxation of vascular smooth muscle
		  • Vasodilation
		
		• Venous dilation decreases preload
		
		• Vasodilation increases blood flow to the myocardium
			• Angina	• Headache
				• Hypotension
				• Increased intracranial pressure
				• Tolerance
				• Cross tolerance

Nitroglycerin (Nitro-Bid, Nitro-Dur, Minitran, Nitrolingual, NitroMist, Rectiv, Nitronal, Nitrostat)	• **A:** Sublingual, PO, IV, ointment, patches • **M:** Hepatic metabolism to active metabolites • **E:** Metabolites excreted in urine			
Isosorbide dinitrate (Isordil, IsoDitrate, Dilatrate)	• **A:** Sublingual, PO • **M:** Hepatic (P450) • **E:** Metabolites excreted in urine and feces			
Isosorbide mononitrate (Imdur)	• **A:** PO • **M:** Hepatic (P450) • **E:** Metabolites excreted in urine			

Continued

ANTIANGINALS: ORGANIC NITRATES, CALCIUM CHANNEL BLOCKERS, AND β-BLOCKER (Continued)

Drug	Pharmacokinetics	Mechanism of Action	Clinical Uses	Side Effects
Nondihydropyridine Calcium Channel Blockers				
Verapamil (Calan, Isoptin, Verelan)	• **A:** PO and IV • **M:** Extensive first pass hepatic (P450) metabolism to active metabolites • **E:** Primarily excreted as metabolites in urine	• Reduce Ca^{2+} influx • Resulting reduction of IC Ca^{2+} leads to smooth muscle relaxation • Result in decreased myocardial contractile force and decreased arterial tone and systemic vascular resistance	• Angina • Supraventricular tachycardia • Ventricular rate control in atrial flutter and fibrillation • Hypertension	• Gingival hyperplasia • Constipation • Hypotension • Inhibits P450 enzymes
Diltiazem (Cardizem, Dilacor, Diltzac, Matzim, Taztia, Tiazac)	• **A:** PO and IV • **M:** Hepatic (P450) • **E:** Parent drug and metabolites excreted in urine and feces		• Angina • Supraventricular arrhythmias • Ventricular rate control in atrial flutter and fibrillation • Hypertension	• Headache • Peripheral edema • Dizziness • First-degree AV block • Inhibits P450 enzymes

Dihydropyridine Calcium Channel Blockers

Nifedipine (Adalat, Afeditab, Procardia, Nifediac, Nifedical)	**A:** PO **M:** Hepatic (P450) **E:** Primarily excreted as metabolites in urine	• Block voltage sensitive calcium channels located primarily in the cardiac muscle and in vascular smooth muscle causing decreased intracellular Ca^{2+} • Block cyclic nucleotide PDE which increases cGMP and decreases Ca^{2+} influx • Results in dilation of peripheral arterioles and venules	• Angina • HTN • HTN in pregnancy	• Flushing • Peripheral edema • Nausea • Dizziness • Inhibits P450 enzymes
Nicardipine (Cardene)	**A:** PO, IV **M:** Hepatic (P450) **E:** Metabolites excreted in urine and feces		• Angina • HTN • Acute HTN	• Flushing • Peripheral edema • Inhibits P450 enzymes
Amlodipine (Norvasc)	**A:** PO **M:** Hepatic (P450) **E:** Parent drug and metabolites excreted in urine		• Angina • HTN	• Peripheral edema • Inhibits P450 enzymes

β-Blockers

Atenolol (Tenormin)	**A:** PO **M:** Hepatic (minimal) **E:** Parent drug excreted in urine, metabolites excreted in feces	• Selective β_1 antagonist	• HTN • Angina • Post MI	• Headache • Fatigue • Dizziness
Metoprolol (Lopressor, Toprol)	**A:** PO, IV **M:** Hepatic (P450) **E:** Metabolites excreted primarily in urine		• HTN • Angina • Rate control in SVT and a fib/flutter • Myocardial infarction	• Hypotension • Diarrhea • Dizziness • Inhibits P450 enzymes

Continued

ANTIANGINALS: ORGANIC NITRATES, CALCIUM CHANNEL BLOCKERS, AND β-BLOCKER (Continued)

Drug	Pharmacokinetics	Mechanism of Action	Clinical Uses	Side Effects
Nadolol (Corgard)	• **A:** PO • **E:** Excreted unchanged in urine	• Nonselective β antagonist	• HTN • Angina	• Sleep disturbances (drowsiness, insomnia)
Pindolol	• **A:** PO • **M:** Hepatic (P450 minor) • **E:** Metabolites excreted in feces and urine		• HTN • Angina	• Edema • Sleep disturbances (drowsiness, insomnia) • Inhibits P450 enzymes
Propranolol (Hemangeol, Inderal, InnoPran)	• **A:** PO, IV • **M:** Hepatic (P450) • **E:** Metabolites excreted primarily in urine		• HTN • Essential tremor • Migraine prophylaxis • Angina • Tachyarrhythmias • IHSS • Pheochromocytoma • Post MI mortality reduction • Class II antiarrhythmic	• Bronchospasm • Hypotension • Inhibits P450 enzymes

EFFECTS OF NITRATES COMBINED WITH β-BLOCKERS

β-Blockers and nitrates are often combined to achieve vasodilation and decreased contractility to relieve angina without causing an increase in HR (reflex tachycardia).

Drug Class	Heart Rate	Arterial Pressure	Contractility
Nitrates	↑	↓ (vasodilation)	↓ then ↑ (reflex tachycardia)
β-Blockers	↓ or ↔	↔	↓
β-Blockers and nitrates	↔	↓	↓ or ↔
☞ Think of this chart as summation vertically:	Heart rate of increase (nitrates) plus decrease (β-blockers) equals no effect (nitrates and β-blockers).	Arterial pressure of decrease plus no effect equals decrease.	Contractility of decrease then increase, plus decrease equals decrease or no effect.

↔, no effect.

MECHANISMS OF ACTION OF ANTIANGINAL DRUGS

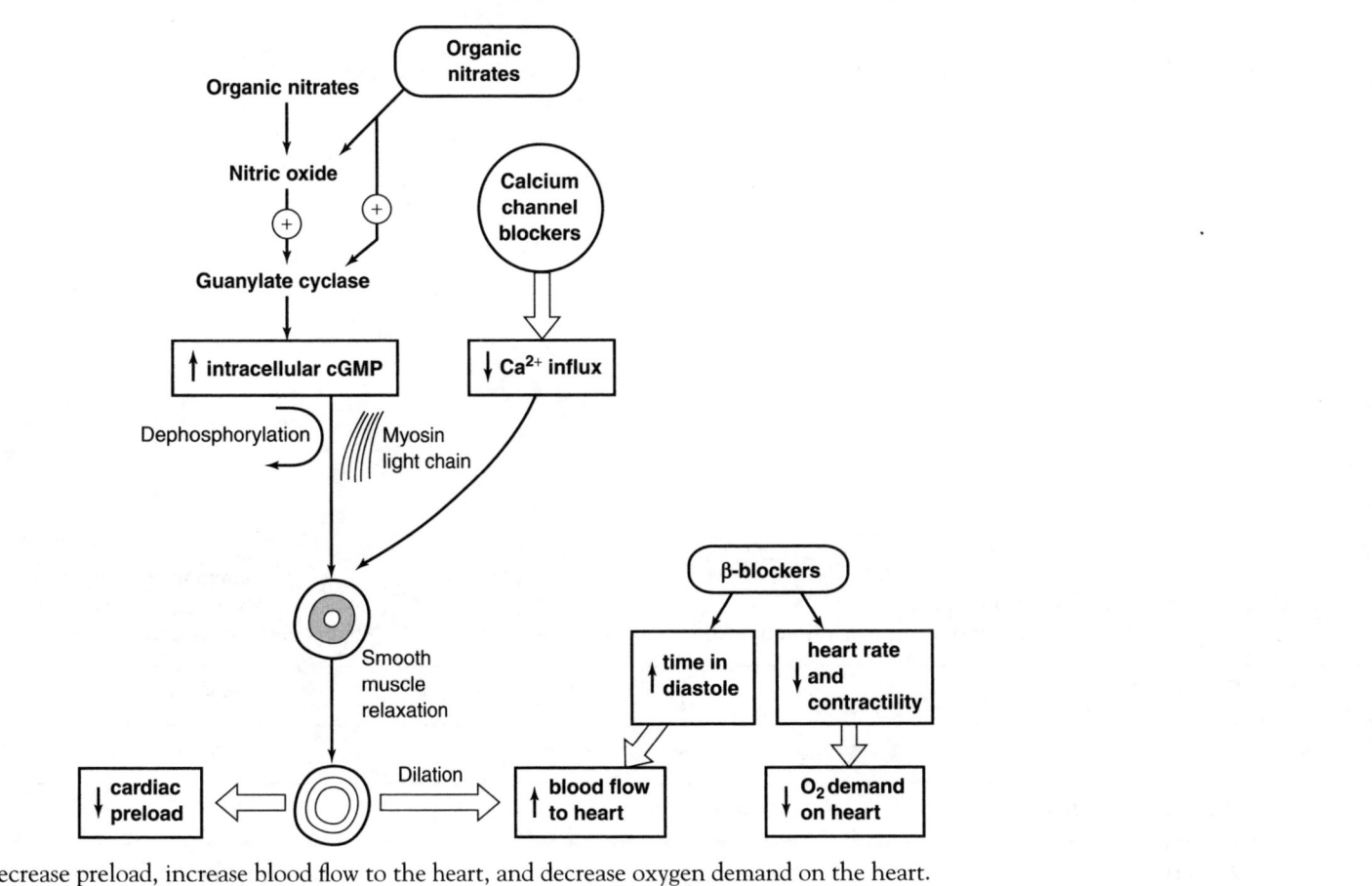

Antianginal drugs function to decrease preload, increase blood flow to the heart, and decrease oxygen demand on the heart.

III. Antiarrhythmics

CLASSIFICATION OF ANTIARRHYTHMIC DRUGS

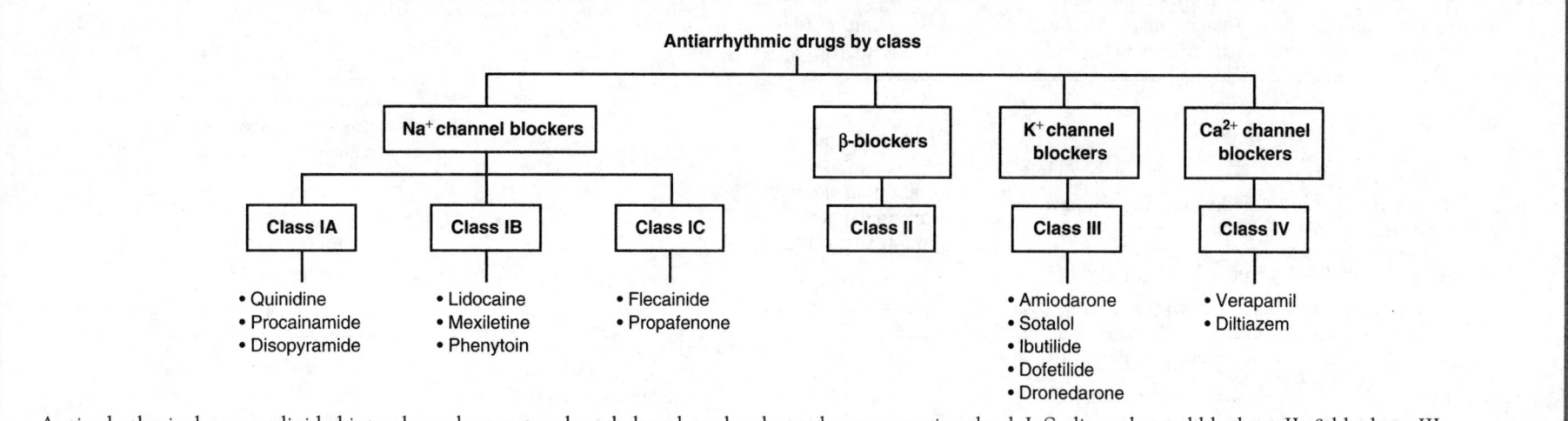

Antiarrhythmic drugs are divided into classes by a system loosely based on the channel or receptor involved: I, Sodium channel blockers; II, β-blockers; III, Potassium channel blockers, and IV, Calcium channel blockers.

Modified from Trevor AJ, Katzung BG, Masters SB: *Katzung & Trevor's Pharmacology Examination & Board Review*, 6th ed, p 120. Originally published by Appleton & Lange. © 2002 by the McGraw-Hill Companies, Inc.

CLASS I ANTIARRHYTHMICS

Drug	Pharmacokinetics	Mechanism of Action	Clinical Uses	Drawbacks and Side Effects
Class IA				
Quinidine	• **A:** PO, IV • **M:** Hepatic (P450) • **E:** Parent drug and metabolites excreted in urine	• Inhibit fast Na^+ channel by blocking activated Na^+ channels • Weakly block K^+ channels (reduces repolarization), which increases AP duration (manifested as lengthening of QT interval)	• All types of arrhythmias • Especially useful for conversion of a fib/flutter to sinus rhythm and maintenance in patients with paroxysmal fib/flutter	• Antimuscarinic activity can suppress vagal tone leading to an increase in AV conduction which may cause tachycardia • Refractory heterogenicity: Depressed conduction can further lead to torsade de pointes and eventual quinidine syncope (due to QT prolongation) • GI irritation (nausea, vomiting, diarrhea) • Increased mortality especially associated with structural heart disease • Inhibits P450 enzymes
Procainamide	• **A:** IM, IV • **M:** Hepatic (P450) metabolism to *N*-acetylprocainamide (NAPA) • **E:** Parent drug and metabolite excreted primarily in urine		• All types of arrhythmias • Especially useful for hemodynamically stable monomorphic VT or preexcited atrial fibrillation	• GI irritation (nausea, vomiting, diarrhea) • Drug-induced lupus-like syndrome • Blood dyscrasias (agranulocytosis, bone marrow suppression, neutropenia, thrombocytopenia, anemia) • Hypotension
Disopyramide (Norpace)	• **A:** PO • **M:** Hepatic (P450) • **E:** Parent drug and metabolite excreted primarily in urine		• Ventricular arrhythmias	• Antimuscarinic activity can suppress vagal tone leading to an increase in AV conduction which may cause tachycardia • Constipation • Xerostomia • Urinary hesitancy

Class IB

Lidocaine (Xylocaine)	• **A:** IV, ET tube • **M:** Hepatic (P450) • **E:** Primarily excreted as metabolites in urine	• Inhibit both inactive and active Na$^+$ channels • Act preferentially on depolarized, arrhythmogenic tissue • Shorten AP duration	• Suppression of recurrent ventricular tachycardia and fibrillation	• CNS side effects (tremor, light-headedness, nausea of central origin, paresthesias) • Inhibits P450 enzymes
Mexiletine	• **A:** PO • **M:** Hepatic (P450) • **E:** Parent drug and metabolites excreted in urine		• Ventricular arrhythmias	• GI side effects (nausea, vomiting) • Neurologic side effects (light-headedness, dizziness, tremor, nervousness)
Phenytoin (Dilantin, Phenytek)	• **A:** PO, IV • **M:** Hepatic (P450) • **E:** Primarily excreted as metabolites in urine		• Ventricular tachycardia and paroxysmal atrial tachycardia	• Cardiovascular collapse (esp with rapid infusion) • Vertigo • Gingivitis gingival hyperplasia • Systemic lupus erythematosus • Induces P450 enzymes

Continued

CLASS I ANTIARRHYTHMICS (Continued)

Drug	Pharmacokinetics	Mechanism of Action	Clinical Uses	Drawbacks and Side Effects
Class IC				
Flecainide (Tambocor)	• **A:** PO and IV; well absorbed • **M:** Hepatic (P450) • **E:** Parent drug and metabolites excreted in urine	• Inhibit fast Na^+ channels • Especially effective in the His-Purkinje system (widens QRS complex) • Usually little effect on AP duration • Prolongation of refractory periods	• Ventricular arrhythmias • Paroxysmal supraventricular arrhythmias	• Proarrhythmic • CNS side effects (dizziness, visual disturbances) • Increased mortality in patients with recent myocardial infarction and non–life-threatening ventricular arrhythmias • Inhibits P450 enzymes
Propafenone (Rythmol)	• **A:** PO and IV • **M:** Hepatic (P450) • **E:** Parent drug and metabolites mainly excreted in urine		• Supraventricular arrhythmias • Ventricular arrhythmias • Prevention of a fib recurrence	• Prolongation of QRS interval • Proarrhythmia • GI side effects (constipation, metallic taste, nausea, vomiting) • Inhibits P450 enzymes

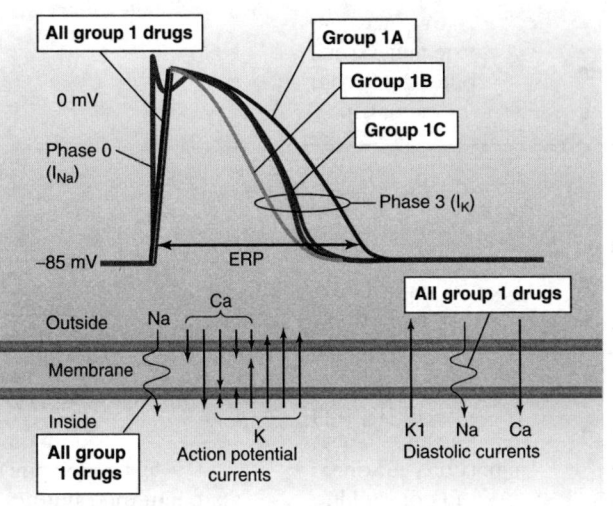

CLASSES II, III, AND IV ANTIARRHYTHMICS

Drug	Pharmacokinetics	Mechanism of Action	Clinical Uses	Side Effects
Class II				
β-Blockers (please see pg 206–208 for complete chart on β blockers)	• **A:** IV or PO	• Block sympathetic effects on the heart • Affect primarily the SA and AV nodes • Decrease SA node automaticity and AV nodal conduction	• Supraventricular arrhythmia • Control of ventricular rate during atrial flutter and fibrillation	• Sudden withdrawal can lead to rebound hypersensitivity
Class III				
Amiodarone (Cordarone, Nexterone, Pacerone)	• **A:** IV and PO; slow GI absorption; long period to reach steady state • **M:** Hepatic (P450) • **E:** Metabolites excreted in urine and feces	• Prolongs AP duration by blocking K^+ channels • Does not affect conduction velocity • Blocks Na^+ channels • Blocks calcium channels • Some β-blocker activity • Coronary and peripheral vasodilator	• Ventricular tachyarrhythmias (especially in post MI and CHF patients) • Atrial fibrillation/flutter • Paroxysmal supraventricular tachycardia • Arrhythmias associated with Wolff-Parkinson-White syndrome	• Pulmonary fibrosis • Hypothyroidism • Paresthesias/tremor • Exacerbation of arrhythmias • Hepatotoxicity • Hypotension • Corneal deposits • Inhibits P450 enzymes
Sotalol (Betapace)	• **A:** PO; well absorbed • **E:** Unchanged in urine	• Prolongs AP duration • Possesses β-blocker and potassium-channel blocking activity		• Bradycardia • Arrhythmias due to QT prolongation • Fatigue

Continued

Drug	Pharmacokinetics	Mechanism of Action	Clinical Uses	Side Effects
Ibutilide (Corvert)	• **A:** IV • **M:** Hepatic • **E:** Primarily excreted as metabolites in urine	• Prolongs AP duration • Exact mechanism of action is unknown	• Atrial fibrillation/flutter	• Arrhythmias • Headache
Dofetilide (Tikosyn)	• **A:** PO • **M:** Hepatic (P450 minor) • **E:** Parent drug and metabolites excreted in urine	• Prolongs AP duration • No effect on Na^+ channels • No α or β activity		
Dronedarone (Multaq)	• **A:** PO • **M:** Hepatic (P450) • **E:** Primarily excreted as metabolites in urine	• Inhibits Na^+, Ca^{2+}, and K^+ channels • Prolongs AP duration and refractory period • β- and α_1-blocker activity		• Increased mortality in patients with symptomatic heart failure and recent decompensation • Inhibits P450 enzymes

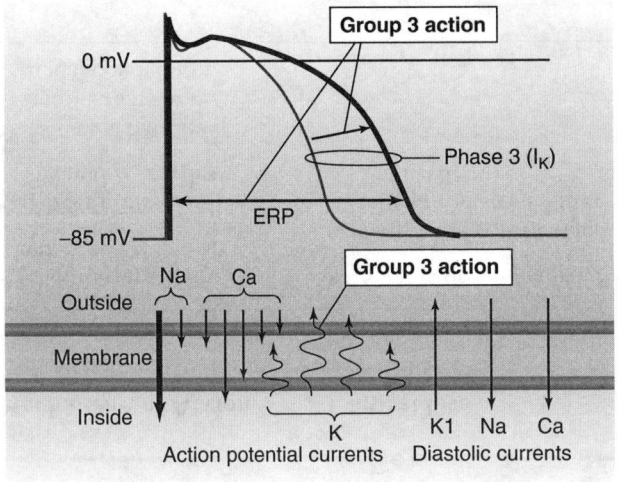

Reproduced, with permission, from Trevor AJ, Katzung BG, Kruidering-Hall MM, Masters SB: *Katzung & Trevor's Pharmacology: Examination & Board Review*, 10th ed. New York: McGraw-Hill Education, 2013.

Class IV

Verapamil (Calan, Isoptin)	• **A:** PO and IV • **M:** Extensive first pass hepatic (P450) metabolism to active metabolites • **E:** Metabolites excreted in urine and feces	• Calcium channel blocker that affects mainly the SA and AV nodes • Reduces SA node automaticity and AV nodal conduction	• Supraventricular arrhythmias • Ventricular rate control in atrial flutter and fibrillation	• Contraindicated with β-blockers • Bradycardia • Constipation • Decreased cardiac contractility • Hypotension • Lassitude • Nervousness • Peripheral edema • Inhibits P450 enzymes
Diltiazem (Cardizem, Dilacor, Diltzac, Matzim, Taztia, Tiazac)	• **A:** PO and IV • **M:** Hepatic (P450) • **E:** Metabolites excreted in urine and feces			• Bradycardia • Decreased cardiac contractility • Hypotension • Inhibits P450 enzymes

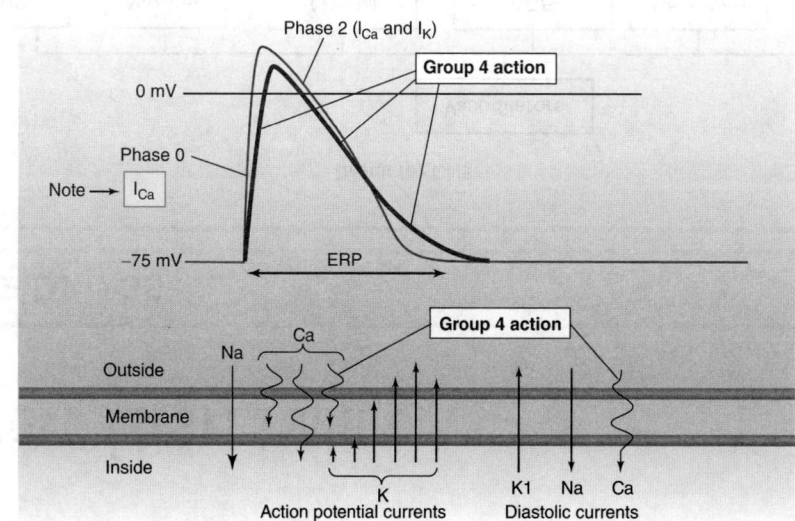

Reproduced, with permission, from Trevor AJ, Katzung BG, Kruidering-Hall MM, Masters SB: *Katzung & Trevor's Pharmacology: Examination & Board Review*, 10th ed. New York: McGraw-Hill Education, 2013.

IV. Managing Congestive Heart Failure

CLASSIFICATION OF CHF DRUGS

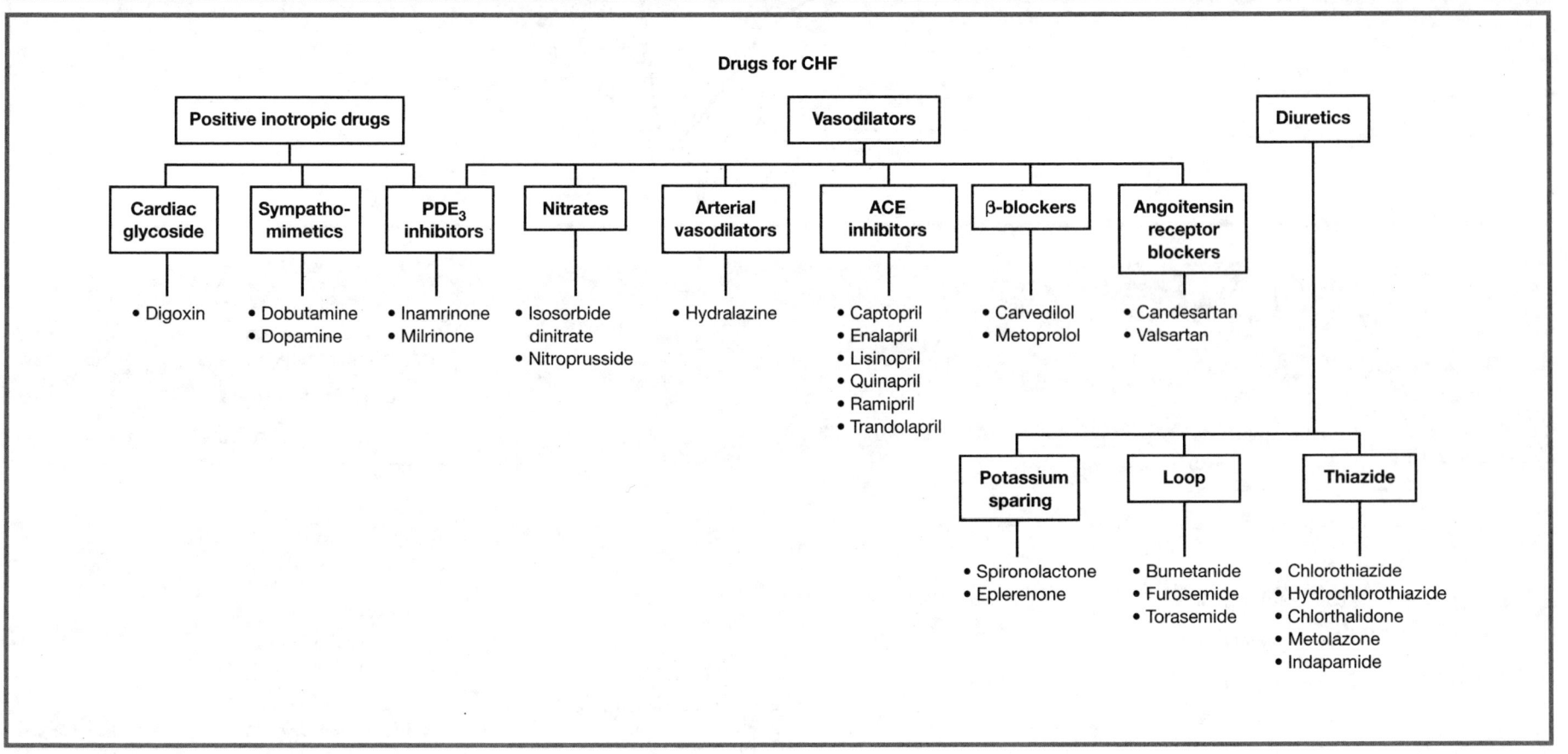

CHF THERAPY: POSITIVE INOTROPIC DRUGS

Drug	Pharmacokinetics	Mechanism of Action	Clinical Uses	Side Effects
Cardiac Glycosides				
Digoxin (Lanoxin, Digox)	• **A:** IV or PO • **M:** Metabolized in stomach and intestine • **E:** Majority excreted unchanged in urine	• Inhibit the Na^+/K^+ ATPase, leading to an increase in IC Na^+ • Increase in IC Na^+ leads to a decrease in activity for the Na^+/Ca^{2+} exchanger, resulting in an increase in IC Ca^{2+} • Increase in IC Ca^{2+} means that the amount of Ca^{2+} present during an AP is higher, leading to a more forceful contraction • Direct electrical effects on the heart include decrease in AP duration, ectopic beats, and arrhythmias	• Treatment of chronic CHF • Therapeutic index is very low (high risk) • Digitalis compounds must be administered slowly and in small doses • Rate control in supraventricular tachyarrhythmias	**Cardiac side effects include:** • AV junctional rhythm • Premature ventricular depolarization • AV blockade **Noncardiac side effects include:** • GI distress (Nausea, Anorexia, Diarrhea) • Color vision abnormality (blurry yellow vision) • Disorientation • Digoxin levels in plasma double when coadministered with quinidine • Hypokalemia can increase the risk of toxicity by worsening arrhythmia • Toxicity treated with Digibind (anti-dig fab fragments)

Continued

CHF THERAPY: POSITIVE INOTROPIC DRUGS (Continued)

Drug	Pharmacokinetics	Mechanism of Action	Clinical Uses	Side Effects
Sympathomimetic				
Dobutamine	• **A:** IV • **M:** Metabolized hepatically and in tissues • **E:** Metabolites excreted in urine	• Leads to an elevation of cAMP and subsequent positive inotropic effects • Low chronotropic activity	• Treatment of acute CHF, decompensated heart failure, and cardiac arrest	• Increased HR • Angina • Increased BP or hypotension
Dopamine (Intropin)	• **A:** IV • **M:** Metabolized in liver, kidneys, and plasma by MAO and COMT • **E:** Metabolites excreted in urine	• Causes release of NE at the heart, which leads to β-adrenergic stimulation • Stimulates β_1-receptors • Inhibits NE release in the periphery causing vasodilation		• Angina • Arrhythmias • Headache • Nausea • Vomiting
PDE3 Inhibitors				
Inamrinone (Inocor) Milrinone	• **A:** IV • **M:** Minor hepatic metabolism • **E:** Parent drug and metabolites excreted in urine	• Inhibition of PDE leads to an elevation of cAMP • Selective for cardiac isoform of PDE • Cause vasodilation and inotropic effects	• Treatment of acute CHF	• Ventricular arrhythmias

CHF THERAPY: DIURETICS AND ACE INHIBITORS

Drug	Pharmacokinetics	Mechanism of Action	Clinical Uses	Side Effects
Potassium-Sparing Diuretic				
Spironolactone (Aldactone)	• **A:** PO • **M:** Hepatic metabolism to active metabolites • **E:** Metabolites excreted in urine and feces	• Competes with aldosterone for receptor sites in the distal renal tubules causing Na^+ and water excretion while retaining K^+ and H^+ ions	• Treatment of severe CHF • Edema • Hypokalemia • Hypertension	• Hyperkalemia (especially with ACE inhibitors) • CNS depression • Tumorigen • Nonanion gap metabolic acidosis • Gynecomastia
Eplerenone (Inspra)	• **A:** PO • **M:** Hepatic (P450) • **E:** Metabolites excreted in urine and feces		• Heart failure • Hypertension	• Hyperkalemia • Hypertriglyceridemia
ACE Inhibitors				
Captopril (Capoten)	• **A:** PO • **M:** Prodrugs metabolized by intestinal wall and liver (P450) to active metabolites (P450) • **E:** Parent drug and metabolites excreted primarily in urine	• Inhibit the formation of the potent vasocontrictor angiotensin II from angiotensin by the inhibition of angiotensin converting enzyme • Decrease peripheral resistance • Reduce the breakdown of bradykinin	• HTN • LV dysfunction following MI • Heart failure with reduced EF	• Angioedema • Cough (due to increased bradykinin) • Hyperkalemia • Renal failure • Contraindicated in pregnancy • Hypotension • Neutropenia

Continued

CHF THERAPY: DIURETICS AND ACE INHIBITORS (Continued)

Drug	Pharmacokinetics	Mechanism of Action	Clinical Uses	Side Effects
Enalapril (Vasotec, Epaned)	• **A:** VI, PO • **M:** Prodrugs metabolized by liver to active metabolite • **E:** Parent drug and metabolites excreted primarily in urine and feces		• HTN • Asymptomatic LV dysfunction • Heart failure with reduced EF	
Lisinopril (Prinivil, Zestril)	• **A:** PO • **E:** Excreted unchanged in urine		• HTN • Heart failure	
Quinapril (Accupril)	• **A:** PO • **M:** Prodrugs metabolized by intestinal wall and liver to active metabolite • **E:** Parent drug and metabolites excreted primarily in urine			
Ramipril (Altace)	• **A:** PO • **M:** Prodrugs metabolized by intestinal wall and liver to active metabolite • **E:** Parent drug and metabolites excreted primarily in urine and feces		• HTN • Heart failure post MI • Reduction in risk of CVA, MI, death	

Drug	Pharmacokinetics	Mechanism	Indications	Adverse Effects
Trandolapril (Mavik)	• **A:** PO • **M:** Prodrugs metabolized by intestinal wall and liver to active metabolite • **E:** Parent drug and metabolites excreted primarily in urine and feces		• HTN • Asymptomatic LV dysfunction • Heart failure with reduced EF	

Angiotensin Receptor Blockers

Drug	Pharmacokinetics	Mechanism	Indications	Adverse Effects
Candesartan (Atacand)	• **A:** PO • **M:** Metabolized to active metabolite via hydrolysis within the intestinal wall and hepatic (P450 minor) • **E:** Primarily excreted unchanged in urine	• Angiotensin II receptor blockade prevents the vasoconstriction caused by angiotensin II	• HTN • Heart failure	• Hyperkalemia • Fatigue • Contraindicated in pregnancy • Inhibits P450 enzymes
Valsartan (Dlovan)	• **A:** PO • **M:** Hepatic • **E:** Parent drug and metabolites excreted primarily in feces		• HTN • Heart failure • Neuropathy in patients with DM and HTN	

β-Blockers

Drug	Pharmacokinetics	Mechanism	Indications	Adverse Effects
Carvedilol	• **A:** PO • **M:** Hepatic (P450) • **E:** Metabolites excreted primarily in feces	• Nonselective β antagonist	• HTN • Heart failure • LV dysfunction following MI	• Hypotension • Fatigue • Dizziness • Weight gain
Metoprolol	• **A:** PO, IV • **M:** Hepatic (P450) • **E:** Metabolites excreted primarily in urine	• Selective β_1 antagonist	• HTN • Angina • Rate control in SVT and a fib/flutter • Myocardial infarction	• Hypotension • Diarrhea • Dizziness • Inhibits P450 enzymes

Continued

CHF THERAPY: DIURETICS AND ACE INHIBITORS (Continued)

Drug	Pharmacokinetics	Mechanism of Action	Clinical Uses	Side Effects
Loop Diuretics				
Bumetanide (Bumex)	• **A:** IV, IM, and PO • **M:** Hepatic (minor) • **E:** Metabolites and parent drug excreted in urine and feces	• Block reabsorption of Na^+ and Cl^- in the cortical and medullary regions of the ascending loop of Henle • Promote Ca^{2+} excretion	• Edema from CHF	• Hyperglycemia (similar effect on pancreas as thiazides) • Hyperuricemia (increased risk for gout) • Hyponatremia • Hypokalemia • Excessive administration can lead to profound diuresis
Furosemide (Lasix)	• **A:** IV, IM, and PO • **M:** Hepatic (minor) • **E:** Metabolites and parent drug excreted in urine		• Edema from CHF • Acute pulmonary edema • HTN	
Torsemide (Demadex)	• **A:** IV, PO • **M:** Hepatic (P450) • **E:** Metabolites and parent drug excreted in urine		• Edema from CHF • Hepatic cirrhosis • HTN	
Thiazide Diuretics				
Chlorothiazide (Diuril)	• **A:** IV, PO • **E:** Excreted unchanged in urine	• Increase urinary and salt output by inhibiting Na^+, Cl^- and water reabsorption in the distal tubule resulting in diuresis	• HTN • Edema	• Hypercalcemia • Hyperglycemia • Hyperlipidemia • Hyperuricemia • Hypomagnesemia • Hypokalemia • Hyponatremia • Metabolic alkalosis • Muscle weakness • Pancreatitis
Chlorthalidone	• **A:** PO • **E:** Excreted unchanged in urine			
Hydrochlorothiazide (HCTZ, Microzide)				
Metolazone (Zaroxolyn)				

Indapamide	• **A:** PO • **M:** Hepatic • **E:** Metabolites excreted in urine			

Nitrates

Isosorbide dinitrate (Isordil, IsoDitrate, Dilatrate)	• **A:** Sublingual, PO • **M:** Hepatic (P450) • **E:** Metabolites excreted in urine and feces	• Converted to nitric oxide intracellularly which activates guanylate cyclase leading to the following cascade of events: • Increase in cGMP • Dephosphorylation of myosin light chain • Relaxation of vascular smooth muscle • Vasodilation • Venous dilation decreases preload • Vasodilation increases blood flow to the myocardium	• Angina	• Headache • Hypotension • Increased intracranial pressure • Tolerance • Cross tolerance
Nitroprusside (Nitropress)	• **A:** IV • **M:** Metabolized in plasma • **E:** Metabolites excreted in urine		• Acute decompensated heart failure • Hypertension	• Hypotension • Cyanide toxicity

Arterial Vasodilators

Hydralazine (Apresoline, Novohylazin, Nu-Hydral)	• **A:** PO, IM, IV • **M:** Extensive first-pass hepatic metabolism; hepatic acetylation (certain patient populations have varying rates of acetylation)	• Arteriole smooth muscle relaxation and vasodilation (probably through action on cAMP and Ca^{2+})	• Hypertension • Hypertensive emergency in pregnancy • Heart failure	• Toxicity in slow acetylators • Tachycardia • Headache • Dizziness • Nausea • Diaphoresis • Flushing • Lupus-like syndrome • Inhibits P450 enzymes

V. Antihyperlipidemic Drugs

CLASSIFICATION OF ANTIHYPERLIPIDEMIC DRUGS

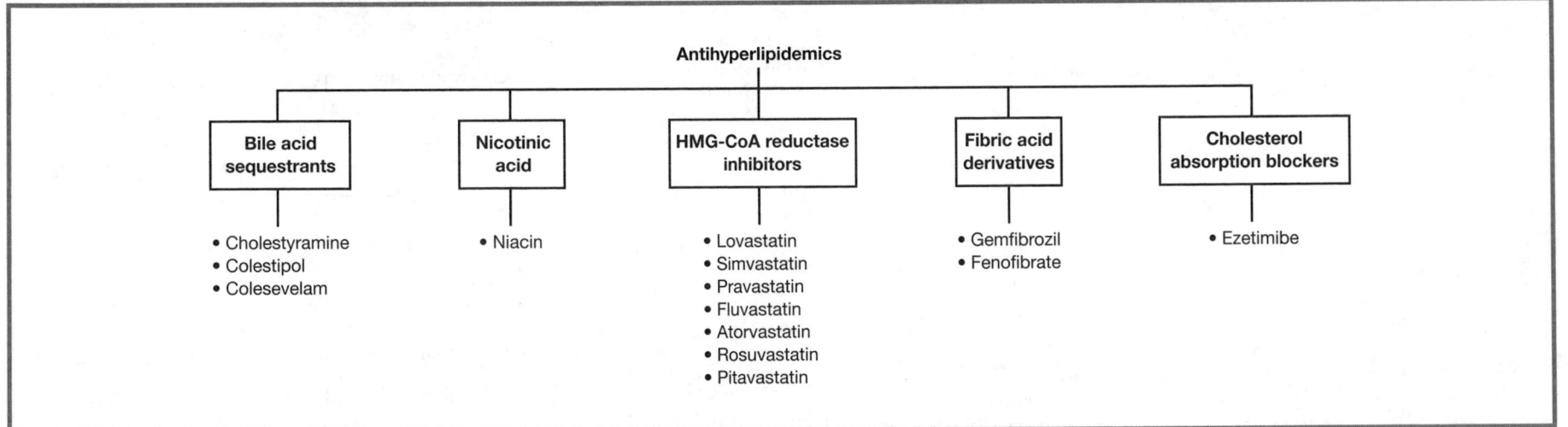

Antihyperlipidemics

Bile acid sequestrants	Nicotinic acid	HMG-CoA reductase inhibitors	Fibric acid derivatives	Cholesterol absorption blockers
• Cholestyramine • Colestipol • Colesevelam	• Niacin	• Lovastatin • Simvastatin • Pravastatin • Fluvastatin • Atorvastatin • Rosuvastatin • Pitavastatin	• Gemfibrozil • Fenofibrate	• Ezetimibe

ANTIHYPERLIPIDEMICS: BILE ACID SEQUESTRANTS AND NICOTINIC ACID

Drug	Pharmacokinetics	Mechanism of Action	Clinical Facts	Side Effects
Bile Acid Sequestrants				
Cholestyramine (Questran, Prevalite, Questran Light) Cholestipol (Cholestid) Colesevelam (Welchol)	• **A:** PO • **E:** Drug/bile acid complex is excreted in feces	• Anion exchange resin that binds bile acids in the intestine and prevents reabsorption • Reduction in bile acid reabsorption results in an increase in production of bile acids from cholesterol in the liver • This increased demand for cholesterol by the liver increases the expression of LDL receptors by the liver • LDL is cleared from the plasma more quickly due to the increased population of receptors	• Treatment of elevated LDL • Greatest effect is seen at lowest doses of the drug • Decrease LDL • Increase HDL • Increase VLDL-TG levels • No effect on Lp(a)	• Abdominal pain • Bloating • Constipation/fecal impaction • Pancreatitis • Interference with absorption of fat soluble vitamins (A, E, D, K) • Decrease absorption of numerous drugs • Avoid in patients with elevated TG
Nicotinic Acid				
Niacin (Niaspan, Niacor)	• **A:** PO; rapidly absorbed • **M:** Extensive first-pass hepatic metabolism • **E:** Metabolites and parent drug excreted in urine	• Decreases hepatic production of VLDL • Increases circulating levels of HDL • Decreases Lp(a) • Inhibits lipolysis in adipose tissue	• Decreases LDL 10–25% • Decreases VLDL-TG 50% • Increases HDL 30–40%	• Acanthosis nigricans/ Hyperpigmentation • Arrhythmias • Cutaneous flushing (can be prevented by pretreatment with aspirin) • Peptic ulcer disease • Glucose intolerance • Hepatitis • Hyperuricemia/Gout

ANTIHYPERLIPIDEMICS

Drug	Pharmacokinetics	Mechanism of Action	Clinical Uses	Side Effects
HMG-CoA Reductase Inhibitors				
Lovastatin (Mevacor, Altoprev) Simvastatin (Zocor) Pravastatin (Pravachol) Fluvastatin (Lescol) Atorvastatin (Lipitor) Rosuvastatin (Crestor) Pitavastatin (Livalo)	• **A:** PO; well absorbed • **M:** Hepatic (P450) • **E:** Parent drug and metabolites excreted in feces > urine	• Inhibit HMG-CoA reductase (the enzyme responsible for cholesterol synthesis) • Increase production of LDL receptors in the liver • Increase uptake of LDL from the plasma • Decrease VLDL secretion	• Decrease VLDL • Decrease TG • Increase HDL	• Elevated hepatic transaminases • Hepatotoxicity • Headaches • Myopathy • Rhabdomyolysis • Immune-mediated necrotic myopathy • Inhibits P450 enzymes (except Rosuvastatin and Pitavastatin)
Cholesterol Absorption Blockers				
Ezetimibe (Zetia)	• **A:** PO • **M:** Hepatic • Metabolites excreted in feces > urine	• Prevents cholesterol absorption at intestinal brush border	• Decreases LDL • No effect on HDL or TG	• Elevated hepatic transaminases • Diarrhea • Myalgias

ANTIHYPERLIPIDEMIC: FIBRIC ACID DERIVATIVES

Drug	Pharmacokinetics	Mechanism of Action	Clinical Uses	Side Effects
Gemfibrozil (Lopid)	• **A:** PO; well absorbed • **M:** Hepatic (P450) • **E:** Parent drug and metabolites excreted in urine	• Agonist for nuclear transcription factor PPARα causing down regulation of Apo-CIII (an inhibitor of lipoprotein lipase) and activating lipoprotein lipase leading to increased lipolysis and elimination of TG-rich particles	• Decrease VLDL • Decrease TG • Increase HDL	• Decreased libido • Cholesterol gallstones • Fatigue • GI distress (dyspepsia, abdominal pain) • Myopathy/rhabdomyolysis • Inhibits P450 enzymes
Fenofibrate (Tricor, Antara, Fenoglide, Lipofen, Triglide) Fenofibric acid (Fibricor, Trilipix)	• **A:** PO • **M:** Metabolized in plasma and tissue by esterases to fenofibric acid which is then hepatically metabolized to inactive form • **E:** Metabolites excreted in urine			• Headache • Increased hepatic transaminases • Myopathy/rhabdomyolysis • Cholesterol gallstones • Inhibits P450 enzymes

EFFECTS OF ANTIHYPERLIPIDEMICS ON LIPOPROTEINS

Drug Class	LDL	HDL	VLDL-TG
Bile acid sequestrants	↓↓	↑	↑
Nicotinic acid	↓↓	↑↑	↓
HMG-CoA reductase inhibitors	↓↓↓	↑	↓ (TG)
Fibric acid derivatives	↓	↑	↓↓↓
Cholesterol absorption blockers	↓↓	—	—

VI. Managing Coagulopathy

CLASSIFICATION OF DRUGS TO REDUCE CLOTTING

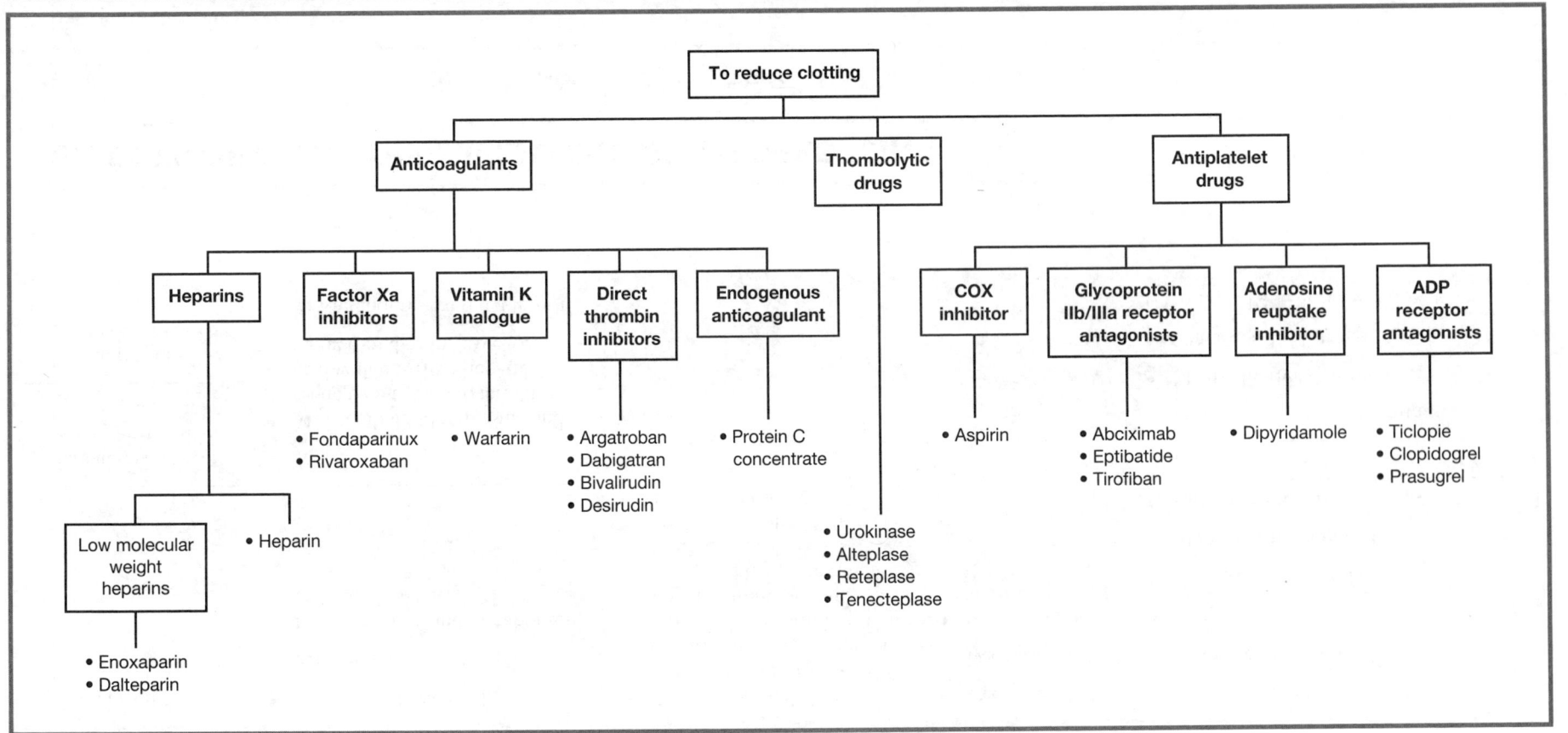

COAGULATION CASCADE

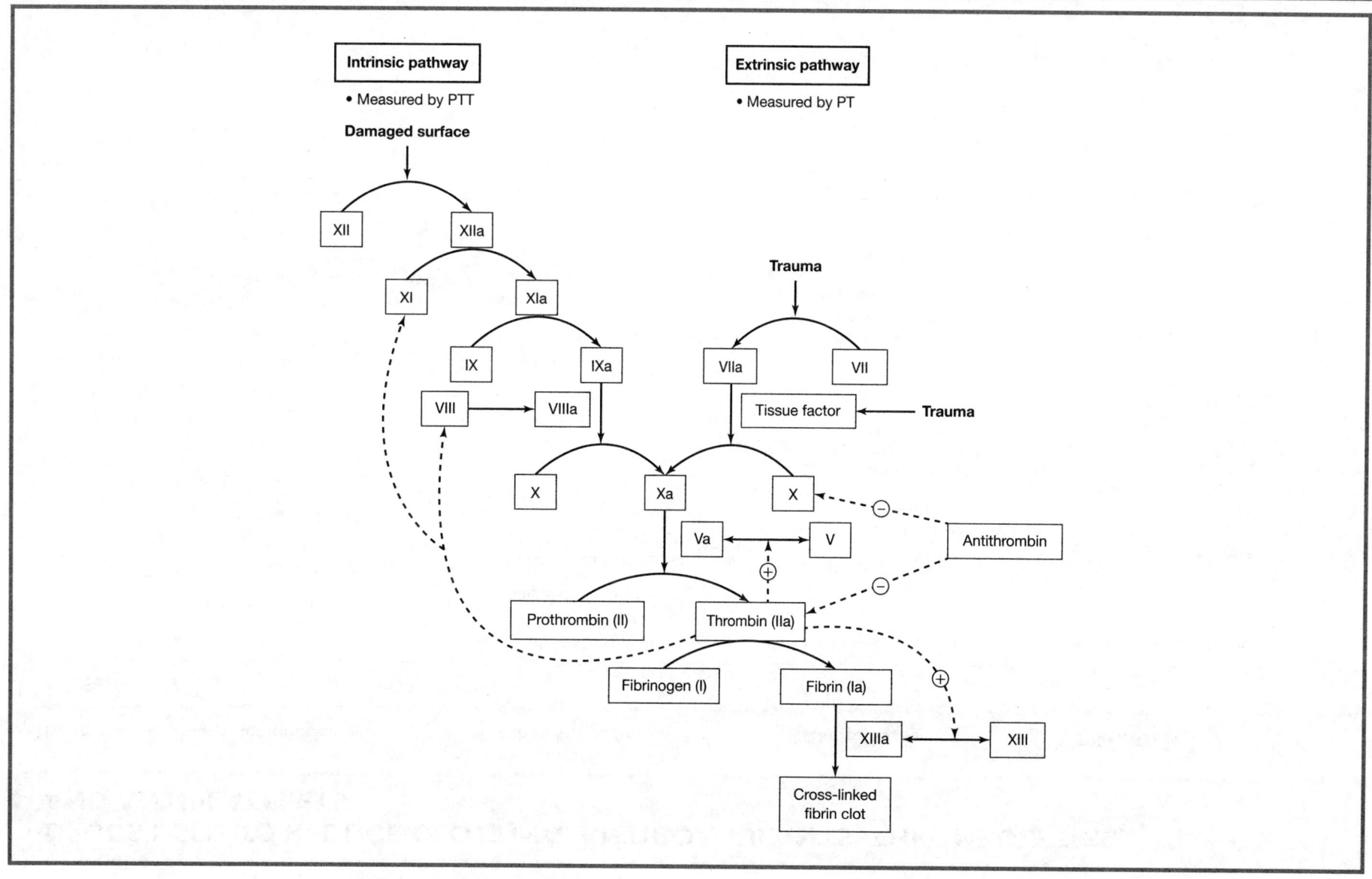

Drug	Pharmacokinetics	Mechanism of Action	Clinical Uses	Side Effects
Anticoagulants				
Warfarin (Coumadin, Jantoven)	• **A:** PO, IV • **B:** 99% protein bound • **D:** Widely distributed; crosses placenta • **M:** Hepatic (P450) • **E:** Excreted primarily as metabolites in urine	• Blocks reduction of vitamin K necessary for carboxylation of coagulation factors • Inhibits synthesis of VII, IX, X, and II as well as proteins C and S	• Reversed with vitamin K and/or factor IX • Effectiveness monitored by PT/INR • Treatment and prevention of thromboembolism • Prevention of embolic complications of a fib or cardiac valve replacements	• Contraindicated in pregnancy • Excessive bleeding • Cutaneous necrosis • Hepatitis • Rarely causes frank infarction of breast, fatty tissues, bowel, or extremities (purple toe syndrome) • Osteoporosis (with LTU)
Protein C (concentrate, ceprotin)	• **A:** IV • **M:** Inactivated by plasma protease inhibitors	• Converted to activated protein C	• Treatment of severe congenital protein C deficiency	• None • Excessive bleeding

| Heparin | • **A:** IV, SC
• **D:** Does not cross the placenta
• **M:** Hepatic; may be partially metabolized by the reticuloendothelial system
• **E:** Urine | • Binds to and activates endogenous antithrombin III, thus inactivating thrombin II, and preventing fibrinogen from being converted to fibrin
• Inhibits clotting factors XII, XI, and X (intrinsic pathway)
• Stimulates the release of lipoprotein lipase | • Acute anticoagulation in ACS and acute thromboembolism
• Treatment and prevention of thromboembolism in pregnancy
• Thromboprophylaxis
• Anticoagulation with percutaneous coronary intervents (cardiac cath)
• Reversed with protamine sulfate
• Effectiveness monitored by PTT level
• New low–molecular-weight (LMW) heparins have longer DOA allowing for once a day dosing | • Heparin-induced thrombocytopenia (HIT) and thrombosis (HIT/T)
• Excessive bleeding
• Alopecia
• LTU can lead to osteoporosis and spontaneous fracture |

Low–Molecular-Weight Heparins

| Enoxaparin (Lovenox) | • **A:** SC, IV
• **M:** Hepatic
• **E:** Parent drug and metabolites excreted in urine | • Inhibits factor Xa | • DVT prophylaxis/treatment
• ACS (unstable angina, NSTEMI, STEMI) | • Excessive bleeding
• Use with caution in patients with recent spinal instrumentation (ie, spinal surgery, epidural catheters) |
| Dalteparin (Fragmin) | | • Inhibits factor Xa and IIa | • DVT prophylaxis/treatment
• ACS (unstable angina, non–Q-wave MI)
• Anticoagulation for hemodialysis | |

Continued

DRUGS USED TO REDUCE CLOTTING: ANTICOAGULANTS, THROMBOLYTICS, AND ANTIPLATELETS (Continued)

Drug	Pharmacokinetics	Mechanism of Action	Clinical Uses	Side Effects
Factor Xa Inhibitors				
Fondaparinux (Arixtra)	• A: SC, IV • E: Primarily excreted unchanged in urine	• Inhibits factor Xa	• DVT/PE treatment • PE postoperative prophylaxis • Stroke prophylaxis in nonvalvular atrial fibrillation	• Excessive bleeding • Use with caution in patients with recent spinal instrumentation (ie, spinal surgery, epidural catheters)
Rivaroxaban (Xarelto)	• A: PO • M: Hepatic (P450) • E: Parent drug and metabolites excreted in urine		• DVT prophylaxis/treatment • PE treatment	
Direct Thrombin Inhibitor				
Argatroban (Acova)	• A: IV • M: Hepatic • E: Parent drug and metabolites excreted primarily in feces	• Direct thrombin inhibitor that reversibly bind to the active site on thrombin preventing conversion of fibrinogen to fibrin	• HIT • PCI	• Excessive bleeding • Hypotension
Dabigatran (Pradaxa)	• A: PO • M: Hepatic • E: Metabolites excreted in urine		• DVT/PE prophylaxis • Stroke prophylaxis in nonvalvular atrial fibrillation	• Use with caution in patients with recent spinal instrumentation (ie, spinal surgery, epidural catheters) • Increased risk of thrombotic events with abrupt discontinuation

Desirudin (Iprivask)	• **A:** SC	• DVT prophylaxis	• Excessive bleeding
	• **E:** Primarily excreted unchanged in urine		• Use with caution in patients with recent spinal instrumentation (ie, spinal surgery, epidural catheters)
Bivalirudin (Angiomax)	• **A:** IV	• STEMI undergoing primary PCT	• Excessive bleeding
	• **M:** Blood proteases	• UA/NSTEMI undergoing early surgical intervention	• Hypotension
	• **E:** Metabolites excreted in urine	• PCI with or without HIT	• Nausea

Continued

DRUGS USED TO REDUCE CLOTTING: ANTICOAGULANTS, THROMBOLYTICS, AND ANTIPLATELETS (Continued)

Drug	Pharmacokinetics	Mechanism of Action	Clinical Uses	Side Effects/Contraindications
Thrombolytics				
Urokinase (Kinlytic)	• A: IV • M: Cleared by kidney and liver	• Human enzyme produced by the kidney that converts plasminogen to plasmin • Plasmin then functions to break up the clot by dissolving fibrin	• PE	Side effects • Excessive bleeding • Cerebral hemorrhage Contraindications • History of intracranial hemorrhage • Significant head trauma, intracranial surgery, or prior stroke within past 2 months • Active intracranial neoplasm • Active or recent internal bleeding within past 6 months • Bleeding diathesis • Uncontrolled severe HTN • Surgery within past 10 days • Thrombocytopenia (<100,000/mm³)
Alteplase (Activase)		• Unmodified human tissue plasminogen activator (t-PA) • Naturally occurring enzyme produced by endothelial cells • Converts fibrin-bound plasminogen to plasmin (clot selective)	• CVA • PE • STEMI • Central line clearance	
Reteplase (Retavase)		• Recombinant plasminogen activator (rPA) • Human t-PA from which several amino acids have been deleted • Converts fibrin-bound plasminogen to plasmin (clot selective)	• STEMI	
Tenecteplase (TNKase)				

Antiplatelet Drugs

COX Inhibitor

Aspirin (Ecotrin, Bayer, Bufferin)	• **A:** PO, PR • **M:** Hepatic (P450 minor) • **E:** Metabolites excreted in urine	• Prevents activation of thromboxane A_2 (a potent stimulator of platelet aggregation) by irreversibly binding to COX	• Prevention of MIs • ACS/CAD/CABG • CVA/TIA • Antipyretic • Anti-inflammatory	• Excessive bleeding • Gastritis/GI bleeding • Tinnitus

Glycoprotein IIb/IIIa Receptor Antagonists

Abciximab (Reopro)	• **A:** IV • **M:** Proteolytic cleavage	• Human monoclonal antibody fragment that binds to the IIb/IIIa receptor complex	• ACS • STEMI • Unstable angina • Percutaneous coronary intervention	• Excessive bleeding • Thrombocytopenia • Hypotension
Eptifibatide (Integrilin)	• **A:** IV • **E:** Parent drug and metabolites excreted in urine	• Reversible blockage of glycoprotein IIb/IIIa receptor		
Tirofiban (Aggrastat)	• **A:** IV • **E:** Excreted primarily as unchanged drug in urine, remainder in feces	• Blocks binding of fibrinogen and VWF to glycoprotein IIb/IIIa receptor		• Excessive bleeding

Continued

DRUGS USED TO REDUCE CLOTTING: ANTICOAGULANTS, THROMBOLYTICS, AND ANTIPLATELETS (Continued)

Drug	Pharmacokinetics	Mechanism of Action	Clinical Uses	Side Effects/Contraindications
ADP Receptor Antagonists				
Clopidogrel (Plavix)	• A: PO; well absorbed • M: Hepatic (P450) • E: Metabolites excreted in urine and feces	• Irreversible inhibition of ADP-mediated platelet aggregation	• Vascular disease (CVA, PAD, MI) • ACS • Atrial fibrillation in patients who are not anticoagulation candidates	• Excessive bleeding • Rash • Inhibits P450 enzymes (except Rosuvastatin and Pitavastatin)
Ticlopidine			• Stroke prevention • Coronary artery stenting	• Excessive bleeding • Hematologic reactions (TTP, aplastic anemia, neutropenia, agranulocytosis) • Diarrhea • Elevated cholesterol • Inhibits P450 enzymes (except Rosuvastatin and Pitavastatin)
Prasugrel (Effient)			• PCI for ACS	• Avoid in elderly secondary to increased risk of ICH • Avoid in patients who may undergo urgent CABG • Excessive bleeding • Hypotension • Elevated cholesterol • Inhibits P450 enzymes (except Rosuvastatin and Pitavastatin)

Adenosine Reuptake Inhibitor				
Dipyridamole (Persantine)	• **A:** IV, PO • **M:** Hepatic • **E:** Metabolites excreted in feces	• Inhibition of RBC reuptake of adenosine thereby inhibiting platelet reactivity • Inhibition of thromboxane A_2	• Adjunctive therapy for prophylaxis of thromboembolism in cardiac valve replacement	• Dizziness • Headache • Exacerbation of angina

CLASSIFICATION OF DRUGS TO FACILITATE CLOTTING/REVERSE ANTICOAGULATION

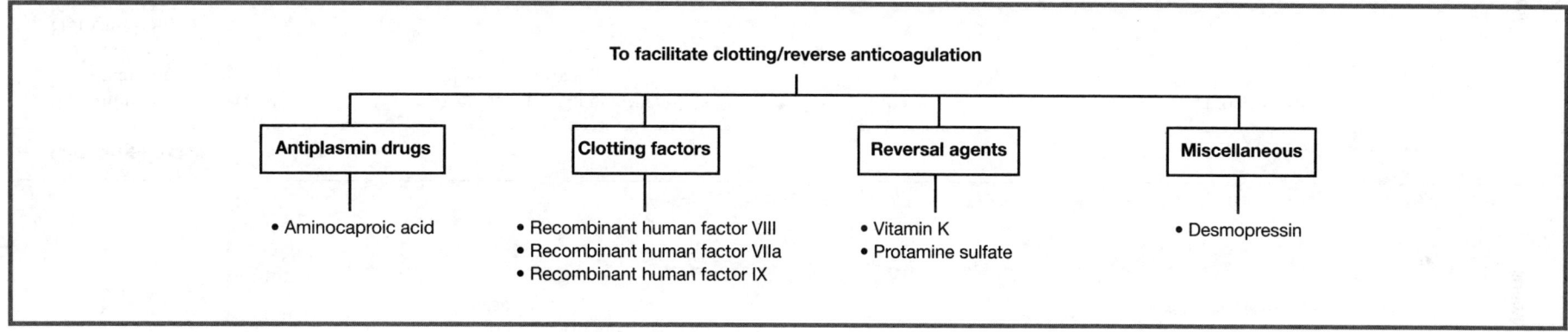

To facilitate clotting/reverse anticoagulation

Antiplasmin drugs
• Aminocaproic acid

Clotting factors
• Recombinant human factor VIII
• Recombinant human factor VIIa
• Recombinant human factor IX

Reversal agents
• Vitamin K
• Protamine sulfate

Miscellaneous
• Desmopressin

DRUGS USED TO FACILITATE CLOTTING/REVERSE ANTICOAGULATION

Drug	Pharmacokinetics	Mechanism of Action	Clinical Uses	Side Effects
Antiplasmin Drugs				
Aminocaproic acid (Amicar)	• A: IV, PO • M: Hepatic (minimal) • E: Primarily excreted unchanged in urine	• Inhibits fibrinolysis via inhibition of plasminogen binding to fibrin and formation of plasmin	• Acute bleeding	• Intravascular thrombosis • Myopathy • Abdominal discomfort
Clotting Factors				
Recombinant human factor VIII (Advate, Helixate FS, Kogenate FS, Recombinate, Xyntha, Xyntha Solofuse)	• A: IV	• Replacement of endogenous clotting factors	• Hemophilia A	• Hypersensitivity reactions
Recombinant human factor VIIa (NovoSeven RT)	• IV		• Hemophilia A/B • Congenital factor VII deficiency • Acquired hemophilia	• Thrombotic events (venous and arterial) • Fever
Recombinant human factor IX (BeneFIX, Rixubis)	• IV		• Hemophilia B	• Headache • Dizziness

Reversal Agents

Vitamin K (Mephyton)	• **A:** PO, IM, IV, SC • **M:** Hepatic • **E:** Metabolites excreted in urine and feces	• Supplementation of endogenous substance responsible for carboxylation of coagulation factors VII, IX, X, and II	• Hemorrhagic disease of the newborn • Reversal of warfarin anticoagulation • Hypoprothrombinemia	• Severe hypersensitivity reactions with parenteral administration
Protamine sulfate	• IV	• Combines with heparin to form a stable salt	• Neutralization of heparin • Heparin overdose	• Hypersensitivity reactions

Miscellaneous

Desmopressin (DDAVP, Stimate)	• **A:** IM, IV, PO, intranasal, SL	• Increases plasma levels of vWF, factor VIII, and tPA	• Hemophilia A • Von Willebrand disease • Diabetes insipidus • Nocturnal enuresis	• Headache • Nausea • Fatigue • Hyponatremia

CHAPTER 7
RESPIRATORY DRUGS

I. COLD MEDICATIONS

Classification of Cold
Medications

Cold Medications: Drug Facts

II. ASTHMA DRUGS

Classification of Asthma and
COPD Drugs

β_2-Adrenergic Agonists

Non–β_2-Adrenergic Agonists

Mechanism of Asthma Drugs
(Theorized)

TERMS TO LEARN

Antitussive	Drug that relieves or prevents cough.
Antihistamine	Drug that counteracts histamine; can be divided into two groups: those that block H_1 histamine receptors and those that block H_2 receptors.
Area Postrema	A region of the brain located in the medulla at the base of the 4th ventricle; location of the chemoreceptive trigger zone where vomiting is triggered.
Churg-Strauss Syndrome	Vasculitis of the small arteries and veins; characterized by extravascular necrotizing granulomas; typically seen in patients with asthma or an allergy history.
Decongestant	Drug that reduces congestion or swelling.
Expectorant	Drug that promotes ejection of mucus or exudate from respiratory tract.

I. Cold Medications

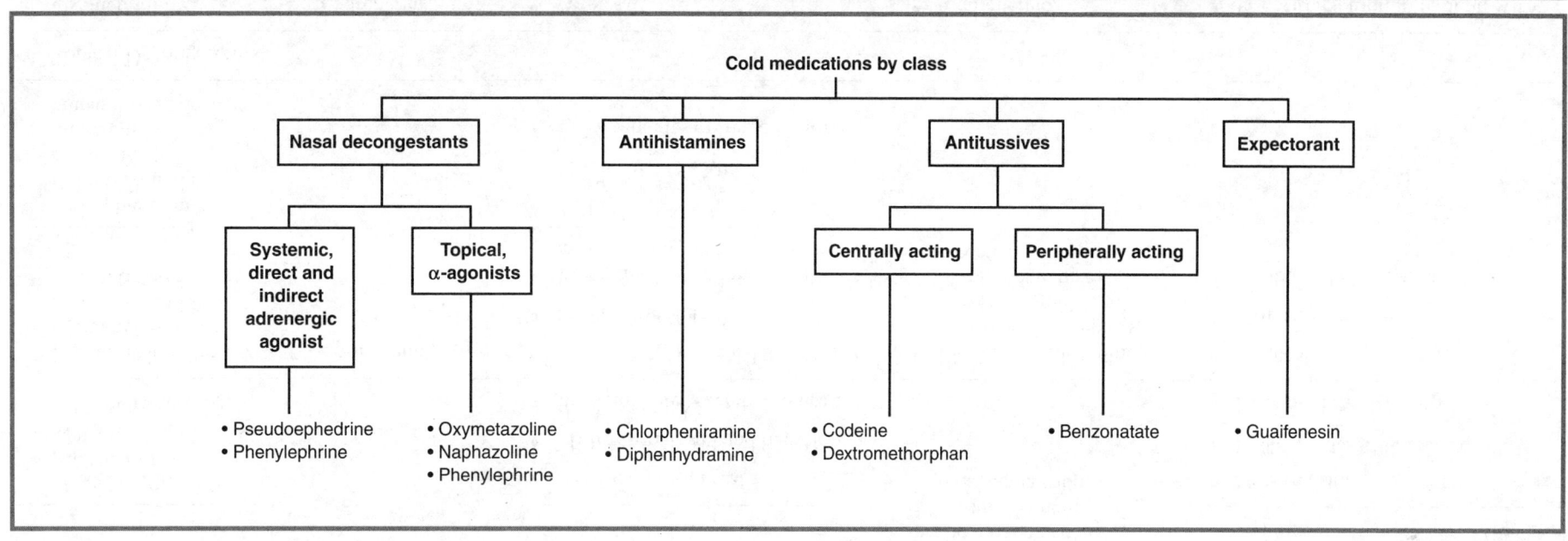

COLD MEDICATIONS: DRUG FACTS

Drug	Class	Pharmacokinetics	Mechanism of Action	Drawbacks/Side Effects
Systemic Decongestants				
Pseudoephedrine (Sudafed as well as numerous other OTC preparations)	• α adrenergic agonist	• A: PO • E: Primarily excreted unchanged in urine	• α adrenergic stimulation in respiratory mucosa leads to vasoconstriction in the nasal mucosa causing decreased nasal congestion	• Hypertension • Palpitations • Restricted access secondary to use in the illicit manufacturing of amphetamines
Phenylephrine (Sudafed PE as well as numerous OTC preparations)		• A: PO, topical, nasal • M: Intestinal wall and hepatic • E: Metabolites excreted in urine		• Hypertension • Reflex bradycardia • Decreased cardiac output
Diphenhydramine (Benadryl as well as numerous OTC preparations)	• Antihistamine	• A: PO, IM, IV, topical • M: Hepatic (P450) • E: Parent drug and metabolites excreted in urine	• Blockade of histamine action of H_1 receptors prevents stimulation of the sneeze reflex receptors	• Sedation • Urinary retention • Inhibits P450 enzymes
Chlorpheniramine (Chlor-Trimeton as well as numerous OTC preparations)		• A: PO • M: Hepatic (P450) • E: Metabolites excreted in urine		
Topical Decongestants				
Oxymetazoline (Afrin as well as numerous other OTC preparations)	• α adrenergic agonist	• A: Nasal • E: Primarily excreted unchanged in urine	• α adrenergic stimulation in respiratory mucosa leads to vasoconstriction in the nasal mucosa causing decreased nasal congestion	• Use with caution in patients with cardiac disease, hyperthyroidism, glaucoma, and diabetes • Rebound nasal congestion following cessation of chronic use

Phenylephrine (Neo-Synephrine)		• **A:** PO, topical, nasal • **M:** Intestinal wall and hepatic • **E:** Metabolites excreted in urine		
Naphazoline (Privine)		• **A:** Nasal • **M:** Unavailable • **E:** Unavailable		
Expectorant				
Guaifenesin (Mucinex, Robitussin)	• Expectorant	• **A:** PO • **M:** Hepatic • **E:** Parent drug and metabolites excreted in urine	• Thought to act as GI irritant triggering increased respiratory secretions therefore creating thinner, more voluminous mucus	• Drowsiness • Renal stone formation with consumption of large quantities
Antitussive				
Codeine	• Centrally acting antitussive • Opioid	• **A:** PO • **M:** Hepatic (P450) • **E:** Primarily excreted as metabolites in urine	• Suppression of cough by action of the μ receptors in the area postrema	• Nausea/vomiting • Constipation • Respiratory depression and death in pediatric patients in the setting of T&A • Histamine release associated with bronchoconstriction, vasodilation, and increased mucus production
Dextromethorphan (Robitussin DM, Delsym as well as numerous other OTC preparations)			• Suppression of cough by action of the δ receptors in the area postrema	• Confusion • Serotonin syndrome • Inhibits P450 enzymes
Benzonatate (Tessalon, Zonatuss)	• Peripherally acting antitussive	• **A:** PO • **M:** Hydrolyzed to PABA by plasma esterases • **E:** Primarily excreted as metabolites in urine	• Topical anesthetic of respiratory stretch receptors	• Confusion • Hypersensitivity reactions

II. Asthma Drugs

CLASSIFICATION OF ASTHMA AND COPD DRUGS

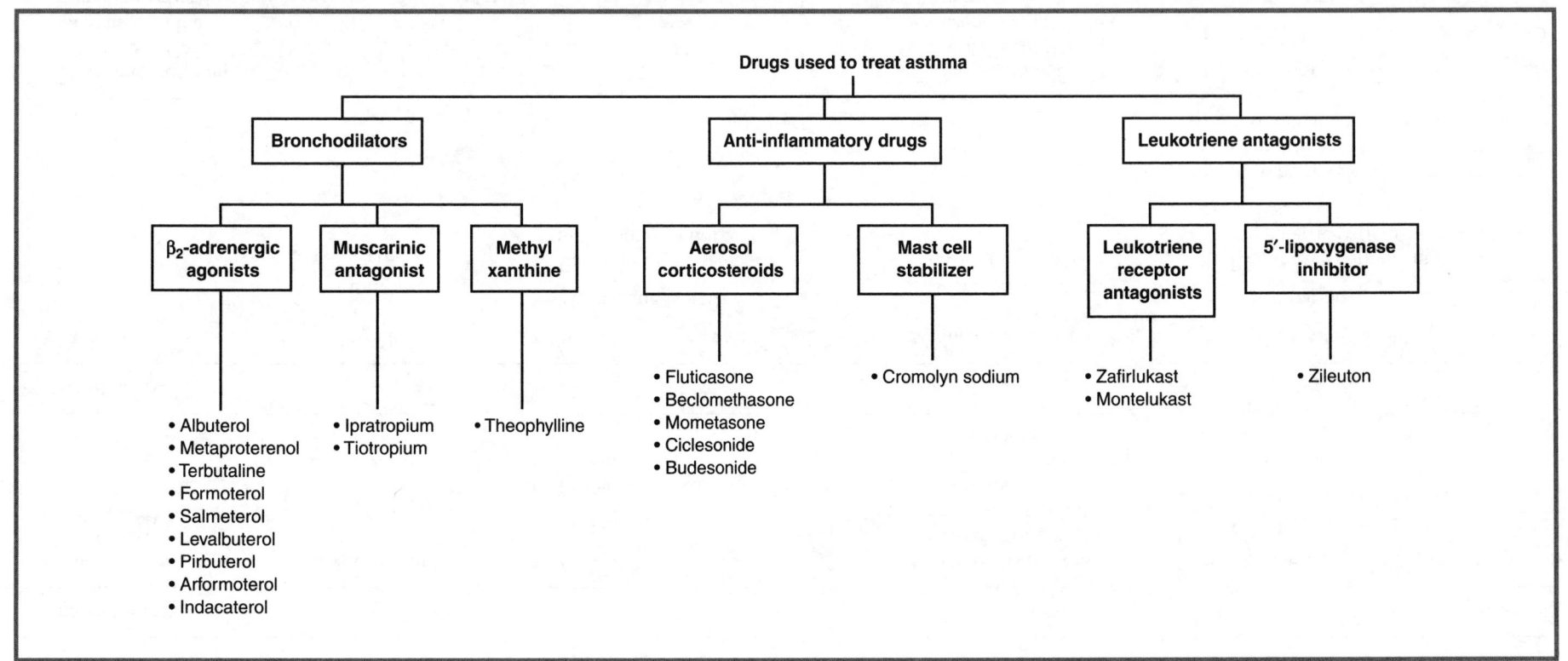

β_2-ADRENERGIC AGONISTS

Drug	Pharmacokinetics	Mechanism of Action	Clinical Uses	Side Effects
Short-Acting β-Agonists (SABA)				
Albuterol (AccuNeb, ProAir, Vospire, Proventil, Ventolin)	• **A:** Inhalation, PO • **M:** Hepatic • **E:** Parent drug and metabolites excreted in urine	• β_2 stimulation leads to increased formation of adenylyl cyclase which causes an increased cAMP in smooth muscle leading to smooth muscle relaxation and subsequent bronchodilation	• Asthma • Bronchoconstriction • COPD • Intracellular shift of K^+ can be monopolized to temporize hyperkalemia • Terbutaline can be used for temporary tocolysis	• Tachycardia • Tremor • Nervousness • Nausea and vomiting • Hypokalemia • Headache
Levalbuterol (Xopenex)	• **A:** Inhalation • **M:** GI tract • **E:** Parent drug and metabolites excreted in urine			
Pirbuterol (Maxair)	• **A:** Inhalation • **M:** Hepatic • **E:** Parent drug and metabolites excreted in urine			
Terbutaline	• **A:** Inhalation, SC, IV, PO • **M:** Hepatic • **E:** Metabolites excreted in urine			
Metaproterenol	• **A:** Inhalation, PO; poorly absorbed • **M:** GI tract • **E:** Parent drug excreted in feces, metabolites primarily excreted in urine			

Continued

β₂-ADRENERGIC AGONISTS (Continued)

Drug	Pharmacokinetics	Mechanism of Action	Clinical Uses	Side Effects
Long-Acting β-Agonists (LABA)				
Arformoterol (Brovana)	• A: Inhalation • M: Hepatic (P450 minor) • E: Primarily excreted as metabolites in urine	• As above	• Bronchoconstriction • COPD maintenance	• As noted above • LABAs associated with increased rate of asthma-related deaths • Increased risk of hospitalization in pediatric and adolescent populations
Indacaterol (Arcapta)	• A: Inhalation • M: Hepatic (P450) • E: Parent drug and metabolites excreted in feces			
Formoterol (Foradil, Perforomist)	• A: Inhalation • M: Hepatic (P450 minor) • E: Parent drug and metabolites excreted in feces			
Salmeterol (Serevent)	• A: Inhalation • M: Hepatic (P450) • E: Parent drug and metabolites excreted in urine and feces			

NON–β_2-ADRENERGIC AGONISTS

Drug	Pharmacokinetics	Mechanism of Action	Clinical Uses	Side Effects
Muscarinic Antagonist				
Ipratropium (Atrovent)	• **A:** Inhaled (highly ionized in alveoli so not well absorbed) and nasal • **M:** Hepatic • **E:** Parent drug and metabolites excreted in urine and feces	• Prevents bronchoconstriction mediated by the action of ACh at muscarinic receptors in bronchial smooth muscle	• Asthma • Bronchospasm associated with COPD	• Headache • Xerostomia
Tiotropium (Spiriva)	• **A:** Inhaled • **M:** Minimally hepatic • **E:** Primarily excreted unchanged in feces			
Methyl Xanthine				
Theophylline (Elixophyllin, Theo-24, Theochron)	• **A:** PO and IV • **M:** Hepatic (P450) • **E:** Parent drug and metabolites excreted in urine	• Inhibits PDE and therefore increases cAMP levels • Leading to bronchodilation inhibits inflammation by activation of histone deacetylase	• Bronchospasm in asthma and other chronic lung diseases	• GI irritant • Inhibits PDE in skeletal muscle causing force of contraction of accessory muscles to be increased • CNS stimulant (can produce seizures) • Enters myocardium and produces β-receptor responses (increased ionotropy and chronotropy) • Inhibits P450 enzymes
Aerosol Corticosteroids				
Fluticasone (Flovent)	• **A:** Inhalation (oral and nasal) • **M:** Hepatic (P450) • **E:** Majority of metabolites excreted in feces			• Churg-Strauss syndrome • Sinusitis • Headache • Oral candidiasis • Arthralgias/myalgias

Continued

NON-β₂-ADRENERGIC AGONISTS (Continued)

Drug	Pharmacokinetics	Mechanism of Action	Clinical Uses	Side Effects
Beclomethasone (QVAR)	• A: Inhalation • M: Hepatic (P450 minor) • E: Majority of metabolites excreted in feces	• Anti-inflammatory, immunosuppressive, and antiproliferative actions	• Asthma	• Headache
Mometasone (Asmanex)	• A: Inhaled, intranasal, topical • M: Hepatic (P450) • E: Excreted as metabolites in feces and urine			• Headache • Arthralgias
Ciclesonide (Alvesco)	• A: Inhaled, intranasal • M: Hepatic (P450) • E: Primarily excreted as metabolites in feces			• Headache • Nasopharyngitis
Budesonide (Pulmicort)	• A: Inhaled, intranasal, and PO • M: Hepatic (P450) • E: Primarily excreted as metabolites in urine			• Otitis media • Rhinitis
Mast Cell Stabilizer				
Cromolyn sodium (Gastrocrom) Nedocromil (Tilade)	• A: PO and inhaled; local effects only due to poor absorption • E: Unchanged in feces and urine	• Prevent release of leukotrienes and histamine from mast cells by inhibition of degranulation following antigen contact • Mastocytosis • Blocks both early- and late-phase responses	• Asthma • Prophylaxis for bronchospasm • Mastocytosis	• Headache

Leukotriene Receptor Antagonist				
Zafirlukast (Accolate)	• **A:** PO • **M:** Hepatic (P450) metabolism by P450 enzymes • **E:** Majority of metabolites excreted in feces	• LTD$_4$- and LTE$_4$-receptor blockers thus blocking • Cysteinyl leukotriene formation which leads to airway edema, smooth muscle constriction, and the inflammatory cascade	• Prophylaxis for acute bronchospastic attacks	• Headache • Churg-Strauss syndrome • Inhibits P450 enzymes
Montelukast (Singulair)				

Inhibitor of 5'-Lipoxygenase				
Zileuton (Zyflo)	• **A:** PO • **M:** Hepatic (P450 minor) and gastrointestinal • **E:** Metabolites excreted in urine	• Prevents formation of leukotrienes via inhibition of metabolism of the 5'-lipoxygenase enzyme		• Dyspepsia • Headache • Inhibits P450 enzymes

MECHANISM OF ASTHMA DRUGS (THEORIZED)

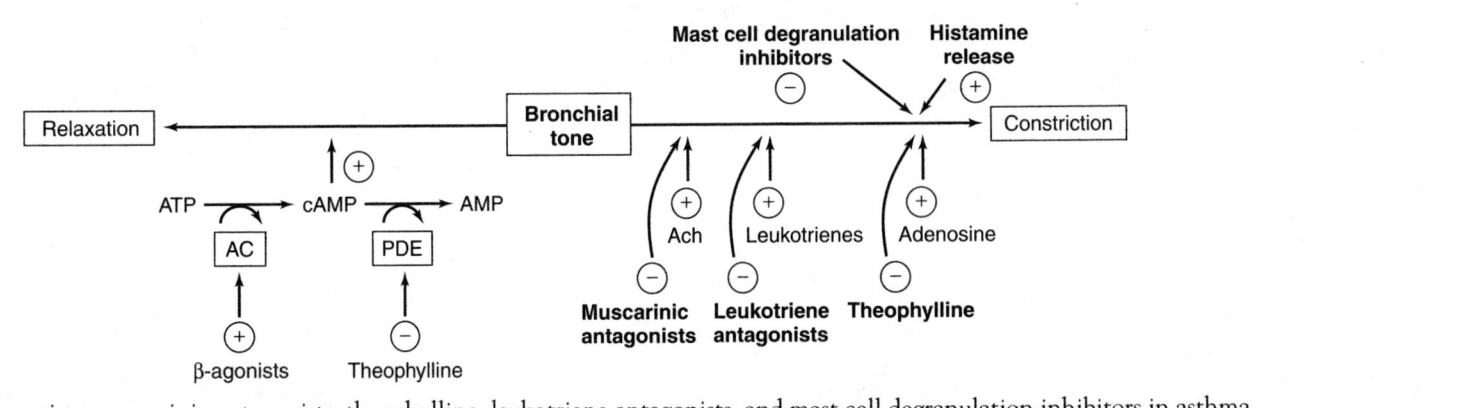

Possible mechanisms of β-agonists, muscarinic antagonists, theophylline, leukotriene antagonists, and mast cell degranulation inhibitors in asthma.

Modified from Trevor AJ, Katzung BG, Masters SB: *Katzung & Trevor's Pharmacology: Examination and Board Review*, 6th ed, p 186. Originally published by Appleton & Lange. © 2002 by the McGraw-Hill Companies, Inc.

CHAPTER 8

GASTROINTESTINAL DRUGS

I. H₂ BLOCKERS

H₂-Receptor Antagonists

II. ANTACIDS AND PROTON PUMP INHIBITORS

Antacids: Drug Facts

Proton Pump Inhibitors: Drug Facts

III. ANTIEMETICS

Other Agents for GI Diseases: Drug Facts

IV. LAXATIVES

Other Agents for GI Diseases: Drug Facts

V. OTHER GI MEDICATIONS

Other Agents for GI Diseases: Drug Facts

Sites of Action of Drugs Used to Treat PUD

TERMS TO LEARN

Anticholelithic	Drug that can dissolve gallstones.
Antiemetic	Prevents or alleviates nausea and vomiting.
Blood Dyscrasias	Disorders of the cellular elements of the blood.
Chemoreceptor Trigger Zone	Part of the brain that induces vomiting; located in the area postrema at the base of the 4th ventricle outside the BBB; it is exposed to medications/toxins in blood and CSF.
Gastroparesis	Paralysis of the stomach.
Gynecomastia	Growth of breast tissue in males.
Zollinger-Ellison Syndrome	Associated with gastrin secreting tumors causing hypergastrinemia and acid hypersecretion; 90% of these patients have PUD.

I. H₂ Blockers

H₂-RECEPTOR ANTAGONISTS

Drug	Pharmacokinetics	Mechanism of Action	Clinical Uses	Side Effects
Cimetidine (Tagamet)	• **A:** PO, IV; oral availability 40–50% • $t_{1/2}$: 1.5–2.3 hours • **M:** Hepatic (partial) • **E:** Metabolites and parent drug excreted in urine	• Decreases gastric acid secretion via competitive inhibition of H₂ receptors on gastric parietal cells	• PUD (heals gastric and duodenal ulcers and prevents their recurrence) • Prophylaxis for duodenal ulcers • Prophylaxis for stress-induced ulcers • GERD • Gastric hypersecretory conditions (ie, Zollinger-Ellison syndrome)	• Headache • Gynecomastia with LTU due to antiandrogenic action (blocks the production and release of testosterone; can be used by transsexuals for breast development) • Inhibits P450 enzymes (except Famotidine)
Famotidine (Pepcid)	• **A:** PO, IV; oral availability 37–45% • $t_{1/2}$: 2.5–4 hours • **M:** Hepatic (partial) • **E:** Most eliminated in urine			• Headache • Dizziness • Diarrhea • Inhibits P450 enzymes (except Famotidine)
Nizatidine (Axid)	• **A:** PO; oral availability 75–100% • $t_{1/2}$: 1.1–1.6 hours • **M:** Hepatic (partial) • **E:** Urine			
Ranitidine (Zantac)	• **A:** PO, IV; oral availability 30–88% • $t_{1/2}$: 1.6–2.4 hours • **M:** Hepatic • **E:** Urine and feces			

II. Antacids and Proton Pump Inhibitors

ANTACIDS: DRUG FACTS

Drug	Pharmacokinetics	Mechanism of Action	Clinical Uses	Side Effects
Aluminum hydroxide (Alternagel)	• **A:** PO; not significantly absorbed • **E:** In feces; absorbed portion excreted in urine	• Weak bases that react with gastric acid to produce salt and water • Increase gastric pH • Pepsin inactivated when gastric pH is >4	• Symptomatic relief of GERD, PUD, esophagitis, and gastric hyperacidity • Safe for use during pregnancy • Better at healing duodenal ulcers than gastric ulcers • Calcium carbonate useful for treatment of hypocalcemia • Magnesium hydroxide useful as a laxative	• Constipation (especially in elderly patients) • Hypophosphatemia • Hypercalcemia • Metabolic alkalosis (milk-alkali syndrome) • Strong laxative effect • Metabolic alkalosis
Calcium carbonate (Caltrate, TUMS)	• **A:** PO; 30% absorbed (vitamin D–dependent) • **E:** Absorbed portion excreted in urine			
Magnesium hydroxide (Phillips' Milk of Magnesia)	• **A:** PO; not significantly absorbed • **E:** Absorbed portion excreted in urine			
Sodium bicarbonate (Brioschi)	• **A:** PO • **E:** Absorbed portion excreted in urine			

Note that these agents are frequently combined to produce other medications (ie, aluminum hydroxide and magnesium hydroxide = Maalox).

PROTON PUMP INHIBITORS: DRUG FACTS

Drug	Pharmacokinetics	Mechanism of Action	Clinical Uses	Side Effects
Esomeprazole (Nexium) Dexlansoprazole (Kapidex) Rabeprazole (AcipHex) Omeprazole (Prilosec) Lansoprazole (Prevacid) Pantoprazole (Protonix)	• **A:** PO (IV form available for esomeprazole and pantoprazole) • **M:** Hepatic metabolism by P450 enzymes • **E:** Metabolites excreted in urine and feces	• Irreversibly inhibits acid secretion (new enzymes required for acid secretion to resume) • Activated when secreted into acidic environment of stomach • Coating on tablet is digested in duodenum and drug is released and absorbed	• GERD • PUD • Esophagitis • NSAID-induced ulcers • Zollinger-Ellison syndrome	• Diarrhea • Nausea • Abdominal pain • Possible increased risk of *Clostridium difficile*-associated diarrhea • Headache • Inhibit P450 enzymes • Induce P450 enzymes (Omeprazole, Lansoprazole and Pantoprazole only)

☞ **Proton** pump inhibitors (PPIs) all end in prazole.

III. Antiemetics

OTHER AGENTS FOR GI DISEASES: DRUG FACTS

Drug	Class	Pharmacokinetics	Mechanism of Action	Side Effects
Ondansetron (Zofran, Zuplenz)	5-HT₃ antagonist	• A: PO, IM, IV • M: Hepatic (P450 minor) • E: Majority excreted as metabolites in urine	• Blocks 5-HT$_3$ receptors both centrally and peripherally • May act to reduce the action of 5-HT in the chemoreceptor trigger zone (CTZ)	• Headache • GI disturbances (ie, constipation, diarrhea) • Cardiac conduction abnormalities (esp, QT prolongation) • Inhibit P450 enzymes (Ondansetron and Dolasetron only)
Dolasetron (Anzemet)		• A: PO, IV • M: Hepatic (P450 minor) • E: Majority excreted as metabolites in urine		
Granisetron (Granisol, Sancuso)		• A: PO, IV, transdermal • M: Hepatic (P450 minor) • E: Majority excreted as metabolites in urine		
Palonosetron (Aloxi)		• A: IV • M: Hepatic (P450 minor) • E: Majority excreted as metabolites in urine		
Prochlorperazine (Compazine, Compro)	• Phenothiazine	• A: PO, IM, IV, rectal • M: Hepatic • E: Fecal	• Block DA receptors in CTZ	• Sedation • EPS • Agitation

Metoclopramide (Reglan)	• DA blocker	• A: PO, IM, IV • M: Hepatic (P450 minor) • E: Metabolites excreted in feces	• Stimulates gastric motility by inhibiting DA-induced gastric smooth muscle relaxation	
Scopolamine	• Anticholinergic agent	• A: IM, IV, SC, transdermal • M: Hepatic • E: Urine	• Antagonist of Ach at parasympathetic sites in smooth muscle, secretory glands, and the CNS; also decreases secretions	• Bradycardia • Hypotension
Dimenhydrinate (Dramamine)	• Antihistamine	• A: PO, IM, IV • M: Hepatic • E: Metabolites excreted in urine	• Competitive antagonist with histamine for the H_1-receptor; muscarinic-blocking effect may be responsible for antiemetic activity	• Sedation
Promethazine (Phenergan)		• A: PO, IM, IV, rectal • M: Hepatic (P450) • E: Metabolites excreted in urine and bile		• Severe tissue associated with extravasation • CNS effects (confusion, EPS, dizziness) • Inhibits P450 enzymes
Dronabinol (Marinol)	• Cannabinoid	• A: PO • M: Hepatic (P450 minor) • E: Majority excreted as metabolites in feces	• May be due to effect on cannabinoid receptors (CB1) within the CNS	• CNS effects (euphoria, dizziness) • Tachycardia
Nabilone (Cesamet)	• Synthetic • Cannabinoid	• A: PO • M: Hepatic (P450 minor) • E: Majority excreted in the feces	• May be due to effect on cannabinoid receptors (CB1) within the CNS	• Sedation • Xerostomia • Visual disturbances
Aprepitant (Emend)	• Substance P/neurokinin-1 receptor antagonist	• A: PO • M: Hepatic (P450) • E: Metabolites excreted in urine and bile	• Prevents vomiting by inhibiting the substance P/neurokinin-1 (NK_1) receptor	• Fatigue • Weakness • Inhibits P450 enzymes • Induces P450 enzymes

IV. Laxatives

OTHER AGENTS FOR GI DISEASES: DRUG FACTS

Drug	Class	Pharmacokinetics	Mechanism of Action	Side Effects
Methylcellulose (Citrucel)	• Bulks-producing laxatives	• Unabsorbed fiber pulls water into GI tract leading to softer, bulkier stool	• Constipation	• None of significance
Polycarbophil (FiberCon, Fiber-Lax, Fiber-Tabs, Equalactin)			• Constipation • Diarrhea	• Abdominal fullness
Psyllium (Metamucil)			• Constipation	• Abdominal cramps • Diarrhea
Lactulose (Enulose, Constulose, Generlac, Kristalose)	• Osmotic laxatives	• Unabsorbed fiber pulls water into GI tract leading to softer, bulkier stool • Degradation of lactulose molecule in the GI tract decreases the pH causing conversion of NH^3 to NH^{4+} which decreases absorption of NH^3 and actually pulls NH^3 from the blood stream	• Laxative • Treatment and prevention of hyperammonemia associated with hepatic encephalopathy	• Electrolyte imbalances
Polyethylene Glycol (Miralax)		• Molecule causes osmotic pull of water into the GI tract	• Constipation	• Abdominal cramps • Bloating • Diarrhea
Sorbitol				• Electrolyte imbalances
Bisacodyl (Dulcolax, Correctol)	• Simulant laxative	• Simulate the smooth muscle of the GI tract causing increased peristalsis		• Abdominal cramps • Bloating
Senna (Ex-Lax, Senokot)		• Increase electrolyte and fluid secretion into the GI tract		• Diarrhea
Docusate (Colace)	• Stool softener	• Increases fat and water content of the stool facilitating bowel movements	• Stool softener	

V. Other GI Medications

OTHER AGENTS FOR GI DISEASES: DRUG FACTS

Drug	Class	Pharmacokinetics	Mechanism of Action	Clinical Uses	Side Effects
Sucralfate (Carafate)	• Aluminum sucrose sulfate	• **A:** PO; minimal absorption • **E:** Majority excreted unchanged in feces	• Mucosal protective agent • Polymerizing gel (polymerizes at pH ≤4) that adheres to bare ulcer crater and protects it to allow healing)	• PUD	• Constipation
Bismuth subsalicylate (Pepto Bismol, Bismatrol, Kaopectate)	• Colloidal bismuth compound	• **A:** PO • **M:** Metabolized in the GI tract • **E:** Metabolites excreted in urine and feces	• Mucosal protective agent • Increases mucus secretion, which forms a barrier to acid diffusion to the ulcer • Causes detachment and lysis of *Helicobacter pylori*	• Diarrhea • Component in *H. pylori* eradication regimen	• Neurotoxicity with overdoze • Discoloration of the tongue • Black stools (neme neg)
Misoprostol (Cytotec)	• Prostaglandin E$_1$ analogue	• **A:** PO • **M:** Hepatic • **E:** Majority of parent drug and metabolites excreted in urine; remainder in feces	• Mucosal protective agent • Suppresses gastric acid secretion	• Prophylaxis for NSAID-induced ulcers • PUD	• Diarrhea • Abdominal pain

Continued

Drug	Class	Pharmacokinetics	Mechanism of Action	Clinical Uses	Side Effects
Chenodiol (Chenodal)	• Bile acid derivatives	• A: PO • M: Hepatic • E: Metabolites excreted in feces	• Inhibits formation of gallstones by reducing the secretion of bile acids from the liver	• Anticholelithic	• Diarrhea
Ursodiol (Actigall)			• Inhibits formation of gallstones via unknown mechanism • May act through inhibition of hepatic cholesterol synthesis and reduced cholesterol absorption allowing cholesterol to be solubilized from existing gallstones		• Back pain • Diarrhea
Mesalamine (Asacol, Pentasa, Rowasa, Canasa, Apriso, Lialda)	• 5-Aminosalicylic acid derivative	• A: PO, rectal • M: Hepatic and GI tract • E: Primarily excreted as metabolites in urine	• Unknown • Thought to modulate the chemical inflammatory response cascade	• Treatment and maintenance of remission of ulcerative colitis • Treatment of ulcerative proctitis	• Headache • Abdominal pain • Pharyngitis
Octreotide (Sandostatin)	• Somatostatin analog	• A: SQ, IM, IV • M: Hepatic • E: Primarily excreted as metabolites in urine	• Mimics somatostatin which inhibits gastrin and VIP release	• Treatment of VIPomas • Treatment of carcinoid tumors	• Bradycardia • Fatigue • Headache

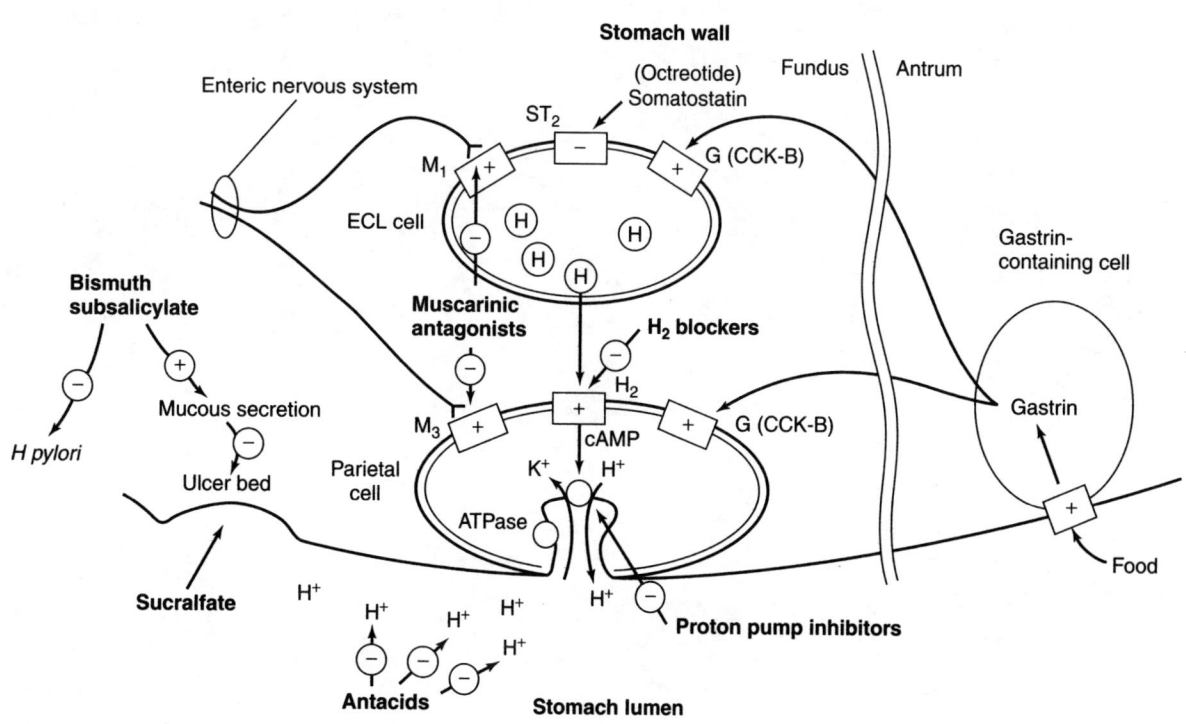

- Misoprostol (not shown here) is thought to reduce acid secretion and increase protective factors such as mucus and bicarbonate.

Modified from Katzung BG, ed: *Basic & Clinical Pharmacology*, 7th ed. Originally published by Appleton & Lange. © 1998 by The McGraw-Hill Companies, Inc.

CHAPTER 9

DRUGS AFFECTING THE ENDOCRINE SYSTEM

I. HYPOTHALAMIC AND PITUITARY HORMONES

Hypothalamic-Pituitary Hormonal Axis

Endogenous and Exogenous Hypothalamic and Pituitary Hormones

Exogenous Hypothalamic and Pituitary Hormones

II. GLUCOCORTICOIDS AND MINERAL-OCORTICOIDS

Exogenous Glucocorticoids (Systemic)

Mineralocorticoids: Agonist and Antagonist

III. THYROID DRUGS

Medications for Treating Thyroid Conditions

Medications for Treating Hypothyroidism

Medications for Treating Hyperthyroidism

IV. MEDICATIONS AFFECTING CALCIUM LEVELS

Medications Affecting Calcium Levels: Drug Facts

V. MEDICATIONS FOR MANAGING DIABETES

Insulin: Drug Facts

Classification of Oral Diabetic Drugs

Oral Diabetic Drugs: Sulfonylureas

Oral Diabetic Drugs: Nonsulfonylureas

VI. DRUGS AFFECTING REPRODUCTIVE HORMONES

Estrogen Preparations: Drug Facts

Antiestrogen Drugs

Estrogen and Progesterone Combinations

Progesterone Preparations

Antiprogesterone Drug

Testosterone Preparations

Antiandrogen Drugs

Antiandrogen Site of Action

TERMS TO LEARN

Acromegaly	Syndrome associated with excessive levels of growth hormone after puberty; symptoms include thickened skin, vocal hoarseness, joint pain, insulin resistance, hypertension, and cardiovascular disease.
Asthenia	Debility or weakness.
Carcinoid Syndrome	Symptoms associated with excessive levels of serotonin secreted by carcinoid tumors; symptoms include facial swelling, diarrhea, bronchial spasm, tachycardia, hypotension, and right-sided valvular disease.
Central Precocious Puberty	Early onset of puberty due to activation of the gonadotropins leading to maturation of the gonads; this early gonadal maturation leads to early secretion of sex hormones and, therefore, early onset of secondary sexual characteristics in adolescents.
Craniosynostosis	Premature closure of the cranial sutures.
Cushing's Disease	Disease associated with excessive glucocorticoid levels most commonly caused by an adrenal cortical adenoma; symptoms include fat redistribution with a characteristic buffalo hump, thin extremities, hypertension, hirsutism, infertility, and amenorrhea.
Diabetes Insipidis	Syndrome due to insufficient levels of ADH (central) or decreased renal response to ADH (peripheral); symptoms resemble the excessive thirst and urination associated with diabetes mellitus.
Endometriosis	Growth of cells of the uterine lining outside of the uterus; symptoms include pelvic pain and infertility.
Hyperprolactinemia	Syndrome associated with excessive levels of prolactin; symptoms include infertility, amenorrhea, galactorrhea, and mastodynia.
Hypogonadotropic Hypogonadism	Inadequate function of the gonads due to insufficient secretion of pituitary gonadotropins.
Kaposi's Sarcoma	Rare skin malignancy characterized by soft blue-black plaques and is typically seen in elderly and immunosuppressed patients; it is caused by human herpes virus 8.
Oligospermia	Low sperm count.

SIADH	Syndrome of inappropriate ADH; numerous causes include trauma, tumors, endocrine disorders, and drugs; excessive levels of ADH lead to hypernatremia.
Steatorrhea	Large amounts of fat in the feces.
Uterine Fibroids	Benign smooth muscle tumors; their growth is related to estrogen.
Virilization	Acquisition of adult male characteristics in women or prepubescent males.

I. Hypothalamic and Pituitary Hormones

HYPOTHALAMIC-PITUITARY HORMONAL AXIS

Hypothalamic hormones regulate the release of anterior pituitary hormones. Oxytocin and vasopressin are produced in the posterior pituitary (an outgrowth of the hypothalamus) where they are released into general circulation. All the endocrine agents listed below are peptides, except for prolactin-inhibiting hormone.

Hypothalamic Hormone	Pituitary Hormone	Target Organ	Target Organ Hormone
Growth hormone-releasing hormone (GHRH)	Growth hormone (GH)	Liver	Somatomedins
Somatostatin[a]			
Thyrotropin-releasing hormone (TRH)	Thyroid-stimulating hormone (TSH)	Thyroid	Thyroxine, triiodothyronine
Corticotropin-releasing hormone (CRH)	Adrenocorticotropic hormone (ACTH)	Adrenal cortex	Glucocorticoids, mineralocorticoids, androgens
Gonadotropin-releasing hormone (GnRH or LHRH)	Follicle-stimulating hormone (FSH) Luteinizing hormone (LH)	Gonads	Estrogen, progesterone, testosterone
Prolactin-releasing hormone (PRH)	Prolactin (PRL)	Lymphocytes	Lymphokines
Prolactin-inhibiting hormone (PIH, dopamine)		Breast	—
Oxytocin		Smooth muscle, especially uterus	—
Vasopressin		Renal tubule, smooth muscle	—

[a]Inhibits GH and TSH release. Also found in GI tissues; inhibits release of gastrin, glucagon, and insulin.

Modified from Trevor AJ, Katzung BG, Masters SB: Katzung & Trevor's Pharmacology Examination and Board Review, 6th ed. Originally published by Appleton & Lange. © 2002 by the McGraw-Hill Companies, Inc.

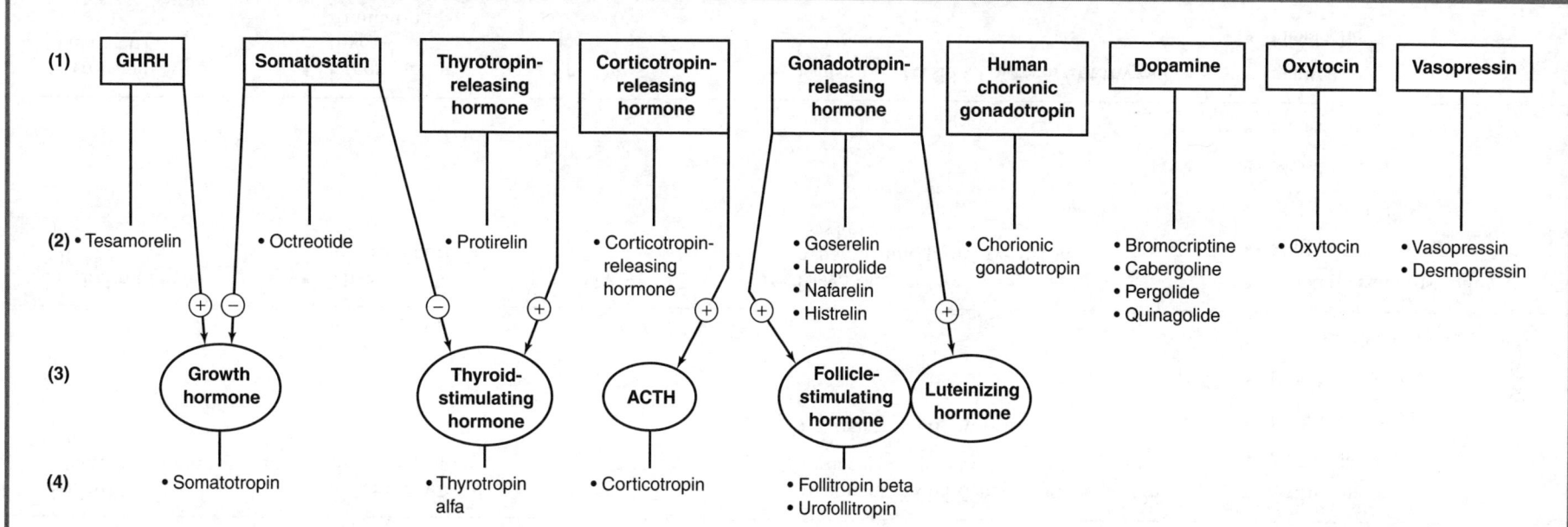

The top row, row 1, shows hypothalamic hormones; row 2 lists drug analogues of the hypothalamic hormones; row 3 is pituitary hormones stimulated by the hypothalamic hormones; and row 4 shows drug analogs of those pituitary hormones.

EXOGENOUS HYPOTHALAMIC AND PITUITARY HORMONES

Drug	Mimicked Hormones	Route of Administration	Clinical Uses	Side Effects
Octreotide (Sandostatin)	• Somatostatin analog	• IM, IV, or SC	• Symptomatic reduction of syndromes from hormone-secreting tumors including acromegaly, carcinoid syndrome, gastrinoma, glucagonoma • Also effective for controlling acute bleeding from esophageal varices	• Nausea • Abdominal pain • Flatulence • Diarrhea • Bradycardia
Tesamorelin (Egrifta)	• GHRH	• SC	• Reduction of excess abdominal fat in HIV patients with lipodystrophy	• Injection site reactions • Arthralgia
Somatotropin (Numerous brand names)	• Recombinant growth hormone	• SC	• Treatment of GH-deficient states (ie, CRI, Turner syndrome, Prader–Willi syndrome) • Treatment of HIV wasting	• Arthralgia • Gynecomastia • Hypothyroidism • Peripheral edema • Scoliosis due to rapid growth
Protirelin (Thyrel TRH)	• Thyrotropin-releasing hormone	• IV	• Diagnostic tool for hypothalamic-pituitary-thyroid axis function	• Blood pressure instability • Flushing • Light-headedness • Metallic taste • Nausea
Thyrotropin Alfa (Thyrogen)	• Recombinant thyroid-stimulating hormone	• IM	• Detection of residual or recurrent thyroid CA	• Nausea • Headache

Corticotropin-releasing hormone	• Exogenous CRH	• IM, IV, and SC	• Diagnostic tool for the differentiation of Cushing's disease from ectopic ACTH secretion	• Facial flushing (transient) • Dyspnea
Corticotropin (ACTH, Acthar, and others)	• Exogenous corticotropin	• IM or SC	• Diagnostic tool to assess adrenocorticol responsiveness	• Rare with doses used for diagnostic evaluations
	• Exogenous gonadotropin-releasing hormone			• Headache • Flushing and light-headedness • Nausea
Goserelin (Zoladex)		• SC implant	• Treatment of endometriosis, breast cancer, and dysfunctional uterine bleeding • Treatment of endometriosis • Palliative treatment of advanced prostate cancer	In women: • Depression • Diminished libido • Headache • Hot flashes and sweats • Vaginal dryness • Peripheral edema
Leuprolide (Lupron, Eligard)		• IM and SC	• Treatment of endometriosis and uterine fibroids • Palliative treatment of advanced prostate cancer • Treatment of central precocious puberty	
Nafarelin (Synarel)		• Nasal	• Treatment of endometriosis • Treatment of central precocious puberty	In men: • Asthenia • Diminished libido • Edema • Gynecomastia • Hot flashes and sweats
Histrelin (Vantas, Supprelin)		• SC implant	• Treatment of central precocious puberty • Palliative treatment of advanced prostate cancer	

Continued

EXOGENOUS HYPOTHALAMIC AND PITUITARY HORMONES (Continued)

Drug	Mimicked Hormones	Route of Administration	Clinical Uses	Side Effects
Follitropin Alfa (Gonal-F) Follitropin Beta (Follistim) Urofollitropin (Bravelle)	• Exogenous follicle-stimulating hormone	• SC • IM and SC • IM and SC	• Treatment of infertility (stimulate ovarian follicle development in women and spermatogenesis in men)	• Headache • Pelvic discomfort • Acne
Chorionic Gonadotropin (Novarel, Pregnyl)	• Exogenous human chorionic gonadotropin	• IM	• Treatment of hypogonadotropic hypogonadism • Induction of ovulation in anovulatory, infertile females	• Depression • Edema • Gynecomastia • Headache • Precocious puberty • Treatment of cryptorchidism • Spermatogenesis induction with follitropin alfa
Bromocriptine (Parlodel, Cycloset)	• Dopamine agonist	• PO	• Treatment of prolactin-secreting adenoma and hyperprolactinemia • Treatment of acromegaly • Treatment of Parkinson's disease • Treatment of 2 diabetes (Cycloset)	• Headache • Fatigue • Dizziness • Nausea • Orthostatic hypotension
Pramipexole (Mirapex)			• Treatment of Parkinson's disease • Treatment of restless legs syndrome	• EPS • Orthostatic hypotension • Dyskinesia

Ropinirole (Requip)				• Somnolence • Dizziness • Nausea
Oxytocin (Pitocin)	• Exogenous oxytocin	• IV and IM	• Induction or augmentation of labor • Control of postpartum uterine hemorrhage • Adjustive therapy in management of abortion	• Hypertensive episodes • Arrtiythmias • Increased risk of uterine rupture
Vasopressin (Pitressin)	• Exogenous vasopressin or antidiuretic hormone	• IM, IV, SC, intranasal, or endotracheal	• Treatment of diabetes insipidus	• Abdominal cramps • Arrhythmias • Vasoconstriction
Desmopressin (DDAVP, Stimate)		• PO, IV, IM, intranasal, and sub-lingual	• Treatment of diabetes insipidus • Treatment of nocturnal enuresis • Control of bleeding in hemophilia A and von Willebrand disease	• Abdominal cramps • Headache • Hyponatremic seizures with overdose

II. Glucocorticoids and Mineralocorticoids

EXOGENOUS GLUCOCORTICOIDS (SYSTEMIC)

Drug	Pharmacokinetics				Clinical Uses	Side Effects
	Route of Administration	t½	Anti-inflammatory Potency*	Mineralocorticoid Potency*		
Hydrocortisone (Cortef, A-Hydrocort)	IM, IV, PO	12 hours	1	1	• Adrenal insufficiency • Anti-inflammatory or immunosuppressive • Status asthmaticus	• Adrenal suppression • Emotional instability • Glucose intolerance • Gastrointestinal hemorrhage or perforation • Cataracts • Pulmonary edema • Arrhythmias
Prednisone	PO	12–24 hours	4	0.8	• ITP • Acute asthma • SLE • RA • Autoimmune hepatitis • PCP pneumonia • Anaphylaxis • Dermatomyositis/polymyositis • Nephrotic syndrome in children	

Triamcinolone (Kenalog, Aristospan)	PO, IM	24 hours	5	0	• Adrenal insufficiency • Nephrotic syndrome • Anti-inflammatory or immunosuppressive • Systemic lupus erythematosus (SLE)
Dexamathasone (Decadron)	PO, IV	36 hours	30	0	• Anti-inflammatory or immunosuppressive • Antiemetic • Multiple myeloma • Cerebral edema • Dexamethasone suppression test • Multiple sclerosis • Treament of shock

*Hydrocortisone is the basis of the potency for the rest of the glucocorticocoids.

MINERALOCORTICOIDS: AGONIST AND ANTAGONIST

Drug	Pharmacokinetics	Mechanism of Action	Clinical Uses	Side Effects
Mineralocorticoid Agonist				
Fludrocortisone (Florinef)	• A: PO • M: Hepatic • E: Metabolites excreted in urine	• Adrenal corticoid steroid with high mineralocorticoid and moderate glucocorticoid activity • Acts at distal tubule to increase K$^+$ and H$^+$ excretion leading to increased Na$^+$ and H$_2$O retention	• Treatment of adrenocortical insufficiency in Addison disease • Treatment of salt-losing adrenogenital syndrome	• CHF • Edema • Hypertension • Hypokalemic alkalosis • Hyperglycemia
Mineralocorticoid Antagonists				
Metyrapone (Metopirone)	• A: PO, well absorbed • M: Hepatic • E: Parent drug and metabolites excreted in urine	• Inhibits enzymatic 11-β hydroxylation of desoxycorticosone leads to decreased production of cortisol and aldosterone; should result in increased CRH and ACTH, which will lead to accumulation of cortisol and aldosterone precursors • Metabolites of these precursors can be measured in urine	• Diagnosis of adrenal insufficiency	• Headache • Abdominal pain • Hypotension • Induces P450 enzymes • Inhibits P450 enzymes
Spironolactone (Aldactone)	• A: PO • M: Hepatic • E: Majority of metabolites excreted in urine; remaining are excreted in feces	• Blocks the effects of aldosterone in the collecting duct leading to Na$^+$ loss and K$^+$ retention • Inhibits the activity of aldosterone at the collecting duct	• Hyperaldosterone states • CHF • Hypokalemia • Hypertension • Nephrotic syndrome • Management of edema excess aldosterone excretion	• Hyperkalemia • Amenorrhea • Confusion • Ataxia • DRESS syndrome
Eplerenone (Inspra)	• A: PO • M: Hepatic (P450) • E: Metabolites excreted in urine > feces	• Blocks mineralocorticoid receptors	• Hypertension • CHF following acute MI	• Hyperkalemia • Hypertriglyceridemia

III. Thyroid Drugs

MEDICATIONS FOR TREATING THYROID CONDITIONS

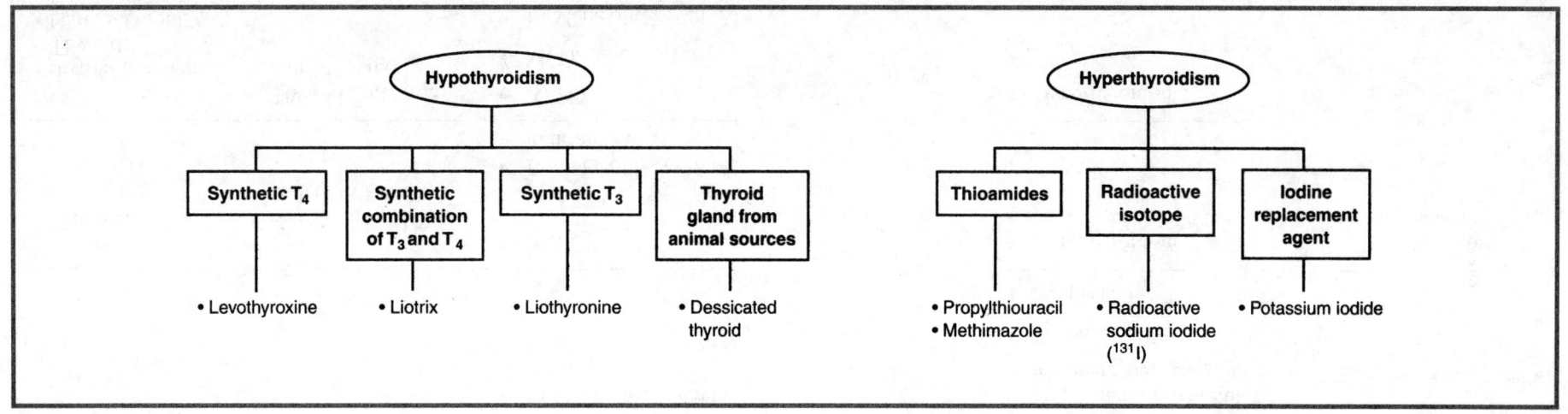

MEDICATIONS FOR TREATING HYPOTHYROIDISM

Drug	Class	Pharmacokinetics	Mechanism of Action	Clinical Uses and General Information	Side Effects
Levothyroxine (Levothroid, Synthroid Levoxyl, Tirosint, Unithroid)	• Synthetic form of T_4	• A: PO, IM, or IV • M: Hepatic • E: Metabolites excreted in urine > feces	• Same mechanism of action as endogenous thyroid hormones	• Hypothyroidism • Myxedema coma • TSH suppression in thyroid CA, benign nodules, and multinodular goiter	• Similar to symptoms of hyperthyroidism • Levoxyl associated with gagging, choking, dysphagia
Liothyronine (Cytomel, Triostat)	• Synthetic form of T_3	• A: PO and IM • M: Hepatic • E: Metabolites excreted in urine		• Hypothyroidism • Myxedema coma • IV preparation is useful for emergency situations • Suppression test • Simple goiter	• Arrhythmias
Liotrix (Thyrolar)	• Synthetic combination of T_3 and T_4 in 1:4 ratio	• A: PO • M: Hepatic • E: Metabolites excreted in urine > feces		• Hypothyroidism	• Similar to symptoms of hyperthyroidism
Desiccated thyroid (Armour Thyroid, Nature-Throid, Westhroid)	• Thyroid gland from animal sources	• A: PO • M: Hepatic • E: Metabolites excreted in urine		• Hypothyroidism	

MEDICATIONS FOR TREATING HYPERTHYROIDISM

Drug	Class	Pharmacokinetics	Mechanism of Action	Clinical Uses and General Information	Side Effects
Propylthiouracil (PTU)	Thioamides	• **A:** PO • **M:** Hepatic • **E:** Parent drug and metabolites excreted in urine	• Inhibits thyroidal peroxidase	• Hyperthyroidism • The thyroid often resumes its normal function after about 2 years of therapy • Safer than methimazole for use during pregnancy • Also inhibits peripheral conversion of T_4 to T_3	• Blood dyscrasias • Nausea • Nephritis • Pruritus • Rash • Weight gain • Hepatic necrosis • Inhibits P450 enzymes (Methimazole only)
Methimazole (Tapazole)		• **A:** PO • **M:** Hepatic • **E:** In urine		• Hyperthyroidism • The thyroid often resumes its normal function after about 2 years of therapy	
Radioactive sodium iodide (I^{131}, Hicon)	Radioactive isotope	• **A:** PO • **E:** In urine (small amounts excreted in feces and saliva)	• Taken up by gland to destroy tissue internally	• Hyperthyroidism • Thyroid carcinoma	• Acute thyroid crisis • Blood dyscrasias
Potassium iodide (Lugol's Solution, Strong Iodide solution)	Iodine replacement agent	• **A:** PO	• Acts as a competitive inhibitor of the radioactive isotopes of iodine • Decreases the activity of an overactive thyroid gland	• Prophylactic treatment of individuals near radioactive accidents • Management of thyrotoxic crisis • Reduction of thyroid vascularity prior to thyroidectomy	• GI upset (diarrhea, nausea) • Hyper/ Hypothyroidism

IV. Medications Affecting Calcium Levels

MEDICATIONS AFFECTING CALCIUM LEVELS: DRUG FACTS

Drug	Pharmacokinetics	Mechanism of Action	Clinical Uses	Side Effects
Selective Estrogen Receptor Modulators				
Tamoxifen (Nolvadex)	• A: PO • M: Hepatic (P450) • E: Majority of metabolites excreted in feces; remainder in urine	• Estrogen agonist/antagonist depending on tissue type • Estrogen antagonist on breast tissue tumors, and other target tissues	• Breast cancer treatment • Risk reduction of breast cancer for high-populations	• Increased incidence of uterine or endometrial cancer • Increased incidence of thromboembolic events (ie, CVA, PE) • Headache • Hepatotoxicity • Hot flashes • Mood disturbance • Inhibits P450 enzymes
Raloxifene (Evista)	• A: PO • M: Hepatic • E: Majority of metabolites excreted in feces; remainder in urine	• Estrogen agonist on bones, increasing bone mineralization and density while decreasing bone loss and fracture	• Risk reduction of breast cancer for high-risk populations • Postmenopausal osteoporosis treatment	• Chest pain • Increased incidence of uterine cancer • Hot flashes • Flu-like symptoms • Increased risk for DVT/PE • Increased risk of death due to stroke in women with CAD • Peripheral edema

Bisphosphonates

Drug	Pharmacokinetics	Mechanism	Indications	Indications	Adverse Effects
Alendronate (Fosamax)	• **A:** PO • **E:** Unchanged in urine; unabsorbed portion excreted unchanged in feces	• Bind to bone hydroxyapatite and inhibit osteoclast activity at the cellular level leading to decreased bone resorption		• Treatment and prevention of osteoporosis in women • Osteoporosis in men • Corticosteroid-induced osteoporosis • Paget's disease	• Esophagitis • GERD
Etidronate (Didronel)	• **A:** PO • **E:** Unchanged in urine			• Paget's disease • Treatment and prophylaxis for heterotropic ossification following hip replacements or spinal cord injuries	• Bone pain • Diarrhea • Nausea
Pamidronate (Aredia)	• **A:** IV • **E:** Unchanged in urine			• Paget's disease • Hypercalcemia associated with malignancy • Osteolytic bone lesions in multiple myeloma and breast cancer	• Hypocalcemia • Leukopenia • Lymphopenia
Risedronate (Actonel, Atelvia)	• **A:** PO • **E:** Unchanged in urine; unabsorbed portion excreted unchanged in feces			• Osteoporosis in postmenopausel women • Osteoporosis in men • Treatment and prevention of corticosteroid-induced osteoporosis • Treatment of Paget's disease	• Glirritation (nausea, abdominal pain, diarrhea, dyspepsia) • Bone pain • Hypertension
Ibandronate (Boniva)	• **A:** IV, PO • **E:** Unchanged in feces and urine			• Treatment and prevention of postmenopausal osteoporosis	• Dyspepsia • Back pain
Zoledronic acid (Reclast, Zometa)	• **A:** IV • **E:** Unchanged in urine		• Treatment of Paget's disease • Hypercalcemia associated with malignancy • Treatment and prevention of osteoporosis	• Treatment and prevention of glucocorticoid-induced osteoporosis • Treatment of multiple myeloma or metastalic bone lesions from solid tumors	• GI (nausea, vomiting, abdominal pain, diarrhea, weight loss) • Anemia • Bone pain • Edema

Continued

MEDICATIONS AFFECTING CALCIUM LEVELS: DRUG FACTS (Continued)

Drug	Pharmacokinetics	Mechanism of Action	Clinical Uses	Side Effects
Gallium nitrate (Ganite)	• A: IV • E: Renal	• Inhibits calcium resorption from bone by inhibition of osteoclast activity	• Treatment of hypercalcemia associated with malignancy	• Nephrotoxicity
Calcitonin (Fortical, Miacalcin)	• A: IV, intranasal • M: Renal, blood, and peripheral tissues • E: Urine	• Molecular similarity to calcitonin with antagonist effects on PTH	• Treatment of Paget's disease • Treatment of hypercalcemia • Treatment of postmenopausal osteoporosis • Treatment of osteoporosis	• Rhinitis

Antineoplastic Agent

Drug	Pharmacokinetics	Mechanism of Action	Clinical Uses	Side Effects
Plicamycin (Mithracin, Mithramycin)	• A: IV • E: Urine	• Reduces serum Ca^{2+} via unknown mechanism (possibly via inhibition of DNA-dependent RNA synthesis that renders the osteoclast unable to respond to PTH)	• Hypercalcemia and hypercalciuria associated with malignancy • Paget's disease • Malignant testicular CA	• Hemorrhage • Hepatotoxicity • Nephrotoxicity • Thrombocytopenia • Severe side-effect profile limits clinical use

Dental Prophylaxis

Drug	Pharmacokinetics	Mechanism of Action	Clinical Uses	Side Effects
Sodium fluoride (Numerous brand name preparations)	• A: PO • E: Urine and feces	• Accumulates in bone where it stabilizes the hydroxyapatite crystal • Promotes remineralization of decalcified enamel	• Prophylaxis for dental caries	• Overdose discolors teeth (dental fluorosis)

V. Medications for Managing Diabetes

INSULIN: DRUG FACTS

Drug	Appearance	Route of Administration	Pharmacokinetics of SC Administration			Clinical Uses	Adverse Reactions
			Onset	Peak	Duration		
Insulin lispro (Humalog)	• Clear	IV, SC	20 min	30 min–2.5 hours	<5 hours	• SC preparations available for routine control of blood sugar in diabetes • IV preparations available for emergent control of hyperglycemia	• Hypoglycemia
Regular (Novolin R, Humulin R)			30 min	2–3 hours	4–8 hours		
Insulin aspart (Novolog)			10 min	1–3 hours	3–5 hours		
Insulin glulisine (Apidra)			20 min	1 hour	3–5 hours		
Insulin glargine (Lantus)		SC	3–4 hours	N/A	11–24 hours	• Routine control of blood sugar in diabetes	
Insulin determir			3–4 hours	3–9 hours	6–23 hours		
NPH (Novolin N, Humulin N)	• Cloudy		2–4 hours	6–10 hours	10–16 hours		
NPH and regular (Humulin 70/30 and 50/50, Novolin 70/30)			30 min–1 hour	2–10 hours (biphasic)	10–20 hours		
Insulin lispro protamine and insulin lispro (Humalog Mic 75/25 and 50/50)			10 min	1–3 hours (biphasic)	10–20 hours		
Insulin aspart protamine and aspart (Novolog Mix 70/30 and 50/50)			15 min	1–4 hours (biphasic)	<24 hours		

CLASSIFICATION OF ORAL DIABETIC DRUGS

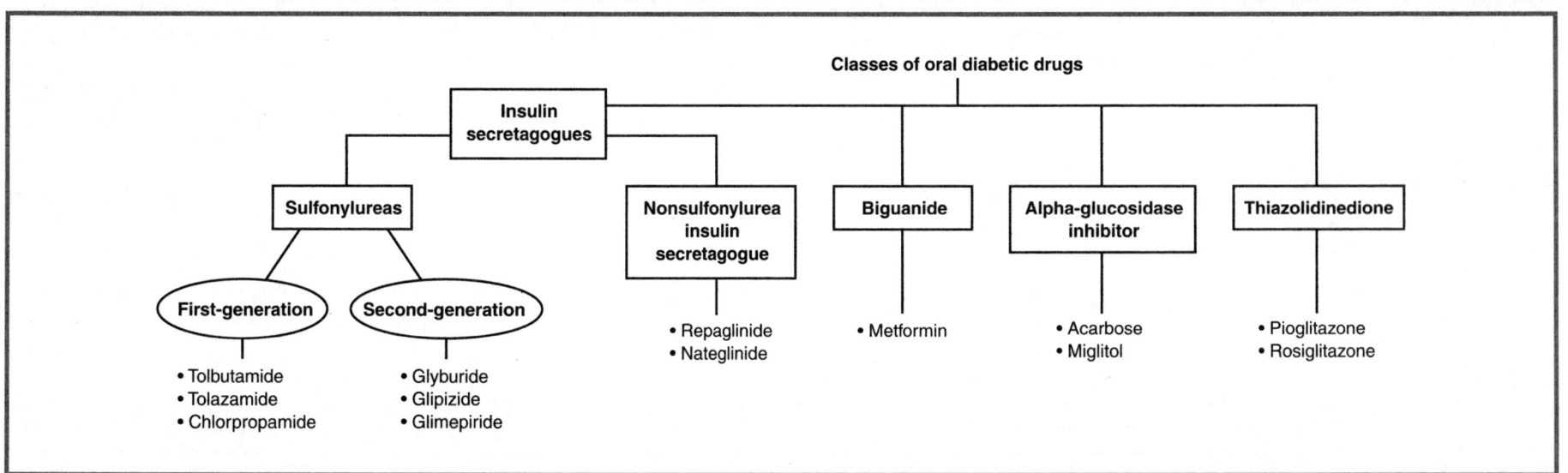

ORAL DIABETIC DRUGS: SULFONYLUREAS

Drug	Pharmacokinetics	Duration of Action	Mechanism of Action	Clinical Uses/ Information	Adverse Reactions
First-generation Sulfonylureas					
Tolbutamide (Orinase)	• **A:** PO • **M:** Hepatic (P450 except Tolazamide) • **E:** Primarily excreted as metabolites in urine	6–24 hours	• Bind to ATP sensitive K^+ channels to block the efflux of K^+ resulting in membrane depolarization thus increasing the Ca^{2+} entering the cell resulting in increase of insulin release from the pancreatic beta cells • Potentiate exocytosis of insulin-containing granules by direct binding to intracellular binding sites • Increase action of insulin on target tissues by increasing the number of insulin receptors • Reduction of glucose release by the liver	• Treatment of NIDDM • Useful when endogenous insulin is being produced • Best results when used in combination with restricted calorie intake and weight reduction	• Refractory hypoglycemia • GI (nausea, vomiting, diarrhea) • Hematologic (pancytopenia, agranulocytosis, thrombocytopenia, hemolytic anemia) • Derm (EM, exfoliative dermatitis) • Hepatic (cholestatic jaundice, hepatitis, liver failure) • CNS (dizziness, headache) • Inhibits P450 enzymes (Tolazamide and Glyburide)
Tolazamide (Tolinase)		10–24 hours			
Chlorpropamide (Diabinese)		24 hours			
Second-generation Sulfonylureas					
Glyburide (DiaBeta, Glynase, PresTab)	• **A:** PO • **M:** Hepatic (P450) • **E:** Metabolites excreted in urine and feces	24 hours			
Glipizide (Glucotrol)		12–24 hours			
Glimepiride (Amaryl)		24 hours			

ORAL DIABETIC DRUGS: NONSULFONYLUREAS

Drug	Pharmacokinetics	Mechanism of Action	Characteristics	Side Effects
Meglitinide Derivatives				
Repaglinide (Prandin)	• DOA: 4–6 hours • M: Hepatic (P450) • E: Majority of metabolites excreted in feces	• Closes an ATP-dependent K+ channel to block the efflux of K+ resulting in membrane depolarization thus increasing the Ca²+ entering the cell resulting in increased insulin release from beta cells	• Effects on blood glucose is similar to sulfonylureas • Acts synergistically with metformin	• Headache • Hypoglycemia • Inhibits P450 enzymes (Nateglinide only)
Nateglinide (Starlix)	• DOA: 4 hours • M: Hepatic (P450) • E: Majority of metabolites excreted in urine			
Biguanide				
Metformin (Glucophage)	• DOA: 10–12 hours • E: Unchanged in the urine	• Increases insulin receptor binding in liver, adipose, and muscle for increased glucose uptake • Inhibits hepatic gluconeogenesis	• Useful in patients with refractory obesity with ineffective insulin action • Used in combination with sulfonylureas and thiazolidinediones	• Diarrhea • Nausea • Weakness
α-Glucosidase Inhibitor				
Acarbose (Precose)	• DOA: 3–4 hours • M: Metabolized by intestinal flora • E: Unabsorbed portion excreted in feces; absorbed metabolites excreted in urine	• Slows carbohydrate digestion and absorption time to prevent exaggerated postprandial rise in blood glucose • Acts as a competitive inhibitor of pancreatic alpha-amylase and alpha-glucosidase delaying hydrolysis of ingested carbohydrates and glucose absorption • Inhibits metabolism of sucrose	• Only decreases postprandial hyperglycemia by 30–50% • Does not cause hypoglycemia in monotherapy	• Abdominal pain • Diarrhea • Flatulence • Hypoglycemia (Combination therapy) • Elevated transaminases with acarbose
Miglitol (Glyset)	• DOA: 2–3 hours • E: Excreted unchanged in urine			

Thiazolidinediones					
Pioglitazone (Actos)	15–24 hours	• **A:** PO • **M:** Hepatic (P450) • **E:** Metabolites excreted in urine and feces	• Peroxisome proliferator-activated receptor gamma (PPAR-gamma) agonists • PPAR-gamma influences the production of proteins involved in glucose and lipid metabolism	• Treatment of NIDDM • Useful for monotherapy or in combination with sulfonylureas and metformin	• CHF exacerbation • Hypoglycemia • Inhibits P450 enzymes • Induces P450 enzymes (Pioglitazone only)
Rosiglitazone (Avandia)	>24 hours				

VI. Drugs Affecting Reproductive Hormones

ESTROGEN PREPARATIONS: DRUG FACTS

Drug	Route of Administration	Clinical Uses and General Information	Drawbacks and Side Effects
Conjugated estrogens (Premarin)	• PO, IM, IV, and vaginal	• Treatment of vasomotor symptoms of menopause	• Nausea and vomiting
Estradiol (Numerous brand names)	• PO, IM, vaginal, topical, and transdermal	• Treatment of vulvar and vaginal atrophy • Treatment of female hypoestrogenism secondary to hypogonadism, castration, or primary ovarian failure • Palliative treatment of advanced breast cancer • Palliative treatment of advanced prostate cancer	• Edema • Headache • Hepatic neoplasms • Breast tenderness
Esterified estrogens (Menest)	• PO	• Used in combination with other therapeutic measures to retard bone loss and progression of osteoporosis in postmenopausal women	• Thromboembolic events especially in smokers • Breakthrough bleeding • Dementia
Estropipate (Ogen)	• PO		• Should be administered with progesterone as unopposed estrogen can cause endometrial hyperplasia and possibly carcinoma
Ethinyl estradiol	• PO	• Estrogen component in most oral contraceptives	
Mestranol	• PO	• Estrogen component in oral contraceptives	

ANTIESTROGEN DRUGS

Drug	Pharmacokinetics	Mechanism of Action	Clinical Uses and General Information	Drawbacks and Side Effects
Clomiphene (Clomid, Serophene)	• **A:** PO • **M:** Hepatic metabolism • **E:** Majority of metabolites excreted in feces	• Estrogen receptor agonist in CNS and GU organs (endometrium, vagina, cervix, and ovary) • Causes preovulatory gonadotropin surge • Blocks estrogen's inhibitory effect on the hypothalamus and pituitary leading to increased FSH/LH levels • Increased LH/FSH levels produce ovulation	• Fertility drug that induces ovulation in anovulatory conditions	• Hot flashes • Ovarian enlargement • Multiple births
Tamoxifen (Soltamox)	• **A:** PO • **M:** Hepatic (P450) • **E:** Majority of metabolites excreted in feces; remainder in urine	• Estrogen antagonist in breast tissue and CNS • Estrogen agonist on endometrium, bone, and lipids	• Used to treat estrogen receptor–negative breast CA in premenopausal women • Can be used prophylactically in women with a history of breast CA • Positive effects on bone density and lipid profile	• Endometrial hyperplasia/carcinoma • Headache • Hepatotoxicity • Hot flashes • Nausea • Inhibits P450 enzymes
Raloxifene (Evista)	• **A:** PO • **M:** Hepatic • **E:** Majority of metabolites excreted in feces; remainder in urine	• Mixed estrogen agonist/antagonist • Estrogen agonist at estrogen receptors on bone, CVS, and CNS	• Prophylaxis and treatment of postmenopausal osteoporosis • Lowers LDL levels • Does not cause endometrial hyperplasia associated with tamoxifen	• Chest pain • Cystitis • Leg cramping • Peripheral edema

ESTROGEN AND PROGESTERONE COMBINATIONS

Estrogen	Progesterone	Examples of Brand Names	Side Effects
Monophasic (various combinations of estrogen and progesterone with constant dose of both)			
• Ethinyl estradiol • Mestranol	• Norethindrone • Norgestrel • Ethynodiol • Norgestimate • Desogestrel • Levonorgestrel • Drospirenone	• Yasmin • Alesse • Ortho-Novum • Lo/Ovral	• Breakthrough bleeding • Headache • Mastalgia • Nausea • Thromboembolic events (especially in smokers) • Weight gain
Biphasic (estrogen and progesterone doses vary)			
• Ethinyl estradiol	• Norethindrone	• Ortho-Novum 10/11 • Necon 10/11	
Triphasic (estrogen and progesterone doses vary)			
• Ethinyl estradiol	• Norethindrone • Desogestrel • Levonorgestrel • Norgestimate	• Ortho Tri-Cyclen • Cyclessa	
Extended Preparations (estrogen dose only varies in Seasonique)			
• Ethinyl estradiol	• Levonorgestrel	• Seasonale • Seasonique • Jolessa	

PROGESTERONE PREPARATIONS

Note that the four progesterone preparations used as contraceptives contain either "nor" or "progesterone" in their names. Megestrol is not used as a contraceptive.

Drug	Route of Administration	Clinical Uses	Side Effects
Etonogestrel (Implanon, Nexplanon)	• SC implant	• Long-term contraception	• Weight gain • Headache • Breakthrough/irregular vaginal bleeding
Hydroxyprogest erone (Makena)	• IM	• Reduction of preterm birth	• Thromboembolic events
Levonorgestrel (Plan B)	• PO	• Emergency contraception	• Breakthrough bleeding
Levonorgestrel (Mirena)	• Intrauterine device	• Long-term contraception • Treatment of heavy vaginal bleeding in patients who desire contraception	• Headache • Mastalgia • Nausea • Thromboembolic events (especially in smokers) • Weight gain
Medroxyprogest erone (Provera)	• PO	• Amenorrhea • Abnormal uterine bleeding • Contraception • Endometriosis • Palliative treatment of recurrent or metastatic endometrial carcinoma • Postmenopausal treatment in combination with estrogen preparations	• Decrease bone density • Breakthrough bleeding • Headache • Mastalgia • Nausea • Weight gain
Medroxyprogest erone (Depo Provera)	• IM		

Continued

PROGESTERONE PREPARATIONS (Continued)

Note that the four progesterone preparations used as contraceptives contain either "nor" or "progesterone" in their names. Megestrol is not used as a contraceptive.

Drug	Route of Administration	Clinical Uses	Side Effects
Norethindrone (Aygestin, Camila, Errin, Heather, Jolivette, Nor-QD, Nora-BE, Micronor)	• PO	• Amenorrhea • Abnormal uterine bleeding • Contraception • Endometriosis	• Breakthrough bleeding • Headache • Mastalgia • Nausea • Thromboembolic events (especially in smokers) • Weight gain
Megestrol (Megace)	• PO	• Weight gain in AIDS-related cachexia • Palliative treatment of endometrial cancer • Palliative treatment of breast cancer	• Hypertension • Headaches • Diarrhea • Hyperglycemia • Impotence

ANTIPROGESTERONE DRUG

Drug	Pharmacokinetics	Mechanism of Action	Clinical Uses	Side Effects
Mifepristone (Mifeprex, Korlym)	• **A:** PO • **M:** Hepatic (P450) • **E:** Metabolites excreted in urine and feces	• Competitive inhibitor at progesterone and glucocorticoid receptors	• Abortifacient agent • Treatment of Type 2 diabetes in patients with endogenous Cushing's syndrome	• Dizziness • Nausea • Headache • Hypokatemia

TESTOSTERONE PREPARATIONS

Drug	Route of Administration	Clinical Uses	Side Effects
Fluoxymesterone (Android)	• A: PO • M: Hepatic • E: Primarily excreted in urine	• Treatment of testosterone deficient states (delayed puberty, hypogonadism) • Palliative treatment of advanced breast CA in women	• Acne • Cholestatic hepatitis • Headache • Gynecomastia • Edema • Labile mood • Oligospermia • Virilization
Methyltestosterone (Android, Testred, Methitest)			
Testosterone enanthate (Delatestryl)	• A: IM		
Testosterone cypionate (Depo-Testosterone)	• A: IM	• Treatment of hypogonadism	
Oxandrolone (Oxandrin)	• A: PO	• Promotes weight gain	

ANTIANDROGEN DRUGS

Drug	Class	Pharmacokinetics	Mechanism of Action	Clinical Uses	Side Effects
Leuprolide (Lupron, Eligard)	• GnRH agonists	• **A:** IM or SC • **M:** Metabolized to smaller peptides (probably in hypothalamus and pituitary) • **E:** Small amounts of metabolites excreted in urine	• Causes down regulation of the receptors in the pituitary subsequently leading to decreased hormonal release	• Treatment of metastatic prostate CA • Other uses include treatment of precocious puberty, endometriosis, and uterine leiomyoma	• Hot flashes in men and women • Amenorrhea • Initial treatment in prostate cancer can cause "tumor flare" (severe pain associated with initial increase in serum testosterone)
Goserelin (Zoladex)		• **A:** SC implant • **E:** Urine (parent drug and metabolites)		• Palliative treatment of prostate cancer • Palliative treatment of breast cancer • Treatment of endometriosis	• Hot flashes • Acne • Decreased libido
Nilutamide (Nilandron)	• Nonsteroidal antiandrogan	• **A:** PO • **M:** Hepatic (P450 Nilutamide and Enzalutamide) • **E:** Primarily in urine as metabolites	• Competitive antagonist at androgen receptor	• Treatment of metastatic prostate cancer	• Hot flashes • Hepatotoxicity • Interstital pneumonitis • Inhibits P450 enzymes
Bicalutamide (Casodex)					• Hot flashes • Hepatitis • Inhibits P450 enzymes
Enzalutamide (Xtandi)			• Acts purely as an androgen antagonist		• Headache • Hot flashes • Fatigue • Inhibits P450 enzymes • Induces P450 enzymes

Continued

ANTIANDROGEN DRUGS (Continued)

Drug	Class	Pharmacokinetics	Mechanism of Action	Clinical Uses	Side Effects
Finasteride (Proscar, Propecia)	5 α-reductase inhibitor	• **A:** PO • **M:** Hepatic (P450) • **E:** Metabolites excreted in feces and urine	• Inhibits the enzyme responsible for the conversion of testosterone to its more potent form dihydrotestosterone	• Treatment of BPH • Treatment of alopecia in male	• Impotence • Orthostatic hypotension
Dutasteride (Avodart)				• Treatment of BPH	• Impotence • Decreased libido
Spironolactone (Aldactone)	17 α-hydroxylase inhibitor	• **A:** PO • **M:** Metabolized to active metabolites • **E:** Majority of metabolites are excreted in urine	• Competitive inhibitor of dihydrotestosterone in target tissues • Inhibits 17 α-hydroxylase activity, thereby decreasing testosterone production	• Treatment of hirsutism in women	• Hepatotoxicity • Gastritis • Gynecomastia • Impotence • Tumorigenic • DRESS

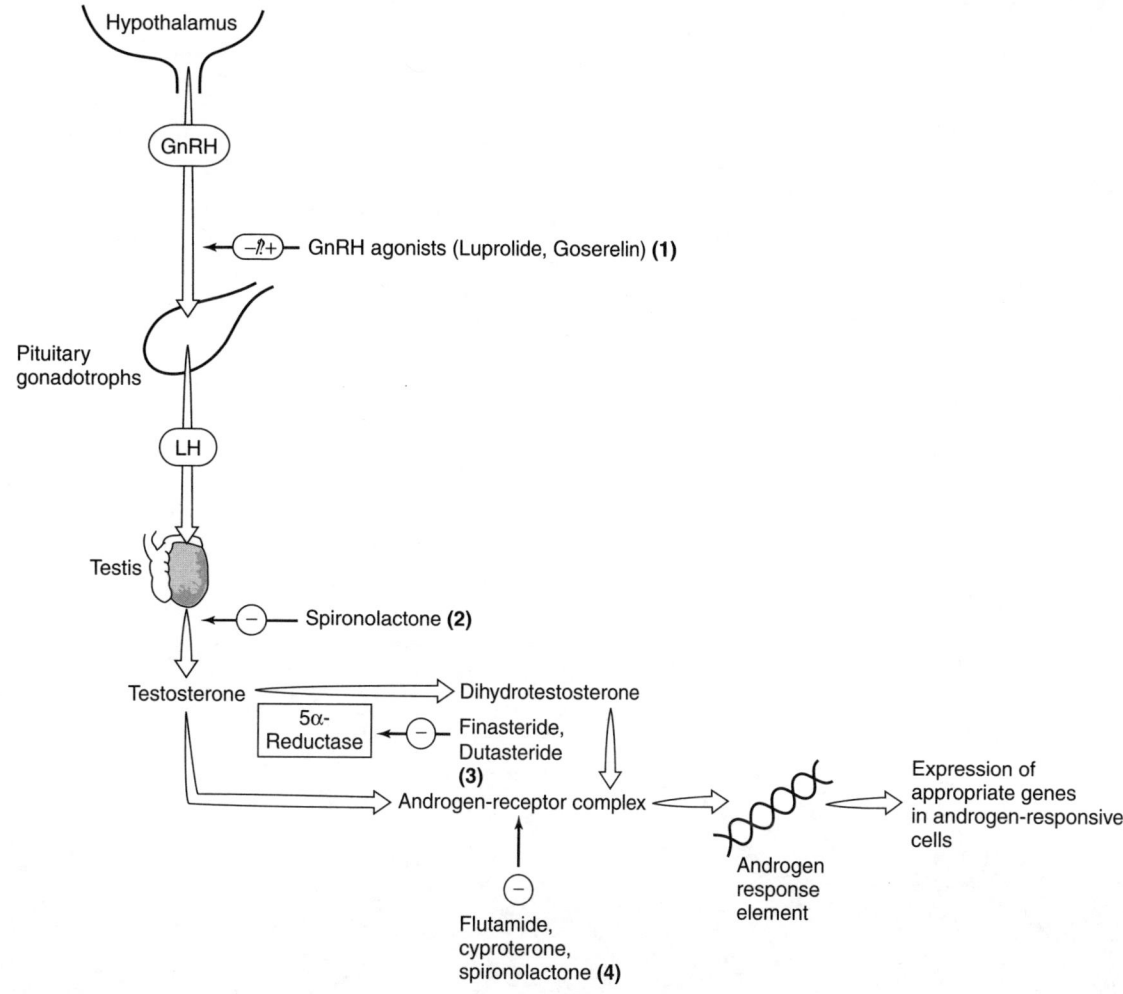

Hypothalamus

GnRH

GnRH agonists (Luprolide, Goserelin) **(1)**

Pituitary gonadotrophs

LH

Testis

Spironolactone **(2)**

Testosterone → Dihydrotestosterone

5α-Reductase ← Finasteride, Dutasteride **(3)**

Androgen-receptor complex

Androgen response element

Expression of appropriate genes in androgen-responsive cells

Flutamide, cyproterone, spironolactone **(4)**

Location (1) shows stimulation (+) or inhibition (−) by GnRH agonists; (2) inhibition of testosterone synthesis by ketoconazole; (3) inhibition of dihydrotestosterone production by finasteride; (4) inhibition of androgen binding at its receptor by flutamide and other drugs.

CHAPTER 10

ONCOLOGIC DRUGS

I. ACTION OF ONCOLOGIC MEDICATIONS

Phases of the Cell Cycle

II. ALKYLATING DRUGS

Alkylating Drug Facts

III. ANTIMETABOLITES

Antimetabolites: Pyrimidine & Purine Analogs, and Folic Acid Antagonists

IV. ANTITUMOR ANTIBIOTICS

Action of Antitumor Antibiotics

Antitumor Antibiotics

V. PLANT ALKALOIDS

Plant Alkaloids by Action and Class

Plant Alkaloids: Drug Facts

VI. HORMONAL ANTICANCER DRUGS

Classification of Hormonal Anticancer Drugs

Hormonal Anticancer Drug Facts

VII. CHEMOTHER-APEUTIC DRUGS

Miscellaneous Chemotherapeutics: Drug Facts

Chemotherapeutics: Monoclonal Antibodies

TERMS TO LEARN

Chronic Myelogenous Leukemia	Bone marrow malignancy involving myeloid cells; it is typically seen in older patients and is associated with poor prognosis.
Ewing's Sarcoma	Malignancy of the bone; seen in young boys.
Gestational Trophoblastic Neoplasms	Group of malignancies stemming from fetal or placental tissue.
Giant Cell Tumors	Benign bone tumor.
Hodgkin's Lymphoma	Malignancy of the lymph nodes; bimodal age distribution (seen in young and old men); associated with a good prognosis with chemotherapy.
Multiple Myeloma	Malignancy of plasma cells; it is characterized by bone pain, "punched out" lytic lesion of the bone, hypercalcemia, and Bence Jones proteinuria.
Neuroblastoma	Most common extracranial solid tumor of childhood; malignancy that arises from the neural crest cells that tends to occur in the abdomen and thorax; it secretes catecholamines.
Non-Hodgkin's Lymphoma	Malignancy of the lymph nodes; more likely to have extranodal primaries (ie, stomach or thyroid) than Hodgkins lymphoma; it is associated with a poorer prognosis than Hodgkin's lymphoma.
Wilms' Tumor	Renal malignancy seen in children; it is associated with hemihypertrophy of the body.

I. Action of Oncologic Medications

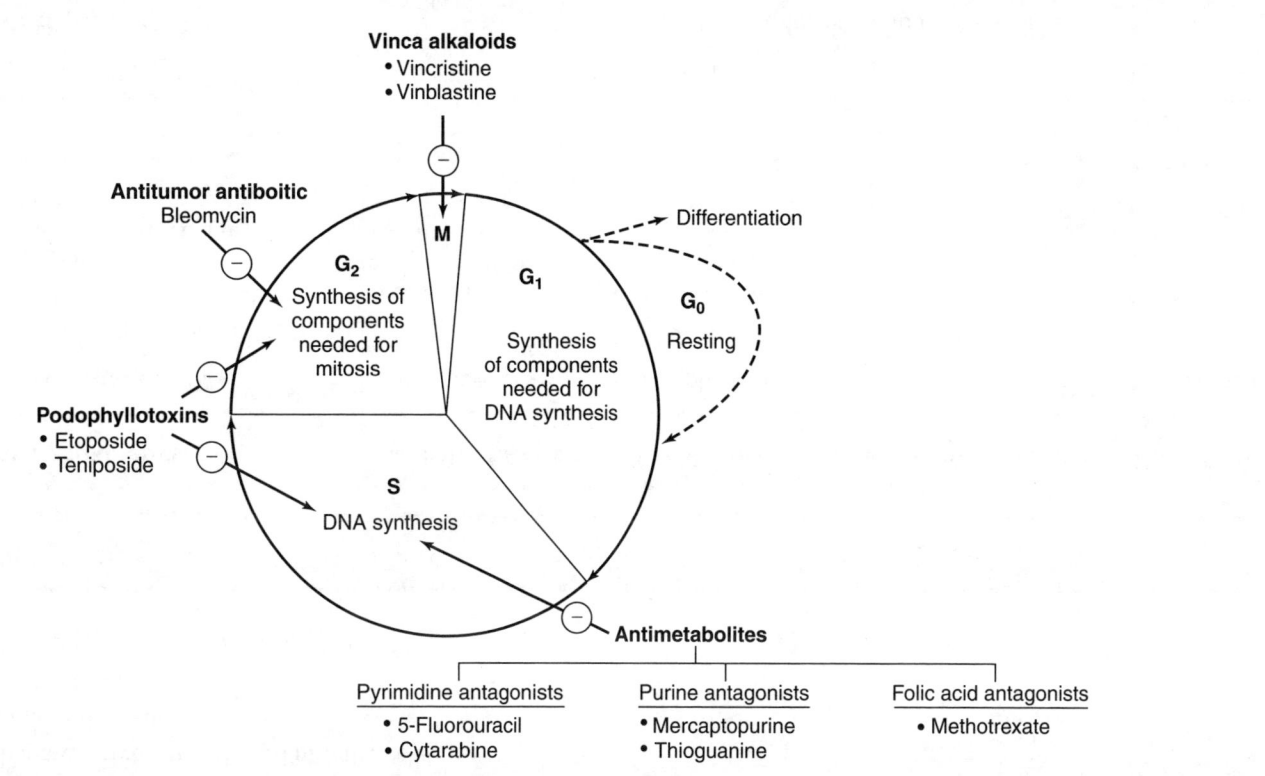

Vinca alkaloids
- Vincristine
- Vinblastine

Antitumor antiboitic
Bleomycin

Differentiation

M

G₂
Synthesis of components needed for mitosis

G₁
Synthesis of components needed for DNA synthesis

G₀
Resting

Podophyllotoxins
- Etoposide
- Teniposide

S
DNA synthesis

Antimetabolites

Pyrimidine antagonists	Purine antagonists	Folic acid antagonists
• 5-Fluorouracil • Cytarabine	• Mercaptopurine • Thioguanine	• Methotrexate

All cells—normal and neoplastic—must traverse these cell cycle phases before and during cell division. CCS drug actions may not be restricted to a specific phase, but tumor cells are usually most responsive to specific drugs (or drug groups) in the phases indicated. Cell cycle-nonspecific (CCNS) drugs act on tumor cells while they are actively cycling and while they are in the resting phase (G_0).

Modified from Katzung BG, ed: *Basic & Clinical Pharmacology*, 8th ed, p 926. Originally published by Appleton & Lange. © 2001 by the McGraw-Hill Companies, Inc.

II. Alkylating Drugs

Mechanism of Action: Alkylating agents have a very reactive chemical moiety that binds to the bases of DNA causing damage that is very difficult to repair and sometimes irreparable.

Resistance Mechanisms: Four resistance mechanisms counteract the effects of alkylating agents:

1. Decreased transport in those that are actively transported into the cells
2. Increased pumping of the drug out of the cell
3. Increased ability to repair the DNA damage
4. Increased glutathione levels to get rid of the reactive species

ALKYLATING DRUG FACTS

Drug	Pharmacokinetics	Mechanism of Action	Clinical Uses and General Information	Side Effects
Mechlorethamine (Mustargen)	• **A:** IV or intracavitary • **M:** Rapid hydrolysis and demethylation in plasma • **E:** Parent drug and metabolites excreted in urine	• Inhibition of DNA and RNA action by various mechanisms resulting in the cross linking of DNA	• Lymphoma (Hodgkin's and non-Hodgkin's) • Malignant effusions • More stable and easier to use than nitrogen mustard	• Bone marrow suppression • Headache • Injection site reaction • Nausea • Vomiting • Sterility • Ototoxicity
Cyclophosphamide (Cytoxan)	• **A:** PO and IV • **M:** Hepatic (P450) to active metabolites • **E:** Parent drug and metabolites excreted in urine		• Breast CA • Lymphoma (Hodgkin's and non-Hodgkin's) • Multiple myeloma • Neuroblastoma • Ovarian adenocarcinoma • Longer acting and more stable analogues of nitrogen mustard	• Bone marrow suppression • Nausea • Vomiting • Hemorrhagic cystitis • Bladder fibrosis/carcinoma • Sterility • Alopecia • Inhibits P450 enzymes • Induces P450 enzymes

Ifosfamide (IFEX)	• **A:** IV • **M:** Hepatic (P450) • **E:** Parent drug and metabolites excreted in urine	• Testicular germ cell tumors	• Alopecia • Encephalopathy • Hemorrhagic cystitis • Nephrotoxicity • Bone marrow suppression • Inhibits P450 enzymes • Induces P450 enzymes
Chlorambucil (Leukeran)	• **A:** PO • **M:** Hepatic • **E:** Parent drug and metabolites excreted in urine	• Chronic lymphocytic leukemia • Lymphoma (Hodgkin's and non-Hodgkin's)	• Allergic reactions (urticaria to hypersensitivity) • Sterility • Bone marrow suppression
Melphalan (Alkeran)	• **A:** PO and IV • **M:** Hepatic • **E:** Majority of parent drug and metabolites excreted in feces; remainder in urine	• Multiple myeloma (palliative) • Ovarian CA	• GI distress
Busulfan (Myleran, Busulfex)	• **A:** PO and IV • **M:** Hepatic • **E:** Metabolites excreted in urine	• Chronic myelogenous leukemia (palliative) • Myeloablation prior to stem cell transplant	• Bone marrow suppression • GI distress • Pulmonary fibrosis
Lomustine (CeeNU)	• **A:** PO • **M:** Hepatic (P450 minor) • **E:** Majority of metabolites excreted in urine	• Brain tumors • Hodgkin's lymphoma	• Bone marrow suppression • GI distress • Hepatotoxicity • Pulmonary fibrosis • Neurotoxicity • Inhibits P450 enzymes

Continued

ALKYLATING DRUG FACTS (Continued)

Drug	Pharmacokinetics	Mechanism of Action	Clinical Uses and General Information	Side Effects
Carmustine (BiCNU, Gliadel)	• **A:** IV and intracranial wafer • **M:** Hepatic • **E:** Majority of metabolites excreted in urine		• Brain tumors • Lymphoma (Hodgkin's and non-Hodgkin's) • Multiple myeloma	• Bone marrow suppression • GI distress • Hepatotoxicity • Pulmonary fibrosis • Nephrotoxicity
Streptozocin (Zanosar)	• **A:** IV • **M:** Hepatic • **E:** Parent drug and metabolites excreted in urine		• Pancreatic CA	
Cisplatin (Platinol)	• **A:** IV • **M:** Nonenzymatic conversion to inactive metabolites • **E:** Majority of metabolites excreted in urine		• Bladder CA (advanced) • Ovarian CA (metastatic) • Testicular CA (metastatic)	• Bone marrow suppression • GI distress • Anaphylaxis • Hepatotoxicity • Nephrotoxicity • Neurotoxicity • Ototoxicity
Carboplatin (Paraplatin)	• **A:** IV • **M:** Hepatic (minor) • **E:** Metabolites excreted in urine		• Ovarian CA (advanced)	• Bone marrow suppression • Anaphylaxis • Neurotoxicity • Vision loss • Ototoxicity • Vomiting

Dacarbazine (Dtic-Dome)	• **A:** IV • **M:** Hepatic (P450) • **E:** Parent drug and metabolites excreted in urine	• Malignant melanoma • Hodgkin's lymphoma	• Bone marrow suppression • Hepatotoxicity • GI distress
Thiotepa	• **A:** IV, intravesicular, intracavitary • **M:** Hepatic • **E:** Metabolites and parent drug excreted in urine	• Ovarian CA • Breast CA • Bladder CA • Malignant effusions	• GI distress • Infertility • Inhibits P450 enzymes
Temozolomide (Temodar)	• **A:** PO, IV • **M:** Hydrolyzed in peripheral tissues • **E:** Majority excreted as metabolites in urine	• Brain tumors (astrocytoma, GBM)	• Peripheral edema • GI distress • Bone marrow suppression
Bendamustine (Treanda)	• **A:** IV • **M:** Hepatic (P450 minor) • **E:** Metabolites excreted in urine	• CLL • NHL	
Procarbazine (Matulane, Natulan)	• **A:** PO • **M:** Hepatic metabolism • **E:** Majority of metabolites excreted in urine	• Hodgkin's lymphoma	• Bone marrow suppression • GI distress • Hepatotoxicity • Neurotoxicity
Altretamine (Hexalen)	• **A:** PO • **M:** Hepatic • **E:** Metabolites excreted in urine	• Ovarian CA (palliative)	• GI distress • Hepatotoxicity • Neurotoxicity

III. Antimetabolites

Pharmacokinetics: Because nucleoside triphosphates, the building blocks of DNA, are too polar to enter the cell, all of these drugs must be taken into the cell as a prodrug and then activated.

Mechanism of Action: All of the antimetabolites are structural analogues of the normal building blocks of DNA. They either are incorrectly incorporated into the DNA—which halts its production—or they inhibit the enzymes involved in the synthesis of DNA building blocks. These only work during the S phase of the cell cycle.

ANTIMETABOLITES: PYRIMIDINE & PURINE ANALOGS, AND FOLIC ACID ANTAGONISTS

Drug	Pharmacokinetics	Mechanisms of Action and Resistance	Clinical Uses	Side Effects
Purine Antagonists				
Mercaptopurine/ 6-MP (Purinethol)	• **A:** PO • **M:** Hepatic and GI mucosa • **E:** Parent drug and metabolites excreted in urine	• Active metabolites decrease de novo purine synthesis and cause DNA strand breaks • Resistance from decreased activity of the enzyme that activates these drugs and increased production of alkaline phosphatases that inactivate the toxic metabolites	• ALL	• GI distress • Hepatotoxicity • Bone marrow suppression
Thioguanine/ 6-TG (Tabloid)			• AML	
Cladribine (Leustatin)	• **A:** IV, SC • **E:** Urine	• Prodrug metabolized to activated to 5′ triphosphate derivative	• Hairy cell leukemia	• Neurotoxicity • Nephrotoxicity • Myelosuppression
Clofarabine (Clolar)	• **A:** IV • **M:** Intracellular enzymatic activation and hepatic (minor) • **E:** Excreted primarily unchanged in urine	• Metabolized to clofarabine 5′ triphosphate	• Acute lymphocytic leukemia	• GI distress • Elevated transaminases • Myelosuppression

Fludarabine (Fludara, Oforta)	• **A:** IV, PO • **M:** Intracellular and plasma dephosphorylation • **E:** Urine	• Inhibits DNA polymerase and ribonucleotide reductase	• Chronic lymphocytic leukemia	• Neurotoxicity • Hematologic emergencies (ITP, hemolytic anemia)
Pentostatin (Nipent)	• **A:** IV • **E:** Primarily excreted unchanged in urine	• Inhibits the enzyme adenosine deaminase (ADA) ultimately leading to cellular toxicity	• Hairy cell leukemia	• GI distress • Myelosuppression • Neurotoxicity • Hepatotoxicity • Pulmonary toxicity • Nephrotoxicity
Nelarabine (Arranon)	• **A:** IV • **M:** Hepatic • **E:** Metabolites excreted primarily in urine	• Metabolized to ara-GTP then incorporated into DNA leading to inhibition of DNA synthesis and apoptosis	• T cell acute lymphocytic leukemia • T cell lymphoblastic lymphoma	• GI distress • Myelosuppression • Neurotoxicity

Pyrimidine Antagonists

5-Fluorouracil/ 5-FU (Adrucil)	• **A:** IV • **M:** Hepatic metabolism to active metabolite • **E:** Metabolites are exhaled and excreted in urine	• Active metabolite inhibits thymidylate synthase • Results in decreased DNA synthesis • Resistance due to decreased activation of 5-FU, increased thymidylate synthase activity, and reduced drug sensitivity of that enzyme	• Colon CA • Breast CA • Rectal CA • Pancreatic CA • Gastric CA	• Alopecia • GI distress • Photosensitivity • Myelosuppression • Inhibits P450 enzymes
Cytosine arabinoside/ Ara-C/ Cytarabine (Cytosar)	• **A:** IV, SC, or intrathecal • **M:** Hepatic • **E:** Metabolites excreted in urine	• Active metabolite inhibits DNA polymerase • Resistance due to decreased conversion to active metabolite and decreased uptake of the drug	• AML induction	• GI distress • Myelosuppression • Neurotoxicity

Continued

ANTIMETABOLITES: PYRIMIDINE & PURINE ANALOGS, AND FOLIC ACID ANTAGONISTS (Continued)

Drug	Pharmacokinetics	Mechanisms of Action and Resistance	Clinical Uses	Side Effects
Gemcitabine (Gemzar)	• **A:** IV, intra-arterial • **M:** Intracellular • **E:** Metabolites excreted in urine	• Inhibits DNA synthesis by inhibiting ribonucleotide reductase • Incorporates into DNA inhibiting DNA polymerase	• Pancreatic CA • Breast CA • Ovarian CA • Non–small cell lung CA	• Hepatotoxicity • GI distress • Myelosuppression
Floxuridine (FUDR)	• **A:** IV • **M:** Hepatic to active metabolites • **E:** Metabolites are exhaled and excreted in urine	• Deoxyribonucleotide of fluorouracil • Fluorinated to pyrimidine antagonist which inhibits DNA and RNA synthesis	• Metastatic colorectal CA • Metastatic gastric CA	• GI distress • Myelosuppression • Inhibits P450 enzymes
Capecitabine (Xeloda)	• **A:** PO • **M:** Hepatic and tissue metabolism • **E:** Metabolites primarily excreted in urine	• Prodrug of 5-FU	• Metastatic breast CA • Metastatic colorectal CA	• Myelosuppression • Hyperbilirubinemia • GI distress • Inhibits P450 enzymes
Decitabine (Dacogen)	• **A:** IV • **M:** Intracellular metabolism to active metabolite, also metabolized in the liver and blood • **E:** Metabolites primarily excreted in urine	• Phosphorylated metabolite is incorporated into DNA • Inhibits DNA methyltransferase causing hypomethylation and cell death	• Myelodysplastic syndrome	• GI distress • Myelosuppression

Azacitidine (Vidaza)	• **A:** IV, SC • **M:** Hepatic • **E:** Excreted primarily in urine	• Inhibits DNA methyltransferase causing hypomethylation and cell death	• Myelodysplastic syndrome	• GI distress • Myelosuppression

Folic Acid Antagonist

| Methotrexate/ MTX (Rheumatrex, Trexall) | • **A:** PO, IV, IM, SC, and intrathecal
• **E:** Majority excreted unchanged in urine | • Substrate for an inhibitor of dihydrofolate reductase, an enzyme in the pathway of purine synthesis
• Resistance from decreased drug accumulation and change in dihydrofolate reductase | • Breast CA
• Head and neck CA
• Non–small cell and small cell lung CA
• Gestational trophoblastic neoplasms
• Leukemias
• Lymphomas
• Choriocarcinoma
• Sarcomas
• Abortion
• Ectopic pregnancy
• RA
• Psoriasis | • GI distress (esp, diarrhea and ulcerative stomatitis)
• Hepatotoxicity
• Bone marrow suppression
• Nephrotoxicity
• Tumor lysis syndrome
• Pneumonitis
• Rash
• Malignant lymphomas |
| Pemetrexed (Alimta) | • **A:** IV
• **E:** Excreted unchanged in urine | • Inhibits multiple enzymes involved in folate metabolism and DNA synthesis | • Malignant mesothelioma
• Non–small cell lung CA | • GI distress
• Myelosuppression |

IV. Antitumor Antibiotics

ACTION OF ANTITUMOR ANTIBIOTICS

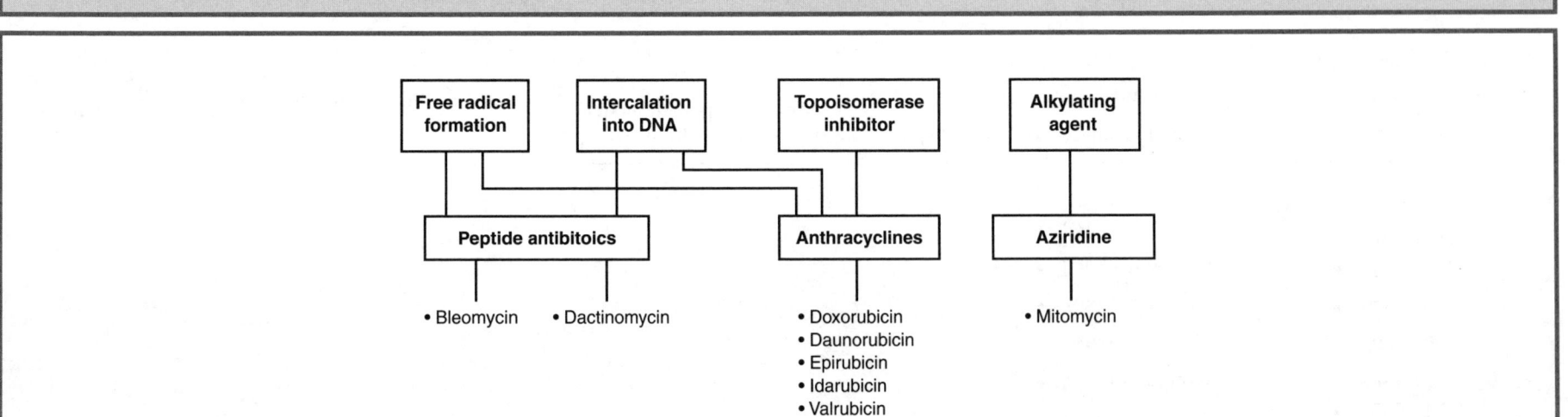

ANTITUMOR ANTIBIOTICS

Drug	Pharmacokinetics	Mechanism of Action	Clinical Uses	Side Effects
Peptide Antibiotics				
Bleomycin (Blenoxane)	• **A:** IV, IM, SC, intrapleural • **M:** Metabolized in tissues throughout the body • **E:** Metabolites excreted in urine	• Inhibit DNA and RNA synthesis causing breaks in double and single strands	• Squamous cell carcinoma (head, neck, penis, cervix, vulva) • Testicular CA • Lymphoma (Hodgkin's and Non-Hodgkin's) • Sclerosing agent for malignancy pleural effusions	• Pulmonary fibrosis • Hypersensitivity reactions
Dactinomycin (Cosmegen)	• **A:** IV • **E:** Majority excreted unchanged in urine	• Inhibit DNA and RNA synthesis by intercalation into DNA base pairs	• Testicular CA • Wilms' tumor • Ewing sarcoma • Rhabdomyosarcoma • Gestational trophoblastic neoplasm	• Myelosuppression • Hepatotoxicity
Anthracyclines				
Doxorubicin (Adriamycin)	• **A:** IV • **M:** Hepatic (P450 Doxorubicin only) • **E:** Metabolites excreted urine and feces	1. Inhibit DNA and RNA synthesis by intercalation into DNA base pairs triggering DNA cleavage 2. Inhibit topoisomerase II which prevents DNA uncoiling thus preventing transcription and replication 3. Generate free radicals that damage proteins, cell membranes, and DNA	• Bladder CA • Breast CA • Gastric CA • Leukemia • Neuroblastoma • Ovarian CA • Small cell lung CA • Thyroid CA • Myeloma • Sarcomas • Hodgkin's lymphoma	• Necrotizing colitis • Myelosuppression • Secondary malignancy (esp, AML) • Myocardial toxicity • Inhibits P450 enzymes • Induces P450 enzymes

Continued

ANTITUMOR ANTIBIOTICS (Continued)

Drug	Pharmacokinetics	Mechanism of Action	Clinical Uses	Side Effects
Daunorubicin (Cerubidine)			• Leukemias (AML & ALL)	• Myelosuppression • Secondary malignancy (esp, AML) • Myocardial toxicity
Epirubicin (Ellence)			• Breast CA	• Amenorrhea • Alopecia • Nausea and vomiting • Myelosuppression • Secondary malignancy (esp, AML) • Myocardial toxicity
Idarubicin (Idamycin)			• AML	• Nausea and vomiting • Elevated bilirubin • Elevated transaminases • Myelosuppression • Myocardial toxicity

Valrubicin (Valstar)	• **A:** Intravesicular • **E:** Excreted unchanged in urine		• BCG refractory bladder CA	• Bladder irritation • Hematuria • Bladder perforation • Myelosuppression • Myocardial toxicity • Secondary malignancy (esp, AML)
Mitoxantrone (Novantrone)	• **A:** IV • **M:** Hepatic • **E:** Excreted in urine and feces		• Multiple sclerosis • Acute nonlymphocytic leukemias • Advanced prostate CA	• Nausea, vomiting, diarrhea • Myelosuppression • Secondary malignancy (esp, AML) • Myocardial toxicity • Inhibits P450 enzymes

Aziridine

Mitomycin (Mutamycin)	• **A:** IV • **M:** Hepatic • **E:** Majority of parent drug and metabolites excreted in urine	• Hepatic metabolism to alkylating agent that cross links DNA	• Adenocarcinomas of the pancreas and stomach	• HUS • TTP • Myelosuppression • Pulmonary fibrosis • Nephrotoxicity

V. Plant Alkaloids

PLANT ALKALOIDS BY ACTION AND CLASS

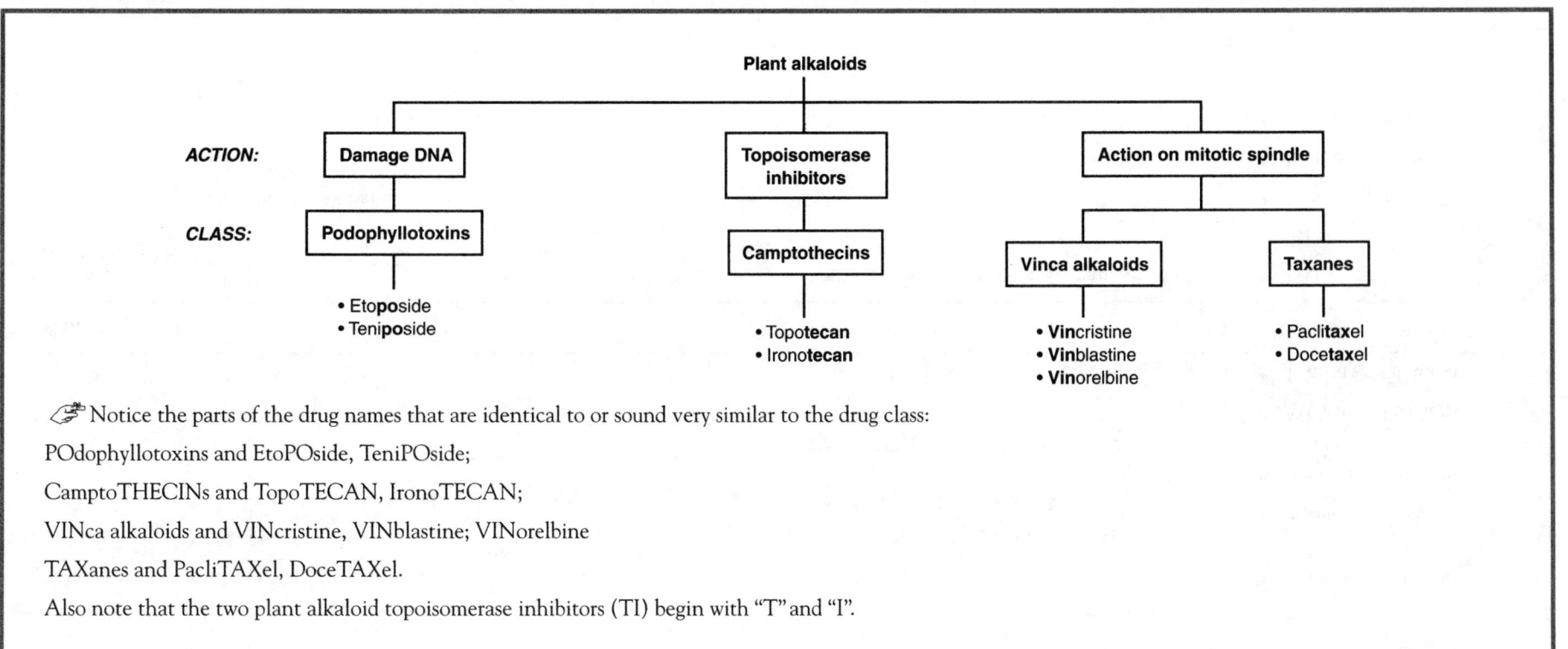

☞ Notice the parts of the drug names that are identical to or sound very similar to the drug class:

POdophyllotoxins and EtoPOside, TeniPOside;

CamptoTHECINs and TopoTECAN, IronoTECAN;

VINca alkaloids and VINcristine, VINblastine; VINorelbine

TAXanes and PacliTAXel, DoceTAXel.

Also note that the two plant alkaloid topoisomerase inhibitors (TI) begin with "T" and "I".

PLANT ALKALOIDS: DRUG FACTS

Drug	Pharmacokinetics	Mechanism of Action	Clinical Uses	Side Effects
Vinca Alkaloids				
Vincristine (Vincasar)	• **A:** IV • **M:** Hepatic (P450) • **E:** Metabolites excreted in feces and urine	• Spindle poisons that bind to the tubulin necessary for midline alignment of chromosomes and separation to the poles in mitosis • Increase apoptosis signals • Most effective during the S and M phases of the cell cycle	• Wilms' tumor • Leukemia • Lymphoma • Neuroblastoma • Rhabdomyosarcoma • Small cell lung CA	• Constipation • Neurotoxicity • GI (constipation, necrosis, paralytic ileus) • Inhibits P450 enzymes
Vinblastine (Velban, Velsar)			• AIDS-related Kaposi's sarcoma • Breast CA • Lymphoma (Hodgkin's and non-Hodgkin's) • Testicular CA	• Alopecia • Constipation • Myelosuppression • Inhibits P450 enzymes • Induces P450 enzymes
Vinorelbine (Navelbine)			• Non–small cell lung CA	• Peripheral neuropathy • Granulocytopenia • Myelosuppression • Inhibits P450 enzymes
Podophyllotoxins				
Etoposide (VP-16, VePesid)	• **A:** IV, PO • **M:** Hepatic (P450) • **E:** Majority of parent drug and metabolites excreted in urine; remainder	• Increases degradation of DNA • Inhibits mitochondrial electron transport • Topoisomerase inhibitor • Most effective during late S and early G2 phases of the cell cycle	• Small cell • Lung CA • Testicular CA	• Alopecia • GI distress • Myelosuppression • Inhibits P450 enzymes

Continued

PLANT ALKALOIDS: DRUG FACTS (Continued)

Drug	Pharmacokinetics	Mechanism of Action	Clinical Uses	Side Effects
Teniposide (Vumon)	• **A:** IV • **M:** Hepatic (P450) • **E:** Parent drug and metabolites primarily excreted in urine		• Leukemia	• GI distress • Myelosuppression • Hypersensitivity reactions • Inhibits P450 enzymes
Camptothecins				
Topotecan (Hycamtin)	• **A:** IV, PO • **M:** pH-dependent hydrolysis in plasma; minor hepatic metabolism • **E:** Majority of parent drug and metabolites excreted in urine; remainder in feces	• Inhibit topoisomerase I • Results in DNA damage	• Metastatic ovarian CA • Small cell lung CA • Cervical CA	• Alopecia • Myelosuppression • GI distress
Irinotecan (Camptosar)	• **A:** IV • **M:** Hepatic (P450) • **E:** Parent drug and metabolites excreted in urine		• Metastatic colorectal CA	• GI distress (especially severe diarrhea) • Hyperbilirubinemia • Myelosuppression

Taxanes				
Paclitaxel (Taxol)	• **A:** IV, intraperitoneal • **M:** Hepatic (P450) • **E:** Majority of parent drug and metabolites excreted in feces; remainder in urine	• Spindle poisons that prevent microtubule disassembly into tubulin monomers • Disrupt mitosis resulting in inhibition of DNA, RNA and protein synthesis	• Metastatic breast CA • AIDS-related Kaposi's sarcoma • Ovarian CA • Non–small cell lung CA	• Hypersensitivity reactions • Peripheral neuropathy • Myelosuppression • Induces P450 enzymes
Docetaxel (Taxotere, Docefrez)			• Breast CA • Non–small cell lung CA • Prostate CA • Gastric adenocarcinoma • Head and neck CA	• Anemia • Neurotoxicity • Neutropenia • Thrombocytopenia • Fluid retention (ascites, pleural effusion) • Hypersensitivity reactions • Inhibits P450 enzymes

VI. Hormonal Anticancer Drugs

CLASSIFICATION OF HORMONAL ANTICANCER DRUGS

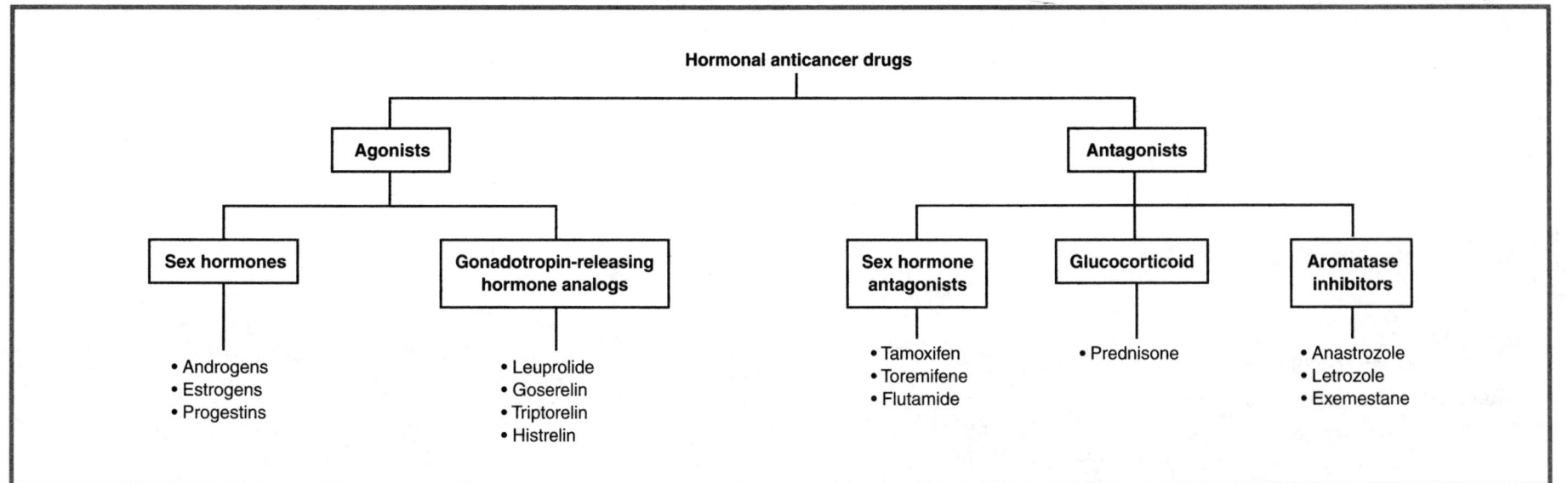

HORMONAL ANTICANCER DRUG FACTS

Drug/Group	Route of Administration	Mechanism of Action	Clinical Uses	Side Effects
Sex Hormones				
Androgens Estrogens Progestins	• Refer to Chapter 9: VI. Drugs Affecting Reproductive Hormones	• Alter hormone balance to not favor tumor growth	• Androgens tend to be used in breast CAs • Estrogens are used in prostate CA	• Varies with hormone
Gonadotropin-Releasing Hormone Analogs				
Leuprolide (Lupron, Eligard)	• SC, IM	• GnRH agonists • Inhibit release of pituitary luteinizing hormone and follicle-stimulating hormone	• Advanced prostate CA	• Bone pain • Gynecomastia • Impotence • Headache • Depression • Insomnia • Nausea and vomiting
Goserelin (Zoladex)	• Implant			
Triptorelin (Trelstar)	• IM			
Histrelin (Supprelin LA, Vantas)	• Implant			

Continued

HORMONAL ANTICANCER DRUG FACTS (Continued)

Drug/Group	Route of Administration	Mechanism of Action	Clinical Uses	Side Effects
Sex Hormone Antagonists				
Tamoxifen (Soltamox)	• PO	• Selective estrogen receptor modulator	• Breast CA	• GI distress (nausea and vomiting) • Hot flashes • Increased incidence of uterine or endometrial CA • Peripheral edema • Vaginal bleeding/discharge
Toremifene (Fareston)			• Breast CA	• Hepatotoxicity • QT prolongation • Hot flashes • Nausea
Flutamide (Eulexin)		• Androgen-receptor antagonist	• Metastatic • Prostate CA	• Gynecomastia • Hot flashes • Hepatotoxicity

Glucocorticoids

| Prednisone (Deltasone) | • PO | • Anti-inflammatory via inhibition of the inflammatory cells
• Exact mechanism unknown
• May trigger apoptosis | • Acute and chronic lymphocytic leukemia
• Hodgkin's lymphoma
• Non-Hodgkin's lymphoma | • Adrenal suppression
• Osteoporosis
• Redistribution of body fat
• Cushing-like symptoms
• Cataracts
• Hypertension
• Ulcers
• Acne |

Aromatase Inhibitors

| Anastrozole (Arimidex)
Letrozole (Femara)
Exemestane (Aromasin) | • PO | • Inhibit aromatase, the enzyme that catalyzes the conversion of androstenedione to estrone | • Advanced breast CA | • Arthralgias
• GI distress (nausea and abdominal pain)
• Hot flashes |

VII. Chemotherapeutic Drugs

MISCELLANEOUS CHEMOTHERAPEUTICS: DRUG FACTS

Drug	Pharmacokinetics	Mechanism of Action	Clinical Uses	Side Effects
Asparaginase (Elspar)	• **A:** IV and IM • **M:** Metabolic fate unknown • **E:** Only trace amounts recovered in urine	• An enzyme that degrades asparagine, an essential amino acid for tumor cell growth	• Acute lymphoblastic leukemia	• Bleeding • Hypersensitivity reactions • Pancreatitis
Mitoxantrone (Novantrone)	• **A:** IV • **M:** Hepatic • **E:** Metabolites excreted in urine and feces	• Incorporates into DNA causing cross links and strand breaks	• Acute non-lymphocytic leukemias • Prostate CA • Relapsing multiple sclerosis	• GI distress (nausea, vomiting, abdominal pain) • Cytopenia • CHF • Severe tissue domage with extravasation • Risk of AML • Inhibits P450 enzymes
Dasatinib (Sprycel)	• **A:** PO • **M:** Hepatic (P450) • **E:** Parent drug and metabolites excreted in feces	• Tyrosine kinase inhibitor which halts leukemia cell proliferation	• Chronic myelogenous leukemia • Philadelphia chromosome+ acute lymphocytic leukemia	• Myelosuppression • Inhibits P450 enzymes
Denileukin (Ontak)	• **A:** IV • **M:** Hepatic	• Fusion protein of amino acid sequences from diphtheria toxin and IL-2 that selectively delivers diphtheria toxin to targeted cells	• Cutaneous T cell lymphoma	• GI distress • Vision loss • Capillary leak syndrome

Erlotinib (Tarceva)	• **A:** PO • **M:** Hepatic (P450) • **E:** Primarily excreted as metabolites in feces	• Tyrosine kinase inhibitor	• Non–small cell lung CA • Pancreatic CA	
Everolimus (Afinitor, Zortress)	• **A:** PO • **M:** Hepatic (P450) • **E:** Primarily excreted as metabolites in feces	• Binds FK-binding protein-12 intracellularly decreasing protein synthesis and cell proliferation • Inhibits vascular endothelial growth factor	• Pancreatic CA • Astrocytoma with tuberous sclerosis • Renal cell CA • Prophylaxis for renal transplants	• Immunosuppression • Increased risk of infection • Increased risk of secondary malignancies • Myelosuppression • GI distress
Bacillus Calmette Guerine/BCG (TheraCys, TICE BCG)	• **A:** Intravesicular • **E:** Excreted unchanged in urine	• Causes a local inflammatory response leading to destruction of superficial tumor cells of the urothelium	• CA in situ of the bladder	• Dysuria • Urinary frequency • Hematuria
Ixabepilone (Ixempra)	• **A:** IV • **M:** Hepatic (P450) • **E:** Primarily excreted as metabolites in feces	• Tubulin polymerizing agent • Binds β tubulin subunit of microtubule	• Breast CA (metastatic or locally advanced)	• Peripheral neuropathy • Myelosuppression • Hepatotoxicity

CHEMOTHERAPEUTICS: MONOCLONAL ANTIBODIES

Drug	Route of Administration	Mechanism of Action	Clinical Uses	Side Effects
Rituximab (Rituxan)	• IV	• A mouse/human chimera • Monoclonal antibody targeted at CD20 antigen on B lymphocytes leading to activation of complement-mediated B cell cytotoxicity	• NHL • CLL • Granulomatosis with polyangiitis	• Fever • Tumor lysis syndrome • Infusion reaction • Mucocutaneous reactions (ie, SJS) • PML secondary to JC viral infection
Trastuzumab (Herceptin)		• Monoclonal Ab against HER-2 protein, a surface protein overexpressed in breast cancer and gastric cancer leading to cellular cytotoxicity of cells with HER-2 protein	• Breast CA • Gastric CA	• Cardiomyopathy • Pulmonary disease (ARDS, pulmonary fibrosis) • GI distress (nausea, vomiting)
Bevacizumab (Avastin)		• Monoclonal Ab that binds and neutralizes vascular endothelial growth factor inhibiting angiogenesis	• Metastatic colorectal cancer • Glioblastoma • Recurrent or metastatic NSC lung cancer • Metastatic renal CA	• Hemorrhage • GI distress • GI perforation • Wound dehiscence • Thromboembolic events
Cetuximab (Erbitux)		• Monoclonal Ab that binds to epidermal growth factor receptor resulting in inhibition of cell growth and induction of apoptosis	• Metastatic colorectal cancer • Head and neck squamous cell carcinoma	• CP arrest • Acneiform rash • GI distress • Fatigue • Hypomagnesemia
Alemtuzumab (Campath)		• Monoclonal Ab that binds to CD52 antigen on B and T lymphocytes triggering T cell lysis	• B cell chronic lymphocytic leukemia	• Infections • Bone marrow suppression

CHAPTER 11
IMMUNOMODULATORS

I. DRUGS THAT INFLUENCE THE IMMUNE RESPONSE

Classification of Immunomodulators

II. IMMUNOSUPPRESSANTS

Immunosuppressants: Drug Facts

Antibody Immunosuppressant Facts

Sites of Action of Immunosuppressive Drugs

III. IMMUNOSTIMULANTS

Immunostimulants: Drug Facts

TERMS TO LEARN

Aplastic Anemia	Low blood count due to defective regeneration of cells.
Erythema Nodosum Leprosum	Painful erythematous subcutaneous nodules seen in patients with a high level of mycobacterial antigens.
Hirsutism	Excessive body and facial hair in women.
Kawasaki Disease	Medium to large vessel vasculitis seen in children; symptoms include conjunctivitis, rash, erythema of the palms and soles, coronary aneurysms, and strawberry tongue.
Malignant Osteopetrosis	Increased skeletal density due to osteoclastic failure.

I. Drugs that Influence the Immune Response

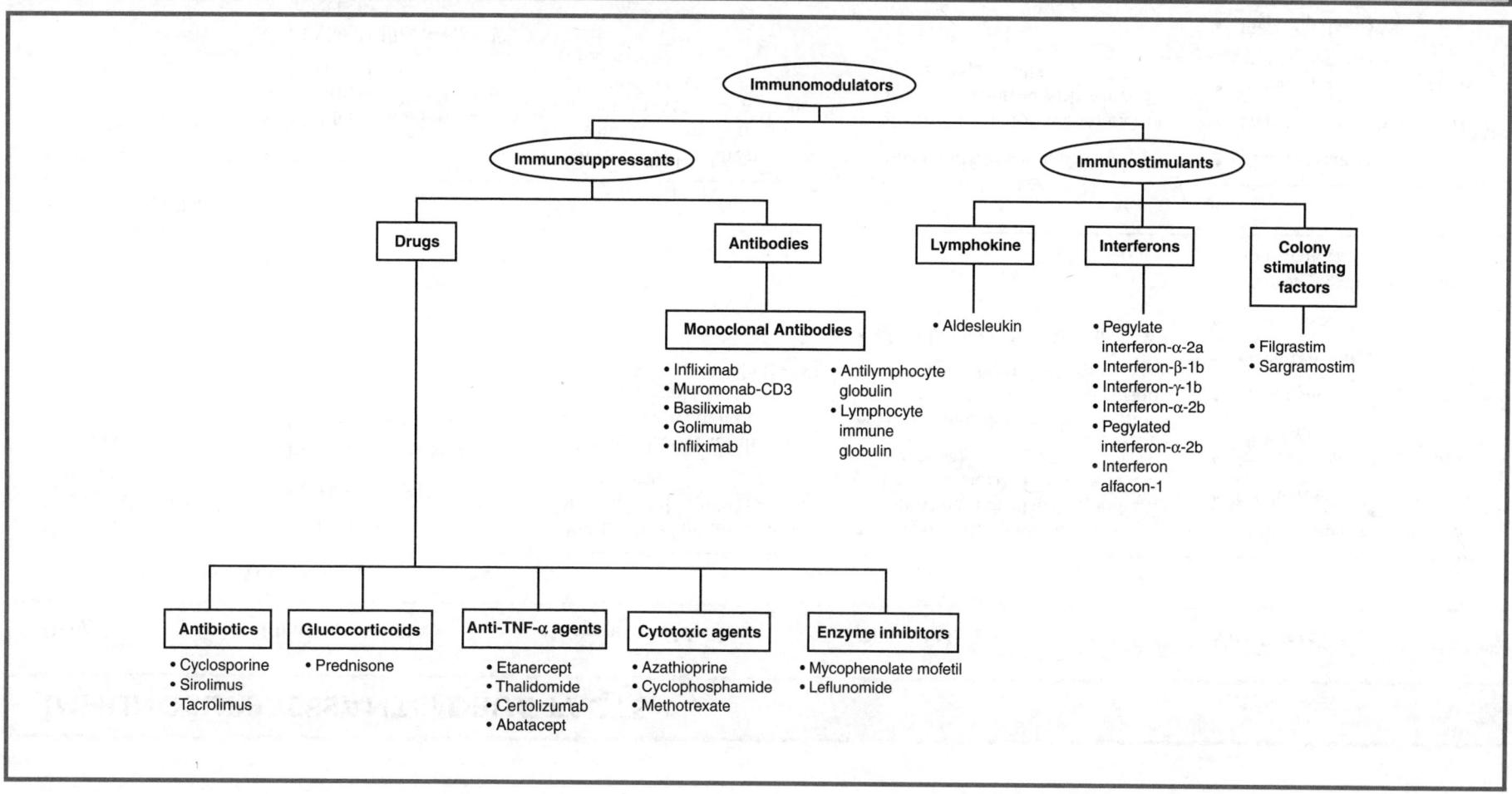

IMMUNOSUPPRESSANTS: DRUG FACTS

Drug	Pharmacokinetics	Mechanism of Action	Clinical Uses	Side Effects
Fungal Cyclic Peptide Antibiotic				
Cyclosporine (Neoral, Gengraf, Sandimmune)	• A: PO or IV • M: Hepatic (P450) • E: Metabolites excreted in feces	• Binds to cyclophilin to form a complex that inhibits calcineurin • Highly selective inhibition of T cell activation by blocking cytokine production (especially IL-2)	• Prophylaxis for organ rejection following transplant (ie, kidney, heart, liver, BMT, lung, and pancreas) • Treatment of graft versus host reactions (often in combination with corticosteroids) • Autoimmune disorders (ie, RA and severe psoriasis)	• Gingival hyperplasia • GI distress • Increased risk of infections and malignancies • Hirsutism • Hypertension • Nephrotoxicity • Neurologic effects (seizures and tremor)
Macrolide Antibiotics				
Sirolimus (Rapamune)	• A: PO • M: Metabolized in intestinal wall and hepatic (P450) • E: Metabolites excreted in feces	• Binds to FK-binding protein, inhibiting the response of T cells to cytokines without affecting cytokine production	• Liver and kidney transplantation • Potentially useful in conjunction with cyclosporine with which it acts synergistically	• Blood dyscrasias • Hepatic artery thrombosis • Increased risk of infections and malignancies • Hyperlipidemia • Hypertension • Rash • Peripheral edema • Inhibits P450 enzymes

Tacrolimus / FK-506 (Prograf, Hecoria)	• **A:** PO or IV • **M:** Hepatic (P450) • **E:** Metabolites excreted in feces	• Binds to FK-binding protein and forms a complex that inhibits calcineurin • Calcineurin regulates the T cells ability to produce interleukins	• 10–100 times more potent immunosuppression than cyclosporine • Liver, cardiac, and kidney transplantation	• Asthenia • Blood dyscrasias • GI (diarrhea, nausea, abdominal pain) • Hyperglycemia due to new onset diabetes • Increased risk of infections and malignancies • Nephrotoxicity • Neurotoxicity • Hyperkalemia • Inhibits P450 enzymes

Glucocorticoid

Prednisone	• **A:** PO • **M:** Metabolized in multiple tissues including the liver (P450 minor) • **E:** Metabolites excreted in urine	• Impaired release of cytokines from macrophages and granulocytes • Suppression of T cell proliferation and activation • Suppression of antibody production • Reduction of accumulation of macrophages • Seems to spare B cell population under normal conditions • Inhibit migration of cells that cause acute rejection of an organ, which is an inflammatory response	• Administered before, during, and after transplant surgery (always used in combination with other immunosuppressants, such as cyclosporine, for organ transplantation) • Autoimmune diseases (eg, RA, SLE, and dermatomyositis) • Treatment of acute graft versus host rejection (suppress secondary [antibody] response via B cell suppression) • Attenuation of allergic reactions • Treatment of asthma • Treatment of PCP pneumonia • Treatment of ITP • Treatment of lupus nephritis and nephrotic syndrome	• Adrenal suppression (cushingoid reactions) associated with an inability to regulate endogenous glucocorticoid levels following use • Osteoporosis (LTU) • Redistribution of body fat • Inhibition of growth • Myopathy • Development of cataracts, glaucoma • Kaposi's sarcoma with prolonged use • Psychiatric disturbances • Inhibits P450 enzymes • Induces P450 enzymes

Continued

IMMUNOSUPPRESSANTS: DRUG FACTS (Continued)

Drug	Pharmacokinetics	Mechanism of Action	Clinical Uses	Side Effects
Anti TNF-α Agents				
Thalidomide (Thalomid)	• **A:** PO • **M:** Undergoes nonenzymatic hydrolysis	• May act as a selective inhibitor of TNF-α but immunologic effect varies on condition	• Treatment and prophylaxis of erythema nodosum leprosum • Treatment of multiple myeloma • Treatment of GVHD	• Dizziness • Drowsiness • GI distress (diarrhea, nausea, constipation, abdominal pain) • Peripheral neuropathy • Edema • Hypocalcemia • Increased risk of thrombosis
Etanercept (Enbrel)	• **A:** SC • **M:** Possibly metabolized by reticuloendothelial system • **E:** Metabolites excreted in urine	• Solution of TNF receptor linked to Fc portion of human IgG1 • Acts as a competitive inhibitor of TNF • Binds TNF and blocks its interaction with the cell surface receptors	• Treatment of RA and juvenile RA	• CNS symptoms suggestive of demyelinating conditions • Increased risk of infections and malignancies

Golimumab (Simponi)	• SC	• Monoclonal antibodies against TNF-α	• Rheumatoid arthritis • Psoriatic arthritis • Ankylosing spondylitis	• Headache • Cardiac arrhythmias • Increased risk for infections and malignancies
Adalimumab (Humira)	• SC		• Rheumatoid arthritis • JRA (Adalimumab only) • Psoriatic arthritis • Ankylosing spondylitis • Plaque psoriasis • Ulcerative colitis • Crohn's disease	• Increased risk for infections and malignancies • GI distress (abdominal pain, nausea, vomiting) • Infusion-related reactions (fevers, chills, pruritis, chest pain, dyspnea, hypotension, myalgia)
Infliximab (Remicade)	• IV			
Certolizumab pegol (Cimzia)	• SC	• Humanized antibody Fab fragment of TNF-α monoclonal antibody that binds to and selectively neutralizes human TNF-α	• Rheumatoid arthritis • Crohn's disease	• Increased risk for infections and malignancies • Nausea
Cytotoxic Agents				
Azathioprine (Imuran, Azasan)	• **A:** PO and IV • **M:** Hepatic, prodrug slowly converted to 6-mercaptopurine • **E:** Metabolites excreted in urine	• Blocks de novo purine synthesis and interferes with DNA synthesis • Somewhat more effect on T cells than B cells	• Autoimmune diseases (ie, RA, SLE) • Prophylaxis of rejection in renal transplants	• Leukopenia • Thrombocytopenia • Rash • GI disturbances • Hepatotoxicity • Increased risk of malignancies

Continued

IMMUNOSUPPRESSANTS: DRUG FACTS (Continued)

Drug	Pharmacokinetics	Mechanism of Action	Clinical Uses	Side Effects
Cyclophosphamide (Cytoxan)	• A: PO, IV, IM, and intracavitary • M: Hepatic (P450) • E: Parent drug and metabolites excreted in urine	• Inhibits DNA and RNA synthesis via cross-linking of these molecules • Destroys any proliferating lymphoid cells (more effective suppression of B cell proliferation)	• Chemotherapy for solid tumor malignancies • Treatment of pediatric nephrotic syndrome	• Hematologic disturbances (anemia, leukopenia, thrombocytopenia) • Severe nausea and vomiting • Hemorrhagic cystitis • Cardiotoxic • Alopecia • Decreased fertility • Inhibits P450 enzymes • Induces P450 enzymes
Methotrexate / MTX (Trexall, Rheumatrex)	• A: PO, IM, IV, and intrathecal • E: Majority excreted unchanged in urine	• Inhibits dihydrofolate reductase blocking synthesis of nucleoside phosphates inhibiting DNA synthesis • Rapidly proliferating cells are destroyed	• Treatment of autoimmune diseases (eg, RA and psoriasis) • Chemotherapy • Combined therapy with cyclosporine with graft versus host reactions following BMT	• GI tract irritation (diarrhea, ulcerative stomatitis) • Hepatotoxicity • Pneumonitis • Bone marrow suppression • Severe rashes • Severe opportunistic infections • Tumor lysis syndrome • Nephrotoxicity

Enzyme Inhibitors				
Mycophenolate Mofetil (Cellcept, Myfortic)	• **A:** PO and IV • **M:** Metabolized presystemically to active metabolite in liver and GI tract • **E:** Metabolites excreted primarily in urine	• Metabolite (MPA) inhibits inosine monophosphate dehydrogenase, an enzyme in the de novo purine synthesis pathway • Blocks de novo purine synthesis • Results in inhibition of B and T lymphocyte proliferation	• Prophylaxis for heart, liver, and kidney transplant rejection • Typically used with cyclosporine and prednisone	• Hypertension • Hyperglycemia • Hypercholesterolemia • Neutropenia • Increased risk of lymphoma and skin malignancies • Increased risk of infection
Leflunomide (Arava)	• **A:** PO • **M:** Hepatic • **E:** Metabolites excreted in urine and feces	• Inhibits dihydroorotate dehydrogenase, an enzyme in the de novo pyrimidine synthesis pathway • Blocks de novo pyrimidine synthesis • Results in inhibition of B and T lymphocyte proliferation	• Treatment of RA	• Alopecia • GI distress (diarrhea, nausea, constipation, abdominal pain) • Hepatotoxicity • Hypertension • Interstitial lung disease • Peripheral neuropathy • Malignancies • Inhibits P450 enzymes
Tofacitinib (Xeljanz)	• **A:** PO • **M:** Hepatic (P450) to active metabolite • **E:** Parent drug and metabolites excreted in urine	• Inhibits Janus kinase enzymes which is involved in hematopoiesis and immune cell function	• RA	• Increased risk for infections and malignancies
Apremilast (Otezla)	• **A:** PO • **M:** Hepatic (P450) • **E:** Metabolites excreted in feces and urine	• Inhibits PDE 4 thus increasing the level of cAMP and thus regulating inflammatory compounds	• Plaque psoriasis • Psoriatic arthritis	• GI distress (nausea, diarrhea)

ANTIBODY IMMUNOSUPPRESSANT FACTS

Drug	Pharmacokinetics	Mechanism of Action	Clinical Uses	Side Effects
Antilymphocyte Globulin / Antilymphocyte Immune Globulin (Atgam)	• IV	• Antibodies that bind to T lymphocytes causing them to be destroyed by complement	• Treatment and prevention of acute rejection following kidney transplants • Treatment of aplastic anemia in patients not suitable for BMT	• Headache • Fever • Rash • Leukopenia • Thrombocytopenia
Immune Globulin Intravenous / IGIV / IVIG	• IV	• Precise mechanism of action unknown • May act via increase of suppressor T cells or diminution of helper T cells	• Treatment of patients with immunodeficiency syndromes • Treatment of Kawasaki syndrome (reduction of systemic inflammation and prevention of coronary aneurysms) • Treatment of severe asthma • Treatment of some autoimmune diseases (eg, ITP, MS, and SLE)	• Dyspnea • Hypersensitivity reactions • Tachycardia
Tocilizumab (Actemra)	• IV	• Monoclonal antibody that acts as an antagonist of IL-6 receptor thereby decreasing activation of inflammatory cascade	• RA and JRA	• Elevated hepatic transaminases • Increased risk of infections and malignancies • Demyelinating disease
Basiliximab (Simulect)	• IV	• Monoclonal antibody that blocks the α chain of the IL-2 receptor on activated T lymphocytes	• Prophylaxis of acute rejection following renal transplants	• Hypertension • Edema • Fever • Tremor

Muromonab-CD3 (Orthoclone OKT3)	• IV	• Monoclonal antibody, directed towards CD3 molecule on the surface of all T cells resulting in inhibition of T cells to function as T lymphocytes	• Treatment of acute rejection following kidney, heart, or liver transplants	• Blood dyscrasias • Cytokine release syndrome (flu-like symptoms) • Photophobia • CNS reactions (encephalopathy, cerebral edema, aseptic meningitis) • Neurologic reactions (headache, seizures)
Ustekinumab (Stelara)	• SC	• Monoclonal antibody that blocks the action of IL13, IL 23 which in turn blocks NK cell activation and CD4 cell activation • Inhibits production of MCP-1, TNF a, IP 10 and IL 8	• Plaque psoriasis • Psoriatic arthritis	• Increased risk for infection • Dermatologic complications (exfoliative dermatitis, erythrodermic psoriasis
Secukinumab (Cosentyx)	• SC	• Monoclonal antibody that binds to and thus blocks the action of IL17A	• Plaque psoriasis	• Increased risk for infection • Nasopharyngitis
Belimimab (Benlysta)	• IV	• Monoclonal antibody that blocks the activity of human B lymphocyte stimulator protein thus preventing B cell survival	• SLE	• GI distress (nausea, diarrhea)
Ofatumumab (Arzerra)	• IV	• Monoclonal antibody that binds to the CD 20 molecule on B lymphocytes causing cell death	• CLL	• Progressive multifocal leukoecephalopathy • Reactivation of Hepatitis B • Increased risk of infection • GI distress (nausea, diarrhea)
Rituximab (Rituxan)	• IV		• CLL • NHL • Granulomatosis with polyangiitis • RA • Microscopic polyangiitis	

Continued

ANTIBODY IMMUNOSUPPRESSANT FACTS (Continued)

Drug	Pharmacokinetics	Mechanism of Action	Clinical Uses	Side Effects
Alemtuzumab (Campath, Lemtrada)	• IV	• Monoclonal antibody that binds to CD52 molecule on B an T cells causing cell death	• B cell CLL • Relapsing MS	• Autoimmune diseases • Cytopenias • Increased risk for infections and malignancies
Natalizumab (Tysabri)	• IV	• Monoclonal antibody that binds to α4 subunit of integrin molecules (a molecule responsible for the adhesion and migration of cells from the vasculature to inflamed tissue)	• MS • Crohn's disease	• Progressive multifocal leukoencephalopathy
Fingolimod (Gilenya)	• A: PO • M: Hepatic (P450) to active metabolite • E: Primarily excreted as metabolites in urine	• Active metabolite blocks the lymphocyte's ability to emerge from the lymph node	• MS	• Headache
Teriflunomide (Aubagio)	• PO	• Inhibits pyrimidine synthesis	• MS	• Hepatotoxicity • Teratogenic effects
Belatacept (Nulojix)	• IV	• Blocks T cell activation by binding to CD80 and CD86	• Prophylaxis for acute renal transplant rejection	• Increased risk for infections and malignancies
Anakinra (Kineret)	• SC	• Blocks IL K1	• RA • Neonatal-onset multisystem inflammatory disease	• Nasopharyngitis • Headache • Increased risk for infection
Abatacept (Orencia)	• IV, SC	• Binds to proteins on antigen presenting cells inhibiting their subsequent activation of T cells	• RA • JRA	• Headache • Nasopharyngitis

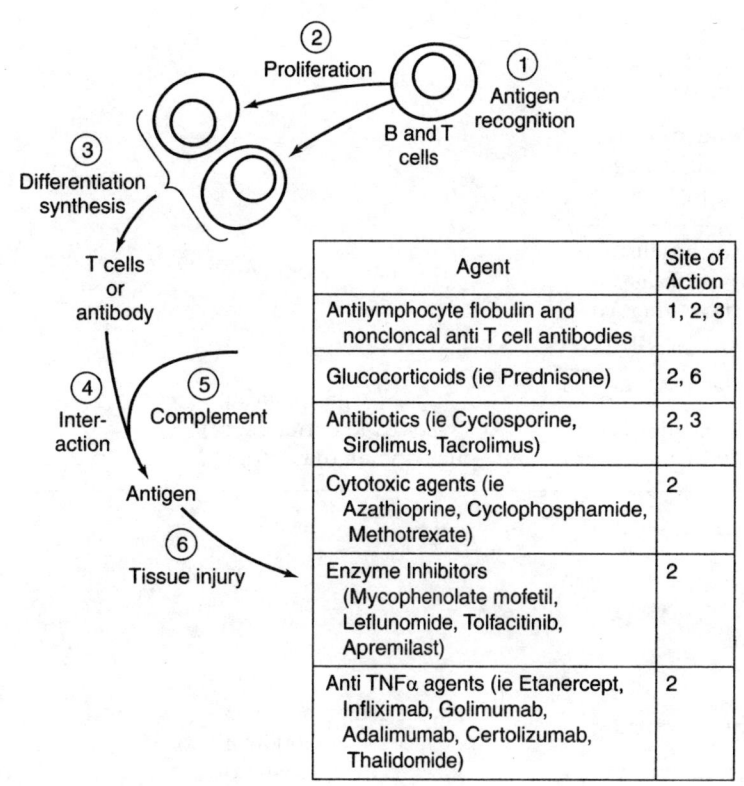

Agent	Site of Action
Antilymphocyte flobulin and noncloncal anti T cell antibodies	1, 2, 3
Glucocorticoids (ie Prednisone)	2, 6
Antibiotics (ie Cyclosporine, Sirolimus, Tacrolimus)	2, 3
Cytotoxic agents (ie Azathioprine, Cyclophosphamide, Methotrexate)	2
Enzyme Inhibitors (Mycophenolate mofetil, Leflunomide, Tolfacitinib, Apremilast)	2
Anti TNFα agents (ie Etanercept, Infliximab, Golimumab, Adalimumab, Certolizumab, Thalidomide)	2

Modified from Katzung BG, ed: *Basic & Clinical Pharmacology*, 8th ed, p 968. Originally published by Appleton & Lange. © 2001 by the McGraw-Hill Companies, Inc.

IMMUNOSTIMULANTS: DRUG FACTS

Drug	Class	Administration	Mechanism of Action	Clinical Uses	Side Effects
Aldesleukin (Proleukin)	• IL-2 lymphokine	• IV	• Increases lymphokine-activated killer cells and helper T cells	• Malignant melanoma • Renal cell carcinoma	• Blood dyscrasias • GI distress (nausea, vomiting, diarrhea) • Hepatotoxicity • Hypotension • Nephrotoxicity • Pulmonary toxicity
Filgrastim (Neupogen)	• Colony stimulating factor	• IV and SC	• Induce proliferation and maturation of various myeloid cells	• Severe chronic neutropenia • BMT recipients • Treatment of cancer patients receiving myelosuppressive chemotherapy	• Skeletal pain • Splenomegaly
Sargramostim (Leukine)				• Neutrophil recovery following induction chemotherapy in AML • Myeloid reconstitution after allogenic BMT	• Arthralgia • Headache • Myalgia • Pericardial effusion

Drug	Route	Mechanism of Action	Indications	Adverse Effects
Pegylated interferon-α-2a (Pegasys)	• SC	• Inhibit cellular growth, alter the state of cellular differentiation, interfere with oncogene expression, alter cell surface antigen expression, increase phagocytic activity of macrophages, and alter cytotoxicity of lymphocytes for target cells	• Chronic hepatitis B and C	• Chest pain • Flu-like symptoms (myalgias, fatigue, fever, chills)
Interferon alfacon-1 (Infergen)	• SC		• Chronic hepatitis C	• Aggravation of neuropsychiatric conditions • Aggravation of autoimmune disorders
Interferon-α-2b (Intron A)	• SC, IM		• Chronic hepatitis B and C • Hairy cell leukemia • Kaposi's sarcoma • Lymphoma • Malignant melanoma • Treatment of condyloma acuminata	• Aggravation of ischemic conditions • Aggravation of infectious illnesses
Pegylated interferon-α-2b (PegIntron, Redipen, Sylatron)	• SC		• Chronic hepatitis C • Melanoma (augmentative therapy)	
Interferon-β-1b (Betaseron, Extavia)	• SC		• Relapsing remitting multiple sclerosis	• Flu-like symptoms (myalgias, fatigue, fever, chills) • Lymphopenia
Interferon-γ-1b (Actimmune)	• SC		• Decrease infections in patients with chronic granulomatous disease • Inhibit disease progression in malignant osteopetrosis	• Flu-like symptoms (myalgias, fatigue, fever, chills) • GI distress (nausea, vomiting, diarrhea, anorexia, abdominal pain)

CHAPTER 12

DRUGS USED TO TREAT INFLAMMATION

I. PROSTAGLANDIN ANALOGS

Prostaglandin Analogs: Drug Facts

II. DRUGS USED IN THE TREATMENT OF GOUT

Managing Gout: Drug Facts

Mechanism of Action of Drugs Used to Treat Gout

III. ANALGESICS

Classification of Analgesics

Aspirin and Related Compounds

NSAIDs

COX-2 Inhibitors

Acetaminophen

Mechanism of Action of Aspirin, NSAIDs, and COX 2 Inhibitors

IV. H₁ BLOCKERS (ANTIHISTAMINES)

Classification of H₁ Blockers (Antihistamines)

First- and Second-Generation H₁ Blockers

TERMS TO LEARN

Abortifacient	An agent that causes an abortion.
Dysmenorrhea	Painful menstruation.
Orthostatic Hypotension	Low blood pressure in the standing position.
Tinnitis	Ringing in the ears.

I. Prostaglandin Analogs

PROSTAGLANDIN ANALOGS: DRUG FACTS

Drug	Pharmacokinetics	Clinical Uses	Side Effects
PGE$_1$ Analogs			
Alprostadil (Prostin, Muse, Caverject)	• **A:** IV, intracavernosal injection, and intraurethral suppository • **M:** Metabolized in the lungs • **E:** Metabolites excreted in urine	• Maintains patent ductus arteriosus in infants with this condition or with congenital heart defects until surgical repair (Prostin) • Erectile dysfunction (Caverject—penile injection; Muse—suppository)	• Flushing • Bradycardia/tachycardia • Hypotension • Diarrhea • May result in gastric obstruction secondary to antral hyperplasia in neonates
Misoprostol (Cytotec)	• **A:** PO • **M:** Hepatic • **E:** Majority of metabolites excreted in urine; remainder in feces	• Treatment and prophylaxis of NSAID-induced gastric ulcer • Abortifacient • Cervical ripening and induction of labor	• GI effects (abdominal pain, diarrhea, constipation, and dyspepsia) • Headache • Vaginal bleeding

Continued

PROSTAGLANDIN ANALOGS: DRUG FACTS (Continued)

Drug	Pharmacokinetics	Clinical Uses	Side Effects
PGE₂ Analog			
Dinoprostone (Prepidil, ProstinE2, Cervidil)	• **A:** Vaginal gel and suppository • **M:** Metabolized in lungs, kidneys, spleen, and other tissues • **E:** Majority of parent drug and metabolites excreted in urine; remainder in feces	• Vaginal suppository to ripen cervix and induce labor (Prepidil—gel) • Induce abortion (Prostin E2—vaginal suppository) • Both indications (Cervidil)	• Chills/shivering • GI effects (abdominal pain, diarrhea, nausea, and vomiting) • Headache
PGI₂ Analog			
Epoprostenol (Flolan)	• **A:** IV • **M:** Hydrolyzed in plasma • **E:** Majority of metabolites excreted in urine; remainder in feces	• Pulmonary hypertension (drug of last resort, not very effective)	• Flushing • GI effects (abdominal pain, diarrhea, nausea, and vomiting) • Headache • Hypotension

II. Drugs Used in the Treatment of Gout

MANAGING GOUT: DRUG FACTS

Drug	Pharmacokinetics	Mechanism of Action	Clinical Uses	Drawbacks and Side Effects
Indomethacin (Indocin)	• **A:** PO, IV, or rectal • **M:** Hepatic (P450 minor) • **E:** Metabolites primarily excreted in urine	• NSAID that inhibits COX • Reduces production of prostaglandins • Inhibits phagocytosis of uric acid crystal by macrophages	• Acute treatment of gouty arthritis	• GI effects (irritation, bleeding, and ulceration) • Renal effects (dysuria, interstitial nephritis, and renal failure) • CNS effects (headache, dizziness) • Hepatic effects (jaundice, cholestatic hepatitis) • Hematologic effects (thrombocytopenia, leukopenia) • Inhibits P450 enzymes
Colchicine	• **A:** PO and IV • **M:** Hepatic (P450) • **E:** Parent drug and metabolites primarily excreted in urine	• Disrupts the inflammatory cycle, which inhibits leukocyte migration and phagocytosis of uric acid crystals	• Acute treatment of gouty arthritis • Low doses useful for chronic treatment of gout	• Narrow therapeutic window so must be carefully titrated to effective dose in each individual • Overdose can lead to nephrotoxicity, hepatotoxicity, or death • Long $t_{1/2}$ in the white blood cells leading to systemic accumulation (must wait 3–4 days between uses) • IV dose must be administered in an indwelling catheter due to irritation • GI side effects (nausea, abdominal discomfort, vomiting, and diarrhea)

Continued

Drug	Pharmacokinetics	Mechanism of Action	Clinical Uses	Drawbacks and Side Effects
Allopurinol (Zyloprim)	• **A:** PO • **M:** Primarily hepatic metabolism; active metabolite formed (oxipurinol) • **E:** Parent drug and metabolites primarily excreted in urine	• Blocks xanthine oxidase thereby decreasing the production of uric acid	• Treatment of chronic gout • Should be initiated 1–2 weeks following gout attack	• Precipitation of gout attack during initiation of therapy • GI upset • Allergic dermatitis • Vasculitis • Peripheral neuritis • Should not be administered with azathioprine or mercaptopurine, which are metabolized by xanthine oxidase
Febuxostat (Uloric)	• **A:** PO • **M:** Hepatic (partial P450) • **E:** Primarily excreted as metabolites in urine	• Blocks xanthine oxidase thereby decreasing the production of uric acid	• Treatment of chronic gout	• Precipitations of gout attack during initiation of therapy • Should not be administistered with azathioprine or mercaptopurine, which are metabolized by xanthine oxidase • Elevated LFTs • Higher rate of cardiovascular thromboembolic events
Rasburicase (Elitek)	• **A:** IV • **M:** Peptide hydrolysis	• Recombinant form of urate oxidase • Catalyzes the conversion of uric acid to allantoin	• Treatment of chronic gout • Prevention and treatment of tumor lysis syndrome	• Contraindicated in patients with G6PD deficiency • Hypersensitivity reactions (ie, anaphylaxis) • Can precipitate methemoglobinemia • GI: diarrhea, abdominal pain • Neuro: HA • Derm: rash, mucositis
Probenecid (Benemid, Probalan)	• **A:** PO • **M:** Hepatic metabolism • **E:** Parent drug and metabolites excreted in urine	• Increases urinary excretion of uric acid (inhibits reabsorption of uric acid in the proximal tubule)		• Allergic dermatitis • Anorexia, nausea, and vomiting • Precipitation of gout attack during initiation of therapy • Renal calculi • Inhibits P450 enzymes

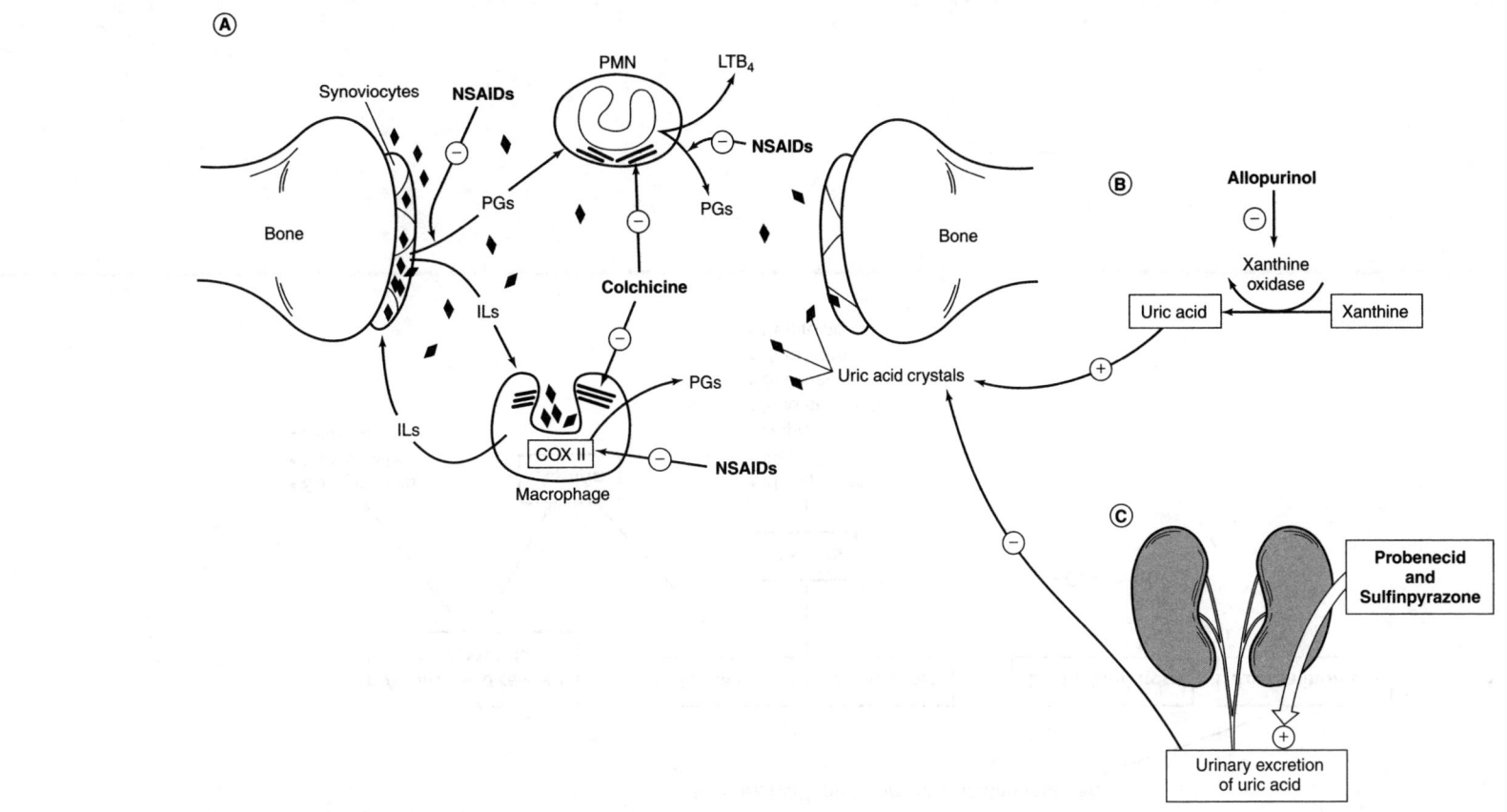

- **A:** Sites of action of some anti-inflammatory drugs in a gouty joint. Synoviocytes damaged by uric acid crystals release prostaglandins (PGs), interleukins (ILs), and other mediators of inflammation. Polymorphonuclear leukocytes (PMNs), macrophages, and other inflammatory cells enter the joint and also release inflammatory substances, including leukotrienes (eg, LTB_4), that attract additional inflammatory cells. Colchicine acts on microtubules in the inflammatory cells. NSAIDs act on COX-2 in all of the cells of the joint.
- **B:** Allopurinol decreases the production of uric acid by inhibiting xanthine oxidase.
- **C:** Probenecid and sulfinpyrazone increase the urinary excretion of uric acid by inhibiting reabsorption of uric acid in the proximal tubule.

Modified from Trevor AJ, Katzung BG, Masters SB: *Katzung & Trevor's Pharmacology Examination & Board Review*, 6th ed. Originally published by Appleton & Lange. © 2002 by the McGraw-Hill Companies, Inc.

III. Analgesics

CLASSIFICATION OF ANALGESICS

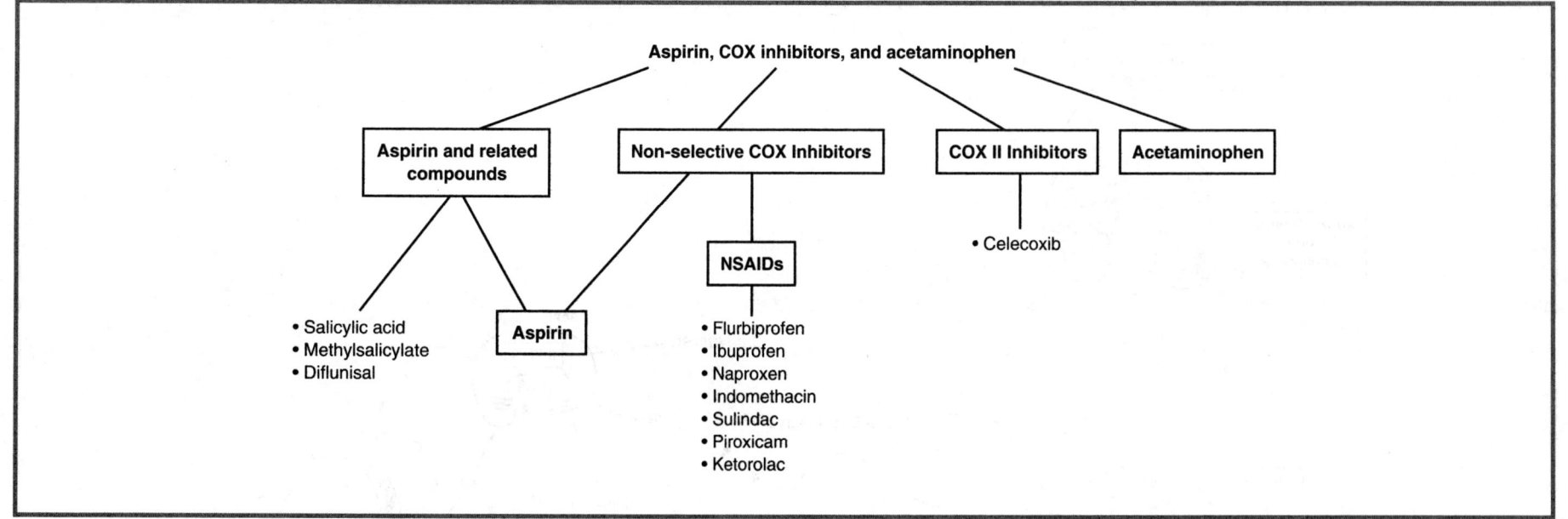

Aspirin, COX inhibitors, and acetaminophen

Aspirin and related compounds

Non-selective COX Inhibitors

COX II Inhibitors

Acetaminophen

• Salicylic acid
• Methylsalicylate
• Diflunisal

Aspirin

NSAIDs

• Flurbiprofen
• Ibuprofen
• Naproxen
• Indomethacin
• Sulindac
• Piroxicam
• Ketorolac

• Celecoxib

ASPIRIN AND RELATED COMPOUNDS

Drug	Pharmacokinetics	Clinical Uses	Drawbacks and Side Effects
Aspirin (Bayer Aspirin)	• **A:** PO and rectal • **M:** Hydrolyzed in liver, GI tract, and plasma; then further hepatic metabolism (partial P450) • **E:** Metabolites excreted in urine	• Fever • Mild to moderate pain relief • Inflammation and pain associated with such disorders as RA and OA • Prophylaxis for thromboembolic events (eg, CVA, MI) because of its action as a platelet aggregate inhibitor	• Contraindicated in children with viral infections • Gastritis • Increased bleeding time • Hypersensitivity • Salicylate poisoning (symptoms include agitation, convulsions, dizziness, drowsiness, fever, hallucinations, nausea, respiratory distress, tinnitus, and vomiting) • Induces P450 enzymes
Salicylic acid	• **A:** Topical	• Acne • Dandruff • Seborrheic dermatitis • Psoriasis • Wart removal	• Skin irritation • Skin erosion • Salicylate poisoning
Methyl-salicylate (Ben-Gay)		• Topical analgesic (draws blood flow to ease myalgias)	• Salicylate poisoning (an especially potent salicylate preparation)

NSAIDs

Drug	Pharmacokinetics	Clinical Uses	Side Effects
Diflunisal (Dolobid)	• **A:** PO • **M:** Hepatic • **E:** Metabolites excreted in urine	• Mild to moderate pain relief • Inflammation and pain associated with such disorders as RA and OA	• GI effects (bleeding, irritation, and ulceration) • Renal effects (dysuria, interstitial nephritis, and renal failure) • CNS effects (headache, dizziness) • Hepatic effects (jaundice, cholestatic hepatitis) • Skin effects (rash, pruritus) • Hematologic effects (thrombocytopenia, leukopenia) • Tinnitus • Blurry vision • Peripheral edema • Inhibits P450 enzymes (Flubiprofen, Ibuprofen and Pirioxicam)
Flurbiprofen (Ansaid)	• **A:** PO and ophthalmic • **M:** Hepatic (P450) • **E:** Parent drug and metabolites excreted in urine	• Inhibition of intraoperative miosis • Inflammation and pain associated with such disorders as RA and OA	
Ibuprofen (Motrin, Advil, and others)	• **A:** PO • **M:** Hepatic (P450 minor) • **E:** Parent drug and metabolites excreted in urine and feces	• Mild to moderate pain relief • Treatment of pericarditis • Inflammation and pain associated with such disorders as RA and OA • Fever	

Naproxen (Naprosyn)	• **A:** PO • **M:** Hepatic (P450 minor) • **E:** Metabolites excreted in urine	• Inflammation and pain associated with such disorders as RA and OA • Dysmenorrhea • Fever
Indomethacin (Indocin)	• **A:** PO, IV, or rectal • **M:** Hepatic (P450 minor) • **E:** Parent drug and metabolites excreted in urine	• Inflammation and pain associated with such disorders as RA, OA, gout, and ankylosing spondylitis • Closure of patent ductus arteriosus (IV form) • Treatment of pericarditis • Dysmenorrhea • Fever • Treatment of shoulder and arm injuries (bursitis, tendinitis)
Sulindac (Clinoril)	• **A:** PO • **M:** Prodrug that undergoes hepatic metabolism to active metabolite • **E:** Parent drug and metabolites excreted in urine and feces	• Treatment of shoulder and arm injuries (bursitis, tendinitis) • Inflammation and pain associated with such disorders as RA, OA, gout, and ankylosing spondylitis
Piroxicam (Feldene)	• **A:** PO • **M:** Hepatic (P450) • **E:** Parent drug and metabolites excreted in urine and feces	• Inflammation and pain associated with such disorders as RA, OA, gout, and ankylosing spondylitis • Dysmenorrhea
Ketorolac (Toradol)	• **A:** PO, IM, and IV • **M:** Hepatic • **E:** Parent drug and metabolites primarily excreted in urine	• Moderate to severe pain (eg, postoperative pain)

COX-2 INHIBITORS

Drug	Pharmacokinetics	Clinical Uses	Drawbacks and Side Effects
Celecoxib (Celebrex)	• **A:** PO • **M:** Hepatic (P450) • **E:** Metabolites excreted in feces and urine	• Inflammation and pain associated with such disorders as RA and OA • Dysmenorrhea • Mild to moderate pain relief • Adjunct for reducing the number of colonic polyps in adults with familial adenomatous polyposis	• GI side effects (gastritis, GI bleeding, and ulceration) • Edema • Skin rash • Bronchitis • Inhibits P450 enzymes

ACETAMINOPHEN

Drug	Pharmacokinetics	Clinical Uses	Drawbacks and Side Effects
Acetaminophen (Tylenol)	• **A:** PO, rectal • **M:** Hepatic (P450 minor) • **E:** Parent drug and metabolites excreted in urine	• Mild to moderate pain relief • Fever • Viral infections in children or persons with aspirin intolerance	• Few side effects • Overdose causes hepatotoxicity due to formation of reactive intermediate, N-acetyl benzoquinone imine • Treatment of overdose by N-acetylcysteine (NAC) • Inhibits P450 enzymes

MECHANISM OF ACTION OF ASPIRIN, NSAIDs AND COX 2 INHIBITORS

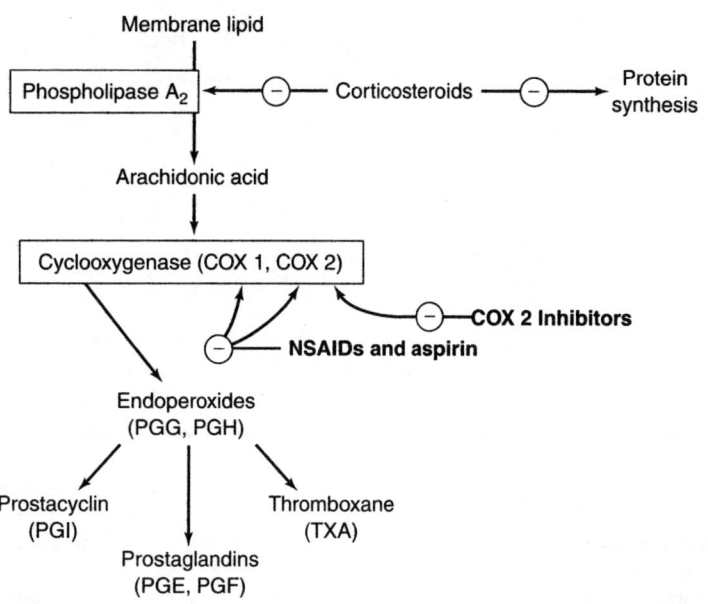

- Aspirin and NSAIDs function via inhibition of COX, which produces prostaglandin.

- **COX 2 inhibitors** function by inhibiting an inducible isoform of this enzyme (allows for baseline enzyme function to be maintained).

- Acetaminophen's mechanism of action remains unknown.

- Corticosteroids inhibit protein synthesis and so indirectly inhibit COX.

Modified from Trevor AJ, Katzung BG, Masters SB: *Katzung & Trevor's Pharmacology Examination & Board Review*, 6th ed. Originally published by Appleton & Lange. © 2002 by the McGraw-Hill Companies, Inc.

IV. H₁ Blockers (Antihistamines)

CLASSIFICATION OF H₁ BLOCKERS (ANTIHISTAMINES)

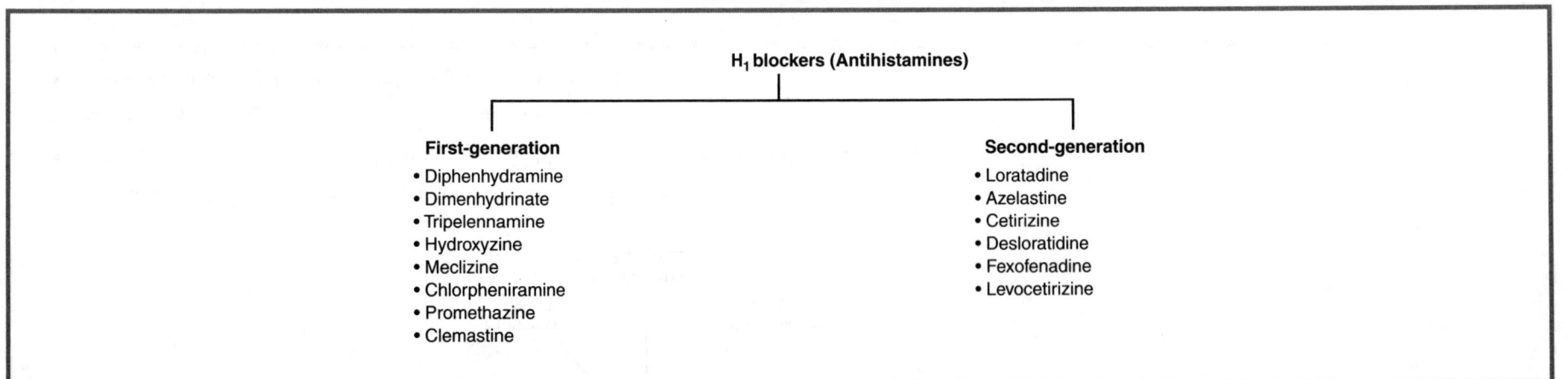

FIRST- AND SECOND-GENERATION H₁ BLOCKERS

Drug	Pharmacokinetics	Mechanism of Action	Clinical Uses	Side Effects
First-Generation H₁ Blocker				
Diphenhydramine (Benadryl)	• **A:** PO, IM, IV • **M:** Hepatic (P450) • **E:** Parent drug and metabolites excreted in urine	• Compete with histamine at H₁ receptors (prevents the action of histamine) • Anticholinergic side effects also result in decrease of nasal congestion	• Allergic reactions associated with histamine release (eg, pruritus associated with transfusions, urticaria, nasal congestion) • Motion sickness	• Sedation (more pronounced in diphenhydramine, hydroxyzine, dimenhydrinate, and tripelennamine) • Orthostatic hypotension due to α-blocker action • Anticholinergic side effects (more pronounced in diphenhydramine, dimenhydrinate, tripelennamine, and clemastine) • Inhibits P450 enzymes (Diphenhydramine, Dimenhydrinate, Hydroxyzine, Promethazine)
Dimenhydrinate (Dramamine)			• Motion sickness	
Tripelennamine (Triplen, Pelamine)	• **A:** PO (hydroxyzine also available in IM form) • **M:** Hepatic (P450) • **E:** Metabolites excreted in urine		• Allergic reactions associated with histamine release (eg, nasal congestion)	
Hydroxyzine (Atarax, Vistaril)			• Pruritis • Anxiety	
Meclizine (Antivert)			• Motion sickness • Diseases associated with vertigo	
Chlorpheniramine (Chlor-Trimeton)			• Allergic reactions associated with histamine release (eg, nasal congestion)	

Continued

FIRST- AND SECOND-GENERATION H₁ BLOCKERS (Continued)

Drug	Pharmacokinetics	Mechanism of Action	Clinical Uses	Side Effects
Promethazine (Phenergan)	• **A:** PO, IM, IV, PR • **M:** Hepatic (P450) • **E:** Primarily excreted as metabolites in urine		• Motion sickness • Antiemetic	
Clemastine (Tavist)	• **A:** PO • **M:** Hepatic • **E:** Primarily excreted as metabolites in urine		• Pruritis • Allergic reactions associated with histamine release (eg, nasal congestion)	
Second Generation H₁ Blockers				
Azelastine (Astelin, Astepro)	• **A:** Nasal spray • **M:** Hepatic (P450) • **E:** Metabolites excreted primarily in feces	• Compete with histamine at the H₁ receptors • Less sedation than first generation	• Allergic reactions associated with histamine release (ie. Allergic rhinitis, urticaria)	• GI: nausea, dry mouth, abdominal pain • Neuro: dizziness, HA, fatigue • Inhibit P450 enzymes (Azelastine, Fexofenadine and Loratidine only)
Desloratidine (Clarinex)	• **A:** PO • **M:** Hepatic • **E:** Metabolites excreted in urine and feces			
Fexofenadine (Allegra)	• **A:** PO • **M:** Hepatic • **E:** Metabolites excreted in urine and feces			
Loratidine (Claritin, Alavert, Tavist ND)	• **A:** PO • **M:** Hepatic (P450) • **E:** Metabolites excreted in urine and feces			
Cetirizine (Zyrtec, Aller-Relief)	• **A:** PO • **M:** Minimal hepatic (P450 minor) • **E:** Primarily excreted unchanged in urine			
Levocetirizine (Xyzal)				

CHAPTER 13
TOXICOLOGY

I. MANAGING POISONINGS

Treating Specific Poisons

II. CHELATORS

Chelators: Drug Facts

TERMS TO LEARN

Neutropenia	Decrease in number of neutrophils in the blood.
Paresthesias	An abnormal touch sensation (such as burning or prickling) often without external stimulus.
Systemic Lupus Erythematous	Autoimmune disorder typically seen in women; characterized by fever, polyarthritis, serositis, endocarditis, and skin rash.
Wilson's Disease	Defect in copper metabolism; leads to hepatic failure, tremor, and psychosis.

I. Managing Poisonings

TREATING SPECIFIC POISONS

Drug	Poison(s)	Mechanism of Action
N-Acetylcysteine/NAC (Mucomyst, Acetadote)	• Acetaminophen	• Glutathione analog that acts as a glutathione surrogate preventing the formation and accumulation of a toxic metabolite
Flumazenil (Romazicon)	• Benzodiazepines	• Direct benzodiazepine antagonist
Oxygen	• Carbon monoxide	• Competitive inhibitor with carbon monoxide for binding sites on hemoglobin
Amyl nitrite and sodium nitrite	• Cyanide	• Induce methemoglobinemia which competes with cyochrome oxidase for cyanide
Sodium thiosulfate (All packaged as cyanide)		• Enhances the conversion of cyanide to thiocyanate which is less toxic
Digoxin-specific antibodies (Digibind)	• Digoxin • Digitoxin	• Antibodies that bind excess digoxin/digitoxin creating a complex that is excreted by the kidneys
Fomepizole (Antizol)	• Methanol • Ethylene glycol	• Competitive inhibitor of alcohol dehydrogenase
Ethanol		
Physostigmine (Antilirium, Eserine)	• Muscarinic antagonists	• Reversible inhibitor of acetylcholinesterase • Results in increased Ach to counteract muscarinic antagonism

Continued

TREATING SPECIFIC POISONS (Continued)

Drug	Poison(s)	Mechanism of Action
Naloxone (Narcan)	• Opiates	• Opiate antagonist
Atropine	• Organophosphates • Carbamates • Anticholinesterases	• Muscarinic antagonist • Prevents muscarinic overactivity caused by inhibition of acetylcholinesterase
Pralidoxime (2-PAM, Protopan)	• Organophosphates	• Reactivates acetylcholinesterase by cleaving the bond between the enzyme and the organophosphate • Reverses Ach overstimulation at both nicotinic and muscarinic receptors
Hydroxocobalamin (Cyanokit)	• Cyanide	• Combines with cyanide to form cyanocobalamin (Vitamin B_{12})
Protamine sulfate	• Heparin	• Neutralizes heparin by formation of a heparin-protamine complex

II. Chelators

CHELATORS: DRUG FACTS

Drug	Pharmacokinetics	Clinical Uses	Side Effects
Dimercaprol (BAL)	• **A:** IM • **M:** Hepatic • **E:** Metabolites excreted in urine	• Arsenic • Gold • Lead • Mercury • Sulfhydryl (–SH) group (good chelators of heavy metals)	• Transient hypertension • Tachycardia • Headache • Abdominal pain, nausea, and vomiting • Paresthesias • Fevers, especially in children
Succimer/DMSA (Chemet)	• **A:** PO; variable absorption • **E:** Absorbed portion excreted unchanged in urine	• Lead • Arsenic • Mercury	• CNS effects • Elevation of liver enzymes • GI distress (nausea, vomiting, diarrhea) • Neutropenia • Skin rash
Edetate calcium disodium (EDTA, Endrate, Versenate)	• **A:** IM and IV • **E:** Unchanged in urine	• All heavy metals, especially lead	• Calcium disodium salt form prevents hypocalcemia • Hypotension • Nausea and vomiting • Nephrotoxicity • Systemic febrile reactions

Continued

CHELATORS: DRUG FACTS (Continued)

Drug	Pharmacokinetics	Clinical Uses	Side Effects
Penicillamine (Cuprimine, Depen)	• **A:** PO • **E:** Unchanged in urine	• Arsenic • Gold • Lead • Copper • Treatment of Wilson's disease	• Nephrotoxicity with proteinuria • Pancytopenia • Autoimmune dysfunction, including systemic lupus erythematosus and hemolytic anemia • Allergic reactions in patients with penicillin allergy
Deferoxamine (Desferel)	• **A:** IM or IV • **E:** Unchanged in urine	• Iron	• Skin reactions • Rapid IV administration may cause histamine release and hypotensive shock • LTU associated with retinal degeneration, hepatic and renal dysfunction, and coagulopathies

DMSA, dimercaptosuccinic acid; EDTA, ethylenediaminetetraacetic acid.

CHAPTER 14
ALTERNATIVE MEDICATIONS

I. HERBAL PREPARATIONS

Herbal and Alternative Remedies: Drug Facts

II. VITAMINS

Water Soluble and Fat Soluble Vitamins

Vitamins: Drug Facts

TERMS TO LEARN

Beriberi	Syndrome associated with thiamine deficiency; symptoms include peripheral neuropathy with CHF (wet beriberi) or without CHF (dry beriberi).
Cheilosis	Noninflammatory condition of the lips; symptoms include chapping and fissuring.
Glossitis	Inflammation of the tongue.
Megaloblastic Anemia	Low blood count with a predominant number of megaloblasts in the bone marrow (enlarged cells); seen in patients with B_{12} deficiency.
Papilledema	Swelling around the optic nerve caused by pressure on the nerve by a tumor or increased intracranial pressure.
Pellagra	Syndrome associated with insufficient niacin; symptoms include dermatitis, diarrhea, dementia, and death.
Torticollis	Excessive tone in the muscles of the neck.
Xerosis	Dryness of the skin, conjunctiva, or mucous membranes.

I. Herbal Preparations

HERBAL AND ALTERNATIVE REMEDIES: DRUG FACTS

Herb	Clinical Uses	Adverse Effects	Drug Interactions and Precautions
Clinical effects of these herbs are not based on evidence in all cases. Because herbal medications are not regulated by the FDA, their presence on the USMLE is negligible; however, they might be covered in a pharmacology course.			
Aloe Vera	• Topical treatment of burns and other inflammatory conditions of the skin • Topical treatment of inflammatory conditions of the skin (ie, psorasis & eczema)	• Skin rash or irritation	• Topical use only recommended • Oral form associated with renal failure, GI cancer and possibly fatal in high doses • Multiple drug interactions with oral form
Capsicum/Cayenne	• Gastroprotective agent against mucosal injury caused by aspirin • Topical treatment of pain associated with neuralgia, RA, and OA	• Stinging or burning at application site • Hypercoagulation • Hypersensitivity reactions	• Avoid contact with eyes or genitalia • Decreases bioavailability of aspirin and salicylic acid • Limit use to 2 days every 2 weeks
Cascara sagrada	• Treatment of constipation	• Arrhythmias • Neuropathies	• Thiazide diuretics, antiarrhythmics, cardiac glycosides, and indomethacin • Bowel obstruction, IBD, or abdominal pain of unknown origin
Chondrotin	• Treatment of OA • Intravesicular administration may relieve symptoms of interstital cystitis	• May worsen asthma symptoms	• May increase INR in patients on Coumadin
Cranberry	• Prevention and treatment of UTIs	• Increases urinary oxalate excretion and the risk of oxalate stones	• Increases bleeding risks in patients on anticoagulants

Continued

HERBAL AND ALTERNATIVE REMEDIES: DRUG FACTS (Continued)

Herb	Clinical Uses	Adverse Effects	Drug Interactions and Precautions
Echinacea	• Decreases duration and intensity of cold symptoms via anti-inflammatory and immunostimulating mechanisms • Treatment of UTIs • Treatment of wounds and burns	• Dizziness • GI upset • Headache • Unpleasant taste	• Immunosuppressant medications • Immunodeficiency syndromes, autoimmune disorders, or TB • Should not be taken for more than 8 weeks
Feverfew	• Decreases frequency and severity of migraine headaches	• Allergic dermatitis • GI upset • Rebound headaches	• Anticoagulants and antiplatelet drugs • May inhibit platelet aggregation
Garlic	• Treatment of hyperlipidemia • Treatment of arteriosclerosis • Treatment of hypertension	• Allergic reactions • Fatigue • GI upset • Headache	• Anticoagulants and antiplatelet drugs • May inhibit platelet aggregation
Ginger	• Treatment of nausea and vomiting (eg, pregnancy, motion sickness)	• Stomach cramps • Neurological (HA, irritation, dizziness) • Reproductive (decreased sperm count, decreased libido, gynecomastia in men)	• Increases bleeding risks in patients on anticoagulants • May increase risk of hypoglycemia in patients on diabetic medications • May increase risk of low BP in patients on antihypertensive medications
Gingko Biloba	• Treatment of cognitive impairment associated with early Alzheimer's disease • Treatment of the symptoms of intermittent claudication • Treatment of vertigo (vascular origin) • Treatment of tinnitus (vascular origin)	• Allergic skin reactions • Bleeding • GI upset • Hypersensitivity reactions • Increased risk for spontaneous intracranial hemorrhage	• Anticoagulants and antiplatelet drugs • May inhibit platelet aggregation • Intracranial hemorrhage

Ginseng	• Treatment of fatigue and debility • May improve mental and physical performance	• Hypertension • Insomnia • Mastalgia • Nervousness • Vaginal bleeding	• MAO inhibitors, loop diuretics, anticoagulants or diabetic medications
Glucosamine	• Treatment of OA	• May trigger reaction in people with shellfish allergy • May increase BP, blood sugar and chloesterol levels	• May increase INR in patients on Coumadin
Goldenseal	• External antiseptic • Treatment of diarrhea caused by numerous GI pathogens • Treatment of trachoma • Treatment of gastric ulcers • Treatment of gallbladder disease	• GI disorders associated with LTU	• Contraindicated in patients with G6PD deficiency • May antagonize the action of heparin
Honey (Medihoney)	• Topical treatment of burns and wound for prevention of infection and healing		
Kava	• Treatment of chronic anxiety states	• Ataxia • Drowsiness • Hepatotoxicity • Sedation • Skin rash • Torticollis	• Barbiturates, alcohol, DA agonists or antagonists • Endogenous depression (increases risk of suicide)

Continued

HERBAL AND ALTERNATIVE REMEDIES: DRUG FACTS (Continued)

Herb	Clinical Uses	Adverse Effects	Drug Interactions and Precautions
Ma-huang (Ephedra)	• Treatment of cough and bronchitis (bronchodilator) • CNS stimulant • Diet aid	• Arrhythmias • CVA • Headache • Hypertension • Insomnia • MI • Nervousness • Tremor • Seizures	• Cardiac glycosides, Guanethidine, MAO inhibitors, or other CNS stimulants
Melatonin	• Treatment of insomnia • Treatment of jet lag		• Increases bleeding risks in patients on anticoagulants • May decrease effectiveness of some antidepressants
Milk thistle	• Treatment of liver and gallbladder disorders • Treatment of dyspepsia • Improves hepatic function in viral hepatitis • Antidote to *Amanita* mushroom poisoning (hepatotoxicity)	• GI upset (nausea, diarrhea, vomiting, abdominal cramping)	• Using milk thistle with typical antipsychotics can alter lipid peroxidation
S-Adenosylmethionine (SAM-e)	• Treatment of depression	• GI irritation (nausea, gas, diarrhea) • Neurological activation (elation, insomnia, dizziness) • Palpitations • Sweating	• May trigger seratonin syndrome when combined with SSRIs • May decrease effectiveness of L-dopa in Parkinson's patients • May change blood sugar levels in patients on diabetes medications

Saw palmetto	• Improves urinary symptoms associated with BPH (no change in gland size) • Treatment of irritable bladder	• Decreased libido • GI upset • Headache • Hypertension	• Hormones or hormone-like medications • May possess androgenic, estrogenic, and α-blocking effects
Soy	• Treatment of hyperlipidemia • Treatment of postmenopausal vasomotor symptoms	• GI upset, constipation, diarrhea	• Increases bleeding risks in patients on anticoagulants • Avoid in patients on MAO inhibitors
St. John's wort	• Treatment of mild to moderate depression • Promotes healing of burns and wounds	• Allergic reactions • Confusion • Dizziness • Dry mouth • Fatigue • GI upset • Photosensitivity	• Antidepressants, such as SSRIs and MAO inhibitors; drugs that cause photosensitivity, such as tetracycline; numerous other drug interactions due to induction of P450 enzymes • Decreases absorption of iron
Valerian	• Treatment of nervousness • Treatment of insomnia	• GI upset	• CNS depressants (such as barbiturates, benzodiazepines, or alcohol) because it has an additive CNS depressive effect
Yohimbe	• Sympatholytic agent • Mydriatic agent • Treatment of impotence with vascular or psychogenic origin	• Dizziness • Headache • Hypertension • Tachycardia • Seizure • Renal failure	• OTC stimulants, alcohol, antidepressants, or antihypertensives • Avoid in liver, heart, or kidney disease • May cause seizures or renal failure

Physicians Desk Reference for Herbal Medicines, 2nd ed.

II. Vitamins

Water Soluble and Fat Soluble Vitamins

Water Soluble Vitamins	Fat Soluble Vitamins
B_1 (Thiamine)	A
B_2 (Riboflavin)	D
B_3 (Niacin)	E
B_5 (Pantothenic acid)	K
B_6 (Pyridoxine)	
B_7 (Biotin)	
B_9 (Folic acid)	
B_{12} (Cobalamin)	
C	

☞ ADEK can be used to remember the fat-soluble vitamins.

All B vitamins function as coenzymes.

Mnemonic for B vitamins "**T**hose **R**eally **N**ice **P**atent **P**umps you **B**ought **F**or **C**hurch".

VITAMINS: DRUG FACTS

Vitamin	Deficiency	Overdose/Side Effects
Vitamin A*	• Xerosis (dry skin) • Night blindness • Blindness (most common type of preventable blindness in children)	• Acute toxicity (increased intracranial pressure, headaches, and papilledema) • Alopecia • Arthralgia • Hepatosplenomegaly
Vitamin B_1 (Thiamine)	• Beriberi (visual disturbances, paralysis, paresthesias of lower extremities, psychosis, and CHF) • Wernicke-Korsakoff syndrome	• None
Vitamin B_2 (Riboflavin)	• Mild symptoms (chelosis, corneal vascularization, angular stomatitis)	• None documented • Possible increase in the risk of stomach cancer
Vitamin B_3 (Niacin)	• Pellagra (diarrhea, dermatitis and dementia—the 3 D's)	• Facial flushing • Hyperuricemia • Liver dysfunction • Pruritus
Vitamin B_5 (Pantothenic acid)	• Alopecia • Dermatitis • GI upset	• None
Vitamin B_6 (Pyridoxine)	• Angular stomatitis • Dermatitis • Glossitis • Peripheral neuropathy • Often associated with isoniazid therapy	• Sensory neuropathy

Continued

VITAMINS: DRUG FACTS (Continued)

Vitamin	Deficiency	Overdose/Side Effects
Vitamin B_7 (Biotin)	• Dermatitis • Enteritis	• None
Vitamin B_9 (Folic Acid)	• Neural tube defects • Megaloblastic anemia	• None
Vitamin B_{12} (Cobalamin)	• Megaloblastic anemia • Glossitis • Neurologic disorders	• None
Vitamin C (Ascorbic acid)	• Scurvy	• GI upset • Kidney stones
Vitamin D*	• Ricket's disease (in children) • Osteomalacia (in adults) • Hypocalcemia	• Hypercalcemia • Mental and growth retardation in children • Kidney failure • Death
Vitamin E*	• Increased fragility of erythrocytes • Peripheral neuropathy (motor and sensory)	• Diarrhea • Fatigue • Kidney stones • Nausea
Vitamin K*	• Bleeding disorders	• Rash • Itching

*Fat soluble vitamins.

INDEX

A

α-adrenergic blockers
  nonselective (irreversible)
    phenoxybenzamine (Dibenzyline), 100
  nonselective (reversible)
    phentolamine, 100
  selective
    alfuzosin (Uroxatral), 101
    doxazosin (Cardura), 101
    prazosin (Minipress), 101
    silodosin (Rapaflo), 101
    tamsulosin (Flomax), 101
    terazosin (Hytrin), 101
Abacavir (Ziagen), 56
Abatacept (Orencia), 360
Abciximab (Reopro), 259
Abortifacient, 366
Abortive antimigraine drugs
  caffeine and ergotamine (Cafergot, Migergot), 172
  ergots
    dihydroergotamine (DHE-45, Migranal), 172
    ergotamine (Ergomar), 172
  5-HT$_{1B/1D}$ receptor agonists
    almotriptan (Axert), 174
    eletriptan (Relpax), 174

frovatriptan (Frova), 174
naratriptan (Amerge), 173
rizatriptan (Maxalt), 173
sumatriptan (Imitrex, Alsuma, Sumavel), 173
zolmitriptan (Zomig), 173
Absence (petite mal) seizures, 163
Acanthosis nigricans, definition of, 199
Acarbose (Precose), 310
Acebutolol (Sectral), 102, 206
ACE (angiotensin-converting enzyme) inhibitors
  benazepril (Lotensin), 215
  captopril (Capoten), 215, 243
  enalapril (Vasotec, Epaned), 216, 244
  fosinopril (Monopril), 215
  lisinopril (Prinivil, Zestril), 215, 244
  moexipril (Univasc), 215
  perindopril (Aceon), 215
  quinapril (Accupril), 215, 244
  ramipril (Altace), 215, 244
  trandolapril (Mavik), 216, 245
Acetaminophen (Tylenol), 376
Acetazolamide (Acetazolam, Diamox), 224
Acetylcholine (Miochol-E), 105
Acetylcholinesterase, definition of, 80
Acromegaly, definition of, 290
Active transport, 7
Acyclovir (Zovirax), 53
Adalimumab (Humira), 355

Adefovir (Hepsera), 56
Adminstration route
  buccal, 8
  inhalation, 8
  intramuscular, 8
  intravenous, 8
  oral, 8
  rectal, 8
  subcutaneous, 8
  sublingual, 8
  topical, 8
  transdermal, 8
ADP receptor antagonists
  clopidogrel (Plavix), 260
  prasugrel (Effient), 260
  ticlopidine, 260
Adrenergic blockers
  β-blockers, 102–103
  α-blockers, 100–101
  classification of, 99
  neuronal blockers, 101
Adrenergic neuronal blockers
  definition of, 80
  guanadrel (Hylorel), 204
  guanethidine (Ismelin), 204
  metyrosine (Demser), 204
  reserpine (Serpasil), 203
Adrenocorticotropic hormone (ACTH), 292–293

Aerosol corticosteroids
    beclomethasone (QVAR), 274
    budesonide (Pulmicort), 274
    ciclesonide (Alvesco), 274
    fluticasone (Flovent), 273
    mometasone (Asmanex), 274
α-glucosidase inhibitor
    acarbose (Precose), 310
    miglitol (Glyset), 310
Agonist
    definition of, 2
    response curve, 6
Albuterol (AccuNeb, ProAir, Vospire, Proventil,
    Ventolin), 271
Albuterol (Proventil, Ventolin), 97
Alcohol, 133
Aldesleukin (Proleukin), 362
Alemtuzmab (Campath, Lemtrada), 360
Alemtuzumab (Campath), 348
Alendronate (Fosamax), 305
Alfentanil (Alfenta), 165, 191
Alfuzosin (Uroxatral), 101
Aliskiren (Tekturna), 217
Alkylating drugs
    altretamine (Hexalen), 329
    bendamustine (Treanda), 329
    busulfan (Myleran, Busulfex), 327
    carboplatin (Paraplatin), 328
    carmustine (BiCNU, Gliadel), 328
    chlorambucil (Leukeran), 327
    cisplatin (Platinol), 328
    cyclophosphamide (Cytoxan), 326
    dacarbazine (Dtic-Dome), 329
    ifosfamide (IFEX), 327
    lomustine (CeeNU), 327
    mechanism of action, 326
    mechlorethamine (Mustargen), 326
    melphalan (Alkeran), 327
    procarbazine (Matulane, Natulan), 329

    resistance mechanisms, 326
    streptozocin (Zanosar), 328
    temozolomide (Temodar), 329
    thiotepa, 329
Allopurinol (Zyloprim), 370
Allylamines
    butenafine (Lotrimin, Mentax), 63
    naftifine (Naftin), 63
    terbinafine (Lamisil, Terbinex), 62
Almotriptan (Axert), 174
Aloe vera, 389
Alopecia, definition of, 199
Alprazolam (Xanax), 146
Alprazolam (Xanax, Niravam), 126
Alprostadil (Prostin, Muse, Caverject), 367
Alteplase (Activase), 258
Alternative medications
    herbal remedies
        aloe vera, 389
        capsicum/cayenne, 389
        cascara sagrada, 389
        chondrotin, 389
        cranberry, 389
        echinacea, 390
        feverfew, 390
        garlic, 390
        ginger, 390
        gingko biloba, 390
        ginseng, 391
        glucosamine, 391
        goldenseal, 391
        honey (medihoney), 391
        kava, 391
        ma-huang (Ephedra), 392
        melatonin, 392
        milk thistle, 392
        S-adenosylmethionine (SAM-e), 392
        saw palmetto, 393
        soy, 393

        St. John's wort, 393
        valerian, 393
        yohimbe, 393
    terms to learn, 388
    vitamins
        A, 395
        B_1 (thiamine), 395
        B_2 (riboflavin), 395
        B_3 (niacin), 395
        B_5 (pantothenic acid), 395
        B_6 (pyridoxine), 395
        B_7 (biotin), 396
        B_9 (folic acid), 396
        B_{12} (cobalamin), 396
        C (ascorbic acid), 396
        D, 396
        E, 396
        K, 396
        water soluble and fat soluble, 394
Altretamine (Hexalen), 329
Aluminum hydroxide (Alternagel), 280
Alzheimer's disease, drugs for
    classification, 144
    donepezil (Aricept), 145
    galantamine (Razadyne), 145
    memantine (Namenda), 145
    rivastigmine (Exelon), 145
    tacrine (Cognex), 145
Amantadine, 50, 139
Amebiasis agents
    iodoquinol (Yodoxin), 69
    metronidazole (Flagyl, Metro), 68
    paromomycin (Humatin), 69
    tinidazole (Tindamax), 69
Amides and other nonesters
    articaine-epinephrine (Articadent, Orabloc,
        Septocaine, Zorcaine), 184
    bupivacaine (Marcaine, Sensorcaine), 183
    lidocaine (Xylocaine), 183

mepivacaine (Carbocaine), 183
prilocaine (Citanest), 184
ropivacaine (Naropin), 184
Amikacin, 36
Amiloride (Midamor), 223
Aminocaproic acid (Amicar), 262
Aminoglycosides, 35–36
amikacin, 36
gentamicin, 35
kanamycin, 36
neomycin (Neo-Fradin), 36
netilmicin (Netromycin), 36
paromomycin, 36
streptomycin, 35
tobramycin (Tobi), 35
Amiodarone (Cordarone, Nexterone, Pacerone), 237
Amitriptyline (Elavil), 118, 175
Amlodipine (Norvasc), 212, 229
Amobarbital (Amytal), 149
Amoxapine, 118
Amoxicillin (Amoxil, Trimox), 17, 21
Amoxicillin and clavulinic acid (Augmentin), 23
Amphetamine-Dextroamphetamine (Adderall), 97
Amphotericin B, 61
Ampicillin (Ampicin), 17, 21
Ampicillin and sulbactam (Unasyn), 23
Amyl nitrate, 227
Amyl nitrite and sodium nitrite, 383
Anakinra (Kineret), 360
Analgesics
acetaminophen (Tylenol, 376
aspirin (Bayer Aspirin), 373
mechanism of action, 377
classification of, 372
cox-2 inhibitors
celecoxib (Celebrex), 376
mechanism of action, 377

methyl-salicylate (Ben-Gay), 373
NSAID
diflunisal (Dolobid), 374
flurbiprofen (Ansaid), 374
ibuprofen (Motrin, Advil), 374
indomethacin (Indocin), 375
ketorolac (Toradol), 375
mechanism of action, 377
naproxen (Naprosyn), 375
piroxicam (Feldene), 375
sulindac (Clinoril), 375
salicylic acid, 373
Anastrozole (Arimidex), 345
Androgens, 343
Anesthesia
components of, 193
general, 186–193. See also General anesthetic drugs
local. See Local anesthetics and adjunctive drugs
stages of, 193
Angina, definition of, 199
Angiotensin action, drugs affecting
ACE inhibitors. See ACE (angiotensin-converting enzyme) inhibitors
angiotensin receptor blockers, 216–217
azilsartan (Edarbi), 217
candesartan (Atacand), 217
eprosartan (Teveten), 217
irbesartan (Avapro), 217
losartan (Cozaar), 216
valsartan (Diovan), 216
functions of angiotensin, 218
renin inhibitors, 217
sympathetic antagonists, 218
Angiotensin receptor blockers
azilsartan (Edarbi), 217
candesartan (Atacand), 217, 245
eprosartan (Teveten), 217
irbesartan (Avapro), 217
losartan (Cozaar), 216

valsartan (Diovan), 216, 245
Anidulafungin (Eraxis), 62
Anisocoria, definition of, 80
Antacids
aluminum hydroxide (Alternagel), 280
calcium carbonate (Caltrate, TUMS), 280
magnesium hydroxide (Phillips' Milk of Magnesia), 280
sodium bicarbonate (Brioschi), 280
Antagonist
chemical, 2
competitive, 2
irreversible, 2
pharmacologic, 2
physiologic, 3
response curve, 6
Anthracyclines
daunorubicin (Cerubidine), 336
doxorubicin (Adriamycin), 335
epirubicin (Ellence), 336
idarubicin (Idamycin), 336
mitoxantrone (Novantrone), 337
valrubicin (Valstar), 337
Antiacetylcholinesterases
carbamates
neostigmine (Prostigmin, Bloxiverz), 89
physostigmine, 88
pyridostigmine (Mestinon, Regonol), 89
organophosphates
echothiophate (Phospholine iodide), 89
malathion (Ovide), 89
parathion, 89
sarin, 89
soman, 89
tabun, 89
quaternary alcohols
donepezil (Aricept), 88
edrophonium (Enlon, Tensilon), 88
tacrine (Cognex), 88

Antiandrogen drugs
  bicalutamide (Casodex), 319
  dutasteride (Avodart), 320
  enzalutamide (Xtandi), 319
  finasteride (Proscar, Propecia), 320
  goserelin (Zoladex), 319
  leuprolide (Lupron, Eligard), 319
  nilutamide (Nilandron), 319
  site of action, 321
  spironolactone (Aldactone), 320
Antianginal drugs
  amyl nitrate, 227
  β-blockers
    atenolol (Tenormin), 229
    effects of nitrates combined with, 231
    metoprolol (Lopressor, Toprol), 229
    nadolol (Corgard), 230
    pindolol, 230
    propranolol (Hemangeol, Inderal, InnoPran), 230
  classification of, 226
  dihydropyridine calcium channel blockers
    amlodipine (Norvasc), 229
    nicardipine (Cardene), 229
    nifedipine (Adalat, Afeditab, Procardia, Nifediac, Nifedical), 229
  isosorbide dinitrate (Isordil, IsoDitrate,Dilatrate), 225
  isosorbide mononitrate (Imdur), 225
  mechanisms of action of, 232
  nitroglycerin (Nitro-Bid, Nitro-Dur, Minitran, Nitrolingual, NitroMist, Rectiv, Nitronal, Nitrostat), 225
  nondihydropyridine calcium channel blockers
    diltiazem (Cardizem, Dilacor, Diltzac, Matzim, Taztia, Tiazac), 228
    verapamil (Calan, Isoptin, Verelan), 228
Antiarrhythmics
  class IA
    disopyramide (Norpace), 234

procainamide, 234
    quinidine, 234
  class IB
    lidocaine (Xylocaine), 235
    mexiletine, 235
    phenytoin (Dilantin, Phenytek), 235
  class IC
    flecainide (Tambocor), 236
    propafenone (Rythmol), 236
  classification of, 233
  class II
    β-blockers, 237
  class III
    amiodarone (Cordarone, Nexterone, Pacerone), 237
    dofetilide (Tikosyn), 238
    dronedarone (Multaq), 238
    ibutilide (Corvert), 238
    sotalol (Betapace), 237
  class IV
    diltiazem (Cardizem, Dilacor), 239
    verapamil (Calan, Isoptin), 239
Antibiotics, mechanisms of action, 16
Antibody immunosuppressants
  abatacept (Orencia), 360
  alemtuzmab (Campath, Lemtrada), 360
  anakinra (Kineret), 360
  antilymphocyte globulin/lymphocyte immune globulin (Atgam), 358
  basiliximab (Simulect), 358
  belatacept (Nulojix), 360
  belimimab (Benlysta), 359
  fingolimod (Gilenya), 360
  immune globulin intravenous, 358
  muromonab-CD3 (Orthoclone OKT3), 359
  natalizumab (Tysabri), 360
  ofatumumab (Arzerra), 359
  rituximab (Rituxan), 359
  secukinumab (Cosentyx), 359

teriflunomide (Aubagio), 360
    tocilizumab (Actemra), 358
    ustekinumab (Stelara), 359
Anticholelithic, definition of, 278
Anticoagulants
  heparin, 255
  protein C (concentrate, ceprotin), 254
  warfarin (Coumadin, Jantoven), 254
Antidepressants
  acute actions of, 117
  classification of, 116
  heterocyclics, 119
  monoamine oxidase inhibitors, 122. See also Monoamine oxidase (MAO) inhibitors
  selective serotonin reuptake inhibitors, 120
  serotonin norepinephrine reuptake inhibitors, 121
  tricyclic, 118
Antiemetics
  aprepitant (Emend), 283
  definition of, 278
  dimenhydrinate (Dramamine), 283
  dolasetron (Anzemet), 282
  dronabinol (Marinol), 283
  granisetron (Granisol, Sancuso), 282
  metoclopramide (Reglan), 283
  nabilone (Cesamet), 283
  ondansetron (Zofran, Zuplenz), 282
  palonosetron (Aloxi), 282
  prochlorperazine (Compazine, Compro), 282
  promethazine (Phenergan), 283
  scopolamine, 283
Antiepileptic drugs, 154–163, 176–179
  carbamazepine (Tegretol,Carbatrol, Epitol, Equetro), 160
  classification of, 154
  clobazam (Onfi), 156
  clonazepam (Klonopin), 157
  clorazepate (Tranxene), 156
  diazepam (Valium, Diastat), 156

ethosuximide (Zarontin), 159
ethotoin (Peganone), 161
ezogabine (Potiga), 159
felbamate (Felbatol), 157
fosphenytoin (Cerebyx), 160
gabapentin (Neurontin, Gralise), 158
lacosamide (Vimpat), 161
lamotrigine (Lamictal), 161
levetiracetam (Keppra), 157
lorazepam (Ativan), 156
methsuximide (Celontin), 159
oxcarbazepine (Trileptal, Oxtellar), 160
perampanel (Fycompa), 159
phenobarbital (Luminal), 155
phenytoin (Dilantin, Phenytek), 160
pregabalin (Lyrica), 158
primidone (Mysoline), 155
rufinamide (Banzel), 161
seizure treatment protocols, 162–163
tiagabine (Gabitril), 155
topiramate (Topamax, Topiragen, Trokendi), 157
valproate (Depacon, Depakene, Stavzor), 158
vigabatrin (Sabril), 155
zonisamide (Zonegran), 159
Antiestrogen drugs
clomiphene (Clomid, Serophene), 313
raloxifene (Evista), 313
tamoxifen (Soltamox), 313
Antifolates, 68
Antifungal agents
allylamines
butenafine (Lotrimin, Mentax), 63
naftifine (Naftin), 63
terbinafine (Lamisil, Terbinex), 62
azoles
clotrimazole (Lotrimin), 63
fluconazole (Diflucan), 63
ketoconazole, 64

miconazole (Monistat, Oravig), 64
posaconazole (Noxafil), 64
voriconazole (Vfend), 65
classification of, 60
echinocandins
anidulafungin (Eraxis), 62
caspofungin (Cancidas), 62
micafungin (Mycamine), 62
mechanisms of action, 60
penicillin derivative
griseofulvin, 65
polyenes
amphotericin B, 61
nystatin (Nyamyc), 61
pyrimidine analog
flucytosine (Ancobon), 65
Antihyperlipidemic drugs
bile acid sequestrants
cholestipol (Cholestid), 249
cholestyramine (Questran, Prevalite, Questran Light), 249
colesevelam (Welchol), 249
cholesterol absorption blockers
ezetimibe (Zetia), 250
classification of, 248
effects on lipoproteins, 251
fibric acid derivatives
fenofibrate (Tricor, Antara, Fenoglide, Lipofen, Triglide), 251
fenofibric acid (Fibricor, Trilipix), 251
gemfibrozil (Lopid), 251
HMG-CoA reductase inhibitors
atorvastatin (Lipitor), 250
fluvastatin (Lescol), 250
lovastatin (Mevacor, Altoprev), 250
pitavastatin (Livalo), 250
pravastatin (Pravachol), 250
rosuvastatin (Crestor), 250
simvastatin (Zocor), 250

nicotinic acid
niacin (Niaspan, Niacor), 249
Antihypertensive drugs
ACE inhibitors
benazepril (Lotensin), 215
captopril (Capoten), 215
enalapril (Vasotec, Epaned), 216
fosinopril (Monopril), 215
lisinopril (Prinivil, Zestril), 215
moexipril (Univasc), 215
perindopril (Aceon), 215
quinapril (Accupril), 215
ramipril (Altace), 215
trandolapril (Mavik), 216
adrenergic neuronal blockers
guanadrel (Hylorel), 204
guanethidine (Ismelin), 202
metyrosine (Demser), 204
reserpine (Serpasil), 203
angiotensin receptor blockers
azilsartan (Edarbi), 217
candesartan (Atacand), 217
eprosartan (Teveten), 217
irbesartan (Avapro), 217
losartan (Cozaar), 216
valsartan (Diovan), 216
β-blockers
acebutolol (Sectral), 206
atenolol (Tenormin), 206
betaxolol (Kerlone), 206
bisoprolol (Zebeta), 206
carvedilol (Coreg), 207
esmolol (Brevibloc), 207
labetalol (Trandate), 207
metoprolol (Lopressor, Toprol), 206
nadolol (Corgard), 207
nebivolol (Brevibloc), 206
penbutolol (Levatol), 207
pindolol, 208

Antihypertensive drugs (*continued*)
propranolol (Hemangeol, Inderal, InnoPran), 208
timolol, 208
calcium channel blockers
amlodipine (Norvasc), 212
clevidipine (Cleviprex), 212
diltiazem (Cardizem), 212
felodipine (Plendil, Renedil), 213
isradipine, 213
nicardipine (Cardene), 213
nifedipine (Adalat, Afeditab, Procardia, Nifediac,Nifedical), 213
nisoldipine (Sular), 213
verapamil (Calan, Isoptin, Verelan), 212
centrally acting α_2 agonists
clonidine (Catapres, Duraclon, Kapvay), 202
guanabenz (Wytensin), 203
guanfacine (Intuniv, Tenex), 203
methyldopa, 202
classification of, 200
diuretics
carbonic anhydrase inhibitor, 224
classification of, 219
loop, 222
mechanism of action, 220
osmotic, 224
potassium-sparing, 223
serum electrolyte effects of, 225
thiazide, 221
vasopressin receptor antagonists, 224
nonselective α-adrenergic blockers
phenoxybenzamine (Dibenzyline), 204
phentolamine (Regitine, Rogitine), 204
renin inhibitors
aliskiren (Tekturna), 217
selective α-adrenergic blockers
doxazosin (Cardura), 205
prazosin (Minipress), 205
terazosin (Hytrin), 205

sympathetic antagonists
clonidine (Catapres), 218
methyldopa (Aldomet), 218
propranolol (Inderal), 218
vasodilators
arterial and venous, 208–209
classification of, 209
hydralazine (Apresoline, NovoHylazin, Nu-Hydral), 211
minoxidil, 211
nitroglycerin (Nitro-Bid, Nitro-Dur,Minitran, Nitro-Time, Nitrolingual, NitroMist, Nitronal, Nitrostat, Rectiv), 210
nitroprusside (Nitropress), 210
Antilymphocyte globulin/lymphocyte immune globulin (Atgam), 358
Antimalarial agents (quinoline derivatives)
chloroquine (Aralen), 67
mefloquine, 68
primaquine, 68
quinidine, 67
quinine (Qualaquin), 67
Antimetabolites
folic acid antagonist
methotrexate (Rheumatrex, Trexall), 333
pemetrexed (Alimta), 333
purine antagonists
cladribine (Leustatin), 330
clofarabine (Clolar), 330
fludarabine (Fludara, Oforta), 331
mercaptopurine-6-MP (Purinethol), 330
nelarabine (Arranon), 331
pentostatin (Nipent), 331
thioguanine-6-TG (Tabloid), 330
pyrimidine antagonists
azacitidine (Vidaza), 333
capecitabine (Xeloda), 332
cytosine arabinoside-ara-C-cytarabine (Cytosar), 331

decitabine (Dacogen), 332
floxuridine (FUDR), 332
5-fluorouracil (Adrucil), 331
gemcitabine (Gemzar), 332
Antimicrobial drugs
antibacterial agents. *See* Antibacterial agents
antifungal agents. *See* Antifungal agents
antiprotozoal agents. *See* Antiprotozoal agents
antiviral agentss. *See* Antiviral agent
classification, 41
daptomycin (Cubicin), 47
nitrofurantoin (Macrobid), 47
30S. *See* 30S antibacterial agents
50S. *See* 50S antibacterial agents
sulfonamides. *See* Sulfonamides
trimethoprim, 41, 44
Antineoplastic agent, 306
Antiplasmin drugs, 262
Antiplatelet drugs, 259
Antiprogesterone drug
mifepristone (Mifeprex, Korlym), 317
Antiprotozoal agents
amebiasis agents
iodoquinol (Yodoxin), 69
metronidazole (Flagyl, Metro), 68
paromomycin (Humatin), 69
tinidazole (Tindamax), 69
antifolates
atovaquone and proguanil (Malarone), 68
antimalarial agents (quinoline derivatives)
chloroquine (Aralen), 67
mefloquine, 68
primaquine, 68
quinidine, 67
quinine (Qualaquin), 67
atovaquone (Mepron), 69
nitazoxanide (Alinia), 69
pentamidine (Pentam, Nebupent), 69
pyrimethamine (Daraprim), 70

therapeutic classification of, 66
trimethoprim/sulfamethoxazole (Bactrim), 70
Antipsychotics
  atypical, 114–115
    aripiprazole (Abilify), 115
    asenapine (Saphris), 115
    clozapine (Clozaril, FazaClo), 114
    iloperidone (Fanapt), 115
    olanzapine (Zyprexa), 115
    paliperidone (Invega), 115
    quetiapine (Seroquel), 115
    risperidone (Risperdal), 114
    ziprasidone (Geodon), 115
  classification of, 112
  typical, 113–114
    butyrophenones, 113
    chlorpromazine (Thorazine), 113
    dibenzoxazepine, 113–114
    diphenylbutylpiperidinesd, 113
    fluphenazine (Prolixin, Permitil), 113
    haloperidol (Haldol), 113
    loxapine (Loxitane), 113–114
    perphenazine, 113
    phenothiazines, 113
    pimozide (Orap), 113
    thioridazine (Mellaril), 113
    trifluoperazine (Stelazine), 113
Antispastic drugs
  baclofen (Lioresal, Gablofen), 177
  botulinum toxin (BoTox), 177
  carisoprodol (Soma), 177
  chlorzoxazone (Parafon Forte, Lorzone), 178
  classification, 176
  cyclobenzaprine (Flexeril, Fexmid, Amrix), 178
  dantrolene (Dantrium, Revonto), 178
  diazepam (Valium), 178
  metaxalone (Skelaxin), 179
  methocarbamol (Robaxin), 179

orphenadrine (Norflex), 179
  tizanidine (Zanaflex), 179
Anti TNF-α agents
  adalimumab (Humira), 355
  certolizumab pegol (Cimzia), 355
  etanercept (Enbrel), 354
  golimumab (Simponi), 355
  infliximab (Remicade), 355
  thalidomide (Thalomid), 354
Antitumor antibiotics
  action of mechanism, 334
  anthracyclines
    daunorubicin (Cerubidine), 336
    doxorubicin (Adriamycin), 335
    epirubicin (Ellence), 336
    idarubicin (Idamycin), 336
    mitoxantrone (Novantrone), 337
    valrubicin (Valstar), 337
  aziridine
    mitomycin (Mutamycin), 337
  peptide antibiotics
    bleomycin (Blenoxane), 335
    dactinomycin (Cosmegen), 335
Antitussive
  benzonatate (Tessalon, Zonatuss), 269
  codeine, 269
  dextromethorphan (Robitussin DM, Delsym), 269
Antiviral agents
  classification of, 48
  guanosine analogs
    ribavirin, 50
  interferons
    interferon alfa-2a, 51
    interferon alfa-2b (Intron-A), 51
    interferon alfacon-1 (Infergen), 51
    interferon alfa-n3 (Alferon N), 51
  major sites of drug action on viral replication, 49

neuraminidase inhibitors
  oseltamivir, 51
  zanamivir (Relenza), 51
non-nucleoside reverse transcriptase inhibitors
  delavirdine (Rescriptor), 57
  efavirenz (Sustiva), 57
  etravirine (Intelence), 57
  nevirapine (Viramune), 57
  rilpivirine (Edurant), 57
nucleoside analogues
  acyclovir (Zovirax), 53
  famciclovir (Famvir), 54
  ganciclovir (Cytovene), 53
  penciclovir (Denavir), 54
  trifluridine (Viroptic), 54
  valcyclovir (Valtrex), 53
  valganciclovir (Valcyte), 53
nucleoside reverse transcriptase inhibitors
  abacavir (Ziagen), 56
  adefovir (Hepsera), 56
  didanosine/DDI (Videx), 55
  emtricitabine (Emtriva), 55
  entecavir (Baraclude), 56
  lamivudine (Epivir), 56
  stavudine (Zerit), 55
  tenofovir (Viread), 55
  zidovudine/AZT (Retrovir), 55
nucleotide analogue
  cidofovir (Vistide), 54
protease inhibitors
  atazanavir (Reyataz), 58
  darunavir (Prezista), 59
  fosamprenavir (Lexiva), 59
  indinavir (Crixivan), 58
  lopinavir and ritonavir (Kaletra), 59
  nelfinavir (Viracept), 58
  ritonavir (Norvir), 58
  saquinavir (Invirase), 58
  tipranavir (Aptivus), 59

Antiviral agents (*continued*)
    pyrophosphonate derivative
        foscarnet (Foscavir), 52
    tricyclic amines
        amantadine, 50
        rimantadine (Flumadine), 50
Anxiety disorders, medications for, 128
Anxiolytics
    antihistamine
        hydroxyzine (Vistaril), 127
    azapirone
        buspirone (Buspar), 126
    benzodiazepines
        alprazolam (Xanax, Niravam, 126
        diazepam (Valium, Diastat), 126
        lorazepam (Ativan), 126
    classification of, 125
    selective serotonin reuptake inhibitors
        escitalopram (Lexapro), 127
    serotonin norepinephrine reuptake inhibitors
        duloxetine (Cymbalta), 127
        venlafaxine (Effexor), 127
Aplastic anemia, 348
Apomorphine (Apokyn), 142
Apraclonidine (Iopidine), 107
Apremilast (Otezla), 357
Aprepitant (Emend), 283
Arformoterol (Brovana), 272
Argatroban (Acova), 256
Aripiprazole (Abilify), 115
Aromatase inhibitors
    anastrozole (Arimidex), 345
    exemestane (Aromasin), 345
    letrozole (Femara), 345
Articaine-epinephrine (Articadent, Orabloc, Septocaine, Zorcaine), 184
Asenapine (Saphris), 115
Asparaginase (Elspar), 346
Aspirin (Bayer Aspirin), 373

Aspirin (Ecotrin, Bayer, Bufferin), 259
Asthenia, definition of, 290
Asthma drugs
    β_2-adrenergic agonists
        long-acting β-agonists (LABA), 272
        short-acting β-agonists (SABA), 271
    classification of, 270
    mechanisms of action, 276
    non-β_2-adrenergic agonists
        aerosol corticosteroids, 273–274
        inhibitor of 5'-lipoxygenase, 275
        leukotriene receptor antagonist, 275
        mast cell stabilizer, 274
        methyl xanthine, 273
        muscarinic antagonist, 273
Atazanavir (Reyataz), 58
Atenolol (Tenormin), 102, 206, 229
Atomoxetine (Strattera), 129
Atorvastatin (Lipitor), 250
Atovaquone (Mepron), 69
Atovaquone and proguanil (Malarone), 68
Atracurium, 196
Atropine, 384
Atropine (Isopto Atropine), 106
Atropine (Sal-Tropine, Isopto Atropine), 91
Attention deficit hyperactivity disorder (ADHD), medications for
    alpha adrenergic agonist
        clonidine (Kapvay), 130
        guanfacine (Intuniv, Tenex), 130
    norepinephrine receptor inhibitor
        atomoxetine (Strattera), 129
    stimulants
        dexmethylphenidate (Focalin), 129
        dextroamphetamine (Dexedrine), 129
        lisdexamfetamine (Vyvanse), 129
        methamphetamine (Desoxyn), 129
        methylphenidate (Concerta, Ritalin, Daytrana, Metadate, Methylin, Quillivant), 129

Atypical antipsychotics, 114–115
    aripiprazole (Abilify), 115
    asenapine (Saphris), 115
    clozapine (Clozaril, FazaClo), 114
    iloperidone (Fanapt), 115
    olanzapine (Zyprexa), 115
    paliperidone (Invega), 115
    quetiapine (Seroquel), 115
    risperidone (Risperdal), 114
    ziprasidone (Geodon), 115
Autonomic nervous system (ANS)
    eye. *See* Eye, pharmacology of medications
        adrenergic blockers, 99–103
        cholinergic agonists, 86–89
        ganglionic blockers, 93–94
        muscarinic antagonists, 90–92
        sympathomimetics, 95–98
    structure
        actions of some drugs, 83
        components, 82
        effects on organ systems, 84–85
        overview of, 83
Azacitidine (Vidaza), 333
Azathioprine (Imuran, Azasan), 355
Azelastine (Astelin, Astepro), 380
Azilsartan (Edarbi), 217
Aziridine, 337
Azithromycin (Zithromax), 39
Azoles
    clotrimazole (Lotrimin), 63
    fluconazole (Diflucan), 63
    ketoconazole, 64
    miconazole (Monistat, Oravig), 64
    posaconazole (Noxafil), 64
    voriconazole (Vfend), 65
Aztreonam (Azactam), 33

B

Bacillus Calmette Guerine-BCG (TheraCys, TICE BCG), 347
Bacitracin, 34
Baclofen (Lioresal, Gablofen), 177
β_2-adrenergic agonists
  long-acting β-agonists (LABA)
    arformoterol (Brovana), 272
    formoterol (Foradil, Performoist), 272
    indacaterol (Arcapta), 272
    salmeterol (Serevent), 272
  short-acting β-agonists (SABA)
    albuterol (AccuNeb, ProAir, Vospire, Proventil, Ventolin), 271
    levalbuterol (Xopenex), 271
    metaproterenol, 271
    pirbuterol (Maxair), 271
    terbutaline, 271
Barbiturates
  methohexital (Brevital), 189
  pentobarbital (Nembutal), 189
  thiopental, 189
Basiliximab (Simulect), 358
β-blockers
  acebutolol (Sectral), 102, 206
  atenolol (Tenormin), 102, 206, 229
  betaxolol (Kerlone), 102, 206
  bisoprolol (Zebeta), 102, 206
  carvedilol, 245
  carvedilol (Coreg), 103, 207
  effects of nitrates combined with, 231
  esmolol (Brevibloc), 102, 207
  labetalol (Trandate), 103, 207
  metoprolol, 245
  metoprolol (Lopressor, Toprol), 206, 229
  metoprolol (Toprol XL, Lopressor), 102
  nadolol (Corgard), 103, 207, 230

nebivolol (Brevibloc), 206
nebivolol (Bystolic, 102
penbutolol (Levatol), 207
pindolol, 208, 230
propranolol (Hemangeol, Inderal, InnoPran), 208, 230
propranolol (Inderal LA), 103
sotalol (Betapace, sorine), 103
timolol, 208
timolol (Blocadren), 103
Beclomethasone (QVAR), 274
Belatacept (Nulojix), 360
Belimimab (Benlysta), 359
Benazepril (Lotensin), 215
Bendamustine (Treanda), 329
Benzocaine, 182
Benzodiazepines
  alprazolam (Xanax), 146
  alprazolam (Xanax, Niravam, 126
  chlordiazepoxide (Librium), 147
  clonazepam (Klonopin), 147
  clorazepate (Tranxene), 148
  diazepam (Valium, Diastat), 126, 148
  estazolam (ProSom), 147
  flurazepam (Dalmane), 148
  lorazepam (Ativan), 126, 147
  midazolam (Versed), 146, 187
  oxazepam (Serax), 146
  quazepam (Doral), 148
  temazepam (Restoril), 147
  triazolam (Halcion), 146
Benzonatate (Tessalon, Zonatuss), 269
Benztropine (Cogentin), 139
Beriberi, definition of, 388
Betaxolol (Betoptic), 107
Betaxolol (Kerlone), 102, 206
Bethanechol (Urecholine), 87
Bevacizumab (Avastin), 348

Bicalutamide (Casodex), 319
Biguanide, 310
Bile acid sequestrants, 251
  cholestipol (Cholestid), 249
  cholestyramine (Questran, Prevalite, Questran Light), 249
  colesevelam (Welchol), 249
Binding, 8
Bioavailability, definition of, 2
Bisacodyl (Dulcolax, Correctol), 284
Bismuth subsalicylate (Pepto Bismol, Bismatrol, Kaopectate), 285
Bisoprolol (Zebeta), 102, 206
Bisphosphonates
  alendronate (Fosamax), 305
  calcitonin (Fortical, Miacalcin), 306
  etidronate (Didronel), 305
  gallium nitrate (Ganite), 306
  ibandronate (Boniva), 305
  pamidronate (Aredia), 305
  risedronate (Actonel, Atelvia), 305
  zoledronic acid (Reclast, Zometa), 305
Bitolterol (Tornolate), 97
Bivalirudin (Angiomax), 257
Blackwater fever, 15
β-lactamase-resistant, 19–20
  cloxacillin, 17
  dicloxacillin, 17, 20
  nafcillin, 17, 20
  oxacillin (Bactocill), 17, 20
β-lactams
  carbapenem, 32–33
    ertapenem (Invanz), 32
    imipenem (Primaxin), 32
    meropenem (Merrem), 32
  monobactam, 33
Bleomycin (Blenoxane), 335
Blepharospasm, definition of, 137

Blood dyscrasias, definition of, 278
Blood-to-gas partition coefficient (B/G coefficient), definition of, 137
Botulinum toxin (BoTox), 177
Brimonidine (Alphagan), 106
Bromocriptine (Parlodel, Cycloset), 142, 296
Buccal adminstration route, 8
Budesonide (Pulmicort), 274
Bumetanide (Bumex), 222, 246
Bupivacaine (Marcaine, Sensorcaine), 183
Buprenorphine (Buprenex, Butrans Subutex), 167
Buprenorphine and naloxone (Suboxone, Zubsolv), 167
Bupropion (Wellbutrin, Zyban, Budeprion, Forfivo, Aplenzin), 119
Buspirone (Buspar), 126, 152
Busulfan (Myleran, Busulfex), 327
Butabarbital (Butisol), 149
Butenafine (Lotrimin, Mentax), 63
Butorphanol (Stadol), 167
Butyrophenones, 113

C

Caffeine, 133
Calcitonin (Fortical, Miacalcin), 306
Calcium carbonate (Caltrate, TUMS), 280
Calcium channel blockers
    amlodipine (Norvasc), 212
    clevidipine (Cleviprex), 212
    dihydropyridine
        amlodipine (Norvasc), 229
        nicardipine (Cardene), 229
        nifedipine (Adalat, Afeditab, Procardia, Nifediac, Nifedical), 229
    diltiazem (Cardizem), 212
    felodipine (Plendil, Renedil), 213
    isradipine, 213
    nicardipine (Cardene), 213

nifedipine (Adalat, Afeditab, Procardia, Nifediac,Nifedical), 213
nisoldipine (Sular), 213
nondihydropyridine
    diltiazem (Cardizem, Dilacor, Diltzac, Matzim, Taztia, Tiazac), 228
    verapamil (Calan, Isoptin, Verelan), 228
    verapamil (Calan, Isoptin, Verelan), 212
Calcium levels, drugs affecting, 304–306
    antineoplastic agent
        plicamycin (Mithracin, Mithramycin), 306
    bisphosphonates
        alendronate (Fosamax), 305
        calcitonin (Fortical, Miacalcin), 306
        etidronate (Didronel), 305
        gallium nitrate (Ganite), 306
        ibandronate (Boniva), 305
        pamidronate (Aredia), 305
        risedronate (Actonel, Atelvia), 305
        zoledronic acid (Reclast, Zometa), 305
    dental prophylaxis
        sodium fluoride, 306
    selective estrogen receptor modulators
        raloxifene (Evista), 304
        tamoxifen (Nolvadex), 304
Camptothecins
    irinotecan (Camptosar), 340
    topotecan (Hycamtin), 340
Candesartan (Atacand), 217, 245
Cannabinoid, 29
Capecitabine (Xeloda), 332
Capsicum/Cayenne, 389
Captopril (Capoten), 215, 243
Carbachol (Isopto Carbachol, Miostat), 87, 105
Carbamates
    neostigmine (Prostigmin, Bloxiverz), 89
    physostigmine, 88
    pyridostigmine (Mestinon, Regonol), 89

Carbamazepine (Tegretol, Carbatrol, Epitol, Equetro), 124, 160
Carbapenem, 32–33
    ertapenem (Invanz), 32
    imipenem (Primaxin), 32
    meropenem (Merrem), 32
Carbenicillin (Geocillin), 17, 22
Carbidopa (Lodosyn), 141
Carbonic anhydrase inhibitor, 224
Carboplatin (Paraplatin), 328
Carcinoid syndrome, definition of, 290
Cardiac and renal function, drugs affecting
    antianginal drugs, 226–232
    antiarrhythmics, 233–239
    antihyperlipidemic drugs, 248–251
    antihypertensive drugs, 200–225
    coagulopathy, management of, 252–263
    congestive heart failure, management of, 240–247
    diuretics. See Diuretics
    terms to learn, 199
Cardiac glycosides, 241
Carisoprodol (Soma), 177
Carmustine (BiCNU, Gliadel), 328
Carteolol (Ocupress), 107
Carvedilol, 245
Carvedilol (Coreg), 103, 207
Cascara sagrada, 389
Caspofungin (Cancidas), 62
Catecholamine (adrenergic agonist), 185
Catecholamines, 95–96
    dobutamine, 96
    dopamine, 95
    epinephrine (Adrenalin, Epipen), 96
    isoproterenol, 96
    norepinephrine (Levophed), 96
    phenylephrine, 96
Celecoxib (Celebrex), 376
Cell wall synthesis inhibitors
    antibiotic mechanisms of action, 16

β-lactams
  carbapenem, 32–33
  monobactam, 33
cephalosporins. *See* Cephalosporins
non-β-lactams, 34
  bacitracin, 34
  cycloserine (Seromycin), 34
  fosfomycin (Monurol), 34
  vancomycin (Vancocin), 34
penicillins. *See* Penicillins
Central precocious puberty, definition of, 290
Cephalosporins
  classification of, 24
  effectiveness against gram-negative and
    gram-positive organisms, 26
  fifth-generation, 25
    ceftaroline (Teflaro), 31
  first-generation, 25, 27
    cefazolin (Ancef, Kefzol), 27
    cephalexin (Keflex), 27
    cephalothin (Keflin), 27
    cephradine (Anspor, Velosef), 27
  fourth-generation, 25
    cefepime (Maxipime), 25, 31
  overview, 25
  second-generation, 25, 28–29
    cefaclor (Ceclor), 28
    cefamandole (Mandol), 28
    cefonicid (Monocid), 28
    cefotetan (Cefotan), 29
    cefoxitin (Mefoxin), 29
    cefuroxime (Ceftin, Zinacef), 28
  third-generation, 25, 30–31
    cefixime (Suprax), 31
    cefoperazone, 30
    cefotaxime (Claforan), 30
    ceftazidime (Tazicef, Fortaz), 30
    ceftizoxime (Cefizox), 30
    ceftriaxone (Rocephin), 31

Certolizumab pegol (Cimzia), 355
Cetirizine (Zyrtec, Aller-Relief), 380
Cetuximab (Erbitux), 348
Cevimeline (Evoxac), 87
Cheilosis, definition of, 388
Chelators
  deferoxamine (Desferel), 386
  dimercaprol (BAL), 385
  edetate calcium disodium (EDTA, Endrate,
    Versenate), 385
  penicillamine (Cuprimine, Depen), 386
  succimer/DMSA (Chemet), 385
Chemical antagonist, definition of, 2
Chemoreceptor trigger zone, definition of, 278
Chemotherapeutic drugs
  alemtuzumab (Campath), 348
  asparaginase (Elspar), 346
  Bacillus Calmette Guerine-BCG (TheraCys, TICE
    BCG), 347
  bevacizumab (Avastin), 348
  cetuximab (Erbitux), 348
  dasatinib (Sprycel), 346
  denileukin (Ontak), 346
  erlotinib (Tarceva), 347
  everolimus (Afinitor, Zortress), 347
  ixabepilone (Ixempra), 347
  mitoxantrone (Novantrone), 346
  rituximab (Rituxan), 348
  trastuzumab (Herceptin), 348
Chenodiol (Chenodal), 286
CHF therapy. *See* Congestive heart failure,
  management of
Chlamydia trachomatis, 15
Chloral hydrate, 152
Chlorambucil (Leukeran), 327
Chloramphenicol, 39
Chlordiazepoxide (Librium), 147
Chloroprocaine (Nesacaine), 181
Chloroquine (Aralen), 67

Chlorothiazide (Diuril), 221, 246
Chlorpheniramine (Chlor-Trimeton), 268, 379
Chlorpromazine (Thorazine), 113
Chlorpropamide (Diabinese), 309
Chlorthalidone, 221, 246
Chlorzoxazone (Parafon Forte, Lorzone), 178
Cholesterol absorption blockers, 250, 251
Cholestipol (Cholestid), 249
Cholestyramine (Questran, Prevalite, Questran Light),
  249
Cholinergic agonists
  classification, 86
  classification of, 86
  direct, 87
  indirect, 88–89
Chondrotin, 389
Chorionic Gonadotropin (Novarel, Pregnyl), 296
Chronic myelogenous leukemia, 324
Ciclesonide (Alvesco), 274
Cidofovir (Vistide), 54
Cimetidine (Tagamet), 279
Cinchonism, 15
Ciprofloxacin (Cipro), 45
Cisatracurium (Nimbex), 196
Cisplatin (Platinol), 328
Citalopram (Celexa), 120
Cladribine (Leustatin), 330
Clarithromycin (Biaxin), 38
Clearance (CL), 11
Clemastine (Tavist), 380
Clevidipine (Cleviprex), 212
Clindamycin (Cleocin), 39
Clobazam (Onfi), 156
Clofarabine (Clolar), 330
Clomiphene (Clomid, Serophene), 313
Clomipramine (Anafranil), 118
Clonazepam (Klonopin), 147, 157
Clonidine (Catapres), 218
Clonidine (Catapres, Duraclon, Kapvay), 202

Clonidine (Kapvay), 130
Clopidogrel (Plavix), 260
Clorazepate (Tranxene), 148, 156
Clotrimazole (Lotrimin), 63
Clotting factors, 262
Cloxacillin, 17
Clozapine (Clozaril, FazaClo), 114
Coagulopathy, management of, 252–263
  adenosine reuptake inhibitor
    dipyridamole (Persantine), 261
  ADP receptor antagonists
    clopidogrel (Plavix), 260
    prasugrel (Effient), 260
    ticlopidine, 260
  anticoagulants
    heparin, 255
    protein C (concentrate, ceprotin), 254
    warfarin (Coumadin, Jantoven), 254
  antiplatelet drugs
    aspirin (Ecotrin, Bayer, Bufferin), 259
  direct thrombin inhibitor
    argatroban (Acova), 256
    bivalirudin (Angiomax), 257
    dabigatran (Pradaxa), 256
    desirudin (Iprivask), 257
  drugs to reduce clotting, classification of, 252
  drugs used to facilitate clotting
    aminocaproic acid (Amicar), 262
    antiplasmin drugs, 262
    classification of, 261
    desmopressin (DDAVP, Stimate), 263
    protamine sulfate, 263
    recombinant human factor IX, 262
    recombinant human factor VIIa, 262
    recombinant human factor VIII, 262
    vitamin K (Mephyton), 263
  factor Xa inhibitors
    fondaparinux (Arixtra), 256
    rivaroxaban (Xarelto), 256

glycoprotein IIb/IIIa receptor antagonists
    abciximab (Reopro), 259
    eptifibatide (Integrilin), 259
    tirofiban (Aggrastat), 259
  low–molecular-weight heparins
    dalteparin (Fragmin), 255
    enoxaparin (Lovenox), 255
  overview, 253
  thrombolytics
    alteplase (Activase), 258
    reteplase (Retavase), 258
    tenecteplase (TNKase), 258
    urokinase (Kinlytic), 258
Cocaine, 182
Cocaine (crack, coke), 133
Codeine, 166, 269
Colchicine, 369
Cold medications
  antitussive
    benzonatate (Tessalon, Zonatuss), 269
    codeine, 267
    dextromethorphan (Robitussin DM, Delsym), 269
  classification of, 267
  expectorant
    guaifenesin (Mucinex, Robitussin), 269
  systemic decongestants
    chlorpheniramine (Chlor-Trimeton), 268
    diphenhydramine (Benadryl), 268
    phenylephrine (Sudafed PE), 268
    pseudoephedrine (Sudafed), 268
  topical decongestants
    naphazoline (Privine), 269
    oxymetazoline (Afrin), 268
    phenylephrine (Neo-Synephrine), 269
Colesevelam (Welchol), 249
Competitive antagonist, definition of, 2
Congestive heart failure, management of
  ACE inhibitors
    captopril (Capoten), 243

    enalapril (Vasotec, Epaned), 244
    lisinopril (Prinivil, Zestril), 242
    quinapril (Accupril), 244
    ramipril (Altace), 244
    trandolapril (Mavik), 245
  angiotensin receptor blockers
    candesartan (Atacand), 245
    valsartan (Dlovan), 245
  arterial vasodilators
    hydralazine (Apresoline, Novohylazin, Nu-Hydral), 247
  β-blockers
    carvedilol, 245
    metoprolol, 245
  classification of drugs, 240
  loop diuretics
    bumetanide (Bumex), 246
    furosemide (Lasix), 246
    torsemide (Demadex), 246
  nitrates
    isosorbide dinitrate (Isordil, IsoDitrate, Dilatrate), 247
    nitroprusside (Nitropress), 247
  positive inotropic drugs
    digoxin (Lanoxin, Digox), 241
    dobutamine, 242
    dopamine (Intropin), 242
    inamrinone (Inocor), 242
    milrinone, 242
  potassium-sparing diuretic
    eplerenone (Inspra), 243
    spironolactone (Aldactone), 243
  thiazide diuretics
    chlorothiazide (Diuril), 246
    chlorthalidone, 246
    hydrochlorothiazide (HCTZ, Microzide), 246
    indapamide, 247
    metolazone (Zaroxolyn), 246

Conivaptan (Vaprisol), 224
Conjugated estrogens (Premarin), 312
Conn's syndrome, 199
Corticotropin (ACTH, Acthar), 295
Corticotropin-releasing hormone (CRH), 292–293, 295
Cox-2 inhibitors, 376
Cranberry, 389
Craniosynostosis, definition of, 290
Cromolyn sodium (Gastrocrom), 274
Cushing's disease, definition of, 290
Cyclobenzaprine (Flexeril, Fexmid, Amrix), 178
Cyclopentolate (Cyclogyl), 106
Cyclophosphamide (Cytoxan), 326, 356
Cycloserine (Seromycin), 34
Cyclosporine (Neoral, Gengraf, Sandimmune), 352
Cyproheptadine (Periactin), 175
Cytosine arabinoside-Ara-C-Cytarabine (Cytosar), 331
Cytotoxic agents
    azathioprine (Imuran, Azasan), 355
    cyclophosphamide (Cytoxan), 356
    methotrexate (Trexall, Rheumatrex), 356

D

Dabigatran (Pradaxa), 256
Dacarbazine (Dtic-Dome), 329
Dactinomycin (Cosmegen), 335
Dalteparin (Fragmin), 255
Dantrolene (Dantrium, Revonto), 178
Daptomycin (Cubicin), 47
Darunavir (Prezista), 59
Dasatinib (Sprycel), 346
Daunorubicin (Cerubidine), 336
Decitabine (Dacogen), 332
Deferoxamine (Desferel), 386
Delavirdine (Rescriptor), 57
Delirium tremens (DTs), 110
Demeclocycline (Declomycin), 37

Denileukin (Ontak), 346
Dental prophylaxis, 306
Desflurane (Suprane), 187
Desiccated thyroid (Armour Thyroid, Nature-Throid, Westhroid), 302
Desipramine (Norparmin), 118
Desirudin (Iprivask), 257
Desloratidine (Clarinex), 380
Desmopressin (DDAVP, Stimate), 263, 297
Desvenlafaxine (Pristiq), 121
Dexamathasone (Decadron), 299
Dexlansoprazole (Kapidex), 281
Dexmedetomidine (Precedex), 190
Dexmethylphenidate (Focalin), 129
Dextroamphetamine (Dexedrine, ProCentra, Zenzedi), 129
Dextromethorphan (Delsym, Robitussin DM), 166
Dextromethorphan (Robitussin DM, Delsym), 269
Diabetes, drugs for management of
    insulin
        determir, 307
        glargine, 307
        glulisine, 307
        lispro, 307
        NPH, 307
        regular, 307
    oral diabetic drugs
        classification of, 308
        nonsulfonylureas, 310–311
        sulfonylureas, 309
Diabetes insipidis, definition of, 290
Diazepam (Valium), 178
Diazepam (Valium, Diastat), 126, 148, 156
Dibenzoxazepine, 113–114
Dicloxacillin, 17, 20
Didanosine/DDI (Videx), 55
Difenoxin (Motofen), 166
Diflunisal (Dolobid), 374
Digoxin (Lanoxin, Digox), 241

Digoxin-specific antibodies (Digibind), 383
Dihydro-ergotamine (DHE-45, Migranal), 172
Dihydropyridine calcium channel blockers
    amlodipine (Norvasc), 229
    nicardipine (Cardene), 229
    nifedipine (Adalat, Afeditab, Procardia, Nifediac, Nifedical), 229
Diltiazem (Cardizem), 212
Diltiazem (Cardizem, Dilacor), 239
Diltiazem (Cardizem, Dilacor, Diltzac, Matzim, Taztia, Tiazac), 228
Dimenhydrinate (Dramamine), 283, 379
Dimercaprol (BAL), 385
Dinoprostone (Prepidil, ProstinE2, Cervidil), 368
Diphenhydramine (Benadryl), 268, 379
Diphenoxylate (Lomotil), 166
Diphenylbutylpiperidinesd, 113
Dipivefrin (Propine), 107
Dipyridamole (Persantine), 261
Direct thrombin inhibitor
    argatroban (Acova), 256
    bivalirudin (Angiomax), 257
    dabigatran (Pradaxa), 256
    desirudin (Iprivask), 257
Disopyramide (Norpace), 234
Distribution, 8
Disulfiram reaction, 15
Diuretics
    carbonic anhydrase inhibitor
        acetazolamide (Acetazolam, Diamox), 224
    classification of, 217
    loop
        bumetanide (Bumex), 222
        ethacrynic acid (Edecrin), 222
        furosemide (Lasix), 222
        torsemide (Demadex), 222
    mechanism of action, 218
    osmotic
        mannitol (Osmitrol), 224

Diuretics (*continued*)
  potassium-sparing
    amiloride (Midamor), 223
    eplerenone (Inspra), 223
    spironolactone (Aldactone), 223
    triamterene (Dyrenium), 223
  serum electrolyte effects of, 225
  thiazide
    chlorothiazide (Diuril), 221
    chlorthalidone, 221
    hydrochlorothiazide (HCTZ), 221
    indapamide, 221
    methyclothiazide, 221
    metolazone (Zaroxolyn), 221
  vasopressin receptor antagonists
    conivaptan (Vaprisol), 224
    tolvaptan (Samsca), 224
Dobutamine, 96, 242
Docetaxel (Taxotere, Docefrez), 341
Docusate (Colace), 284
Dofetilide (Tikosyn), 238
Dolasetron (Anzemet), 282
Donepezil (Aricept), 88, 145
Dopamine, 95
Dopamine agonists
  apomorphine (Apokyn), 142
  bromocriptine (Parlodel, Cycloset), 142
  pramipexole (Mirapex), 142
  ropinirole (Requip), 142
  rotigotine (Neupro), 142
Dose-response curve
  comparison of, 5
  graded, 4–5
  quantal, 4–5
  time action, 4–5
Dosing, 12
Doxacurium (Nuromax), 196
Doxazosin (Cardura), 101, 205

Doxepin (Silenor), 118
Doxorubicin (Adriamycin), 335
Doxycycline (Vibramycin), 37
Dronabinol (Marinol), 283
Dronedarone (Multaq), 238
Drug movement, within body, 7
Drugs of abuse
  cannabinoid
    marijuana (Mary Jane, Weed, Pot), 131
  hallucinogens
    lysergic acid diethylamide (LSD), 132
    phencyclidine (PCP, wet), 132
  opiates
    heroin, 132
  sedatives
    alcohol, 133
  stimulants
    caffeine, 133
    cocaine (crack, coke), 133
    methamphetamine (crystal meth), 133
    3,4-methylenedioxy-*N*-methylamphetamine (MDMA, Ecstasy), 133
    nicotine, 133
Drug solubility, 7
Duloxetine (Cymbalta), 121, 127
Dutasteride (Avodart), 320
Dyskinesias, definition of, 110
Dysmenorrhea, 366
Dysphagia, definition of, 137
Dystonia, definition of, 110

E

EC$_{50}$, definition of, 2
Echinacea, 390
Echinocandins
  anidulafungin (Eraxis), 62
  caspofungin (Cancidas), 62
  micafungin (Mycamine), 62

Echothiophate (Phospholine iodide), 89
Echothiophate iodide (Phospholine Iodide), 105
ED$_{50}$, definition of, 2
Edetate calcium disodium (EDTA, Endrate, Versenate), 385
Edrophonium (Enlon, Tensilon), 88
Efavirenz (Sustiva), 57
Effector, definition of, 2
Efficacy, definition of, 2
Eletriptan (Relpax), 174
Elimination
  first-order, 10
  zero-order, 10
Elimination disorders, medications for, 128
Emtricitabine (Emtriva), 55
Enalapril (Vasotec, Epaned), 216, 244
Endocrine system, drugs affecting
  calcium levels, drugs affecting, 304–306
  diabetes, drugs for management of, 307–311
  exogenous glucocorticoids
    dexamathasone (Decadron), 299
    hydrocortisone (Cortef, A-Hydrocort), 298
    prednisone, 298
    triamcinolone (Kenalog, Aristospan), 299
  hypothalamic and pituitary hormones, 292–297
  mineralocorticoid agonist, 300
  mineralocorticoid antagonists, 300
  terms to learn, 290–291
  thyroid drugs, 301–303. *See also* Thyroid drugs
Endometriosis, definition of, 290
Enflurane (Ethrane), 188
Enhances physiological tremor, treatment of, 143
Enoxaparin (Lovenox), 255
Entacapone (Comtan), 141
Entecavir (Baraclude), 56
Enzalutamide (Xtandi), 319
Enzyme inhibitors
  apremilast (Otezla), 357
  leflunomide (Arava), 357

mycophenolate Mofetil (Cellcept, Myfortic), 357
  tofacitinib (Xeljanz), 357
Ephedrine, 97
Epinephrine, 185
Epinephrine (Adrenalin,Epipen), 96
Epinephrine (Epifrin, Glaucon), 106
Epirubicin (Ellence), 336
Eplerenone (Inspra), 223, 243, 300
Epoprostenol (Flolan), 368
Eprosartan (Teveten), 217
EPS. *See* Extrapyramidal syndrome (EPS)
Eptifibatide (Integrilin), 259
Ergotamine (Ergomar), 172
Ergotamine and caffeine (Cafergot, Migergot), 172
Ergotism, definition of, 137
Ergots
  dihydroergotamine (DHE-45, Migranal), 172
  ergotamine (Ergomar), 172
Erlotinib (Tarceva), 347
Ertapenem (Invanz), 32
Erythema nodosum leprosum, 350
Erythromycin (Erythrocin), 38
Escitalopram (Lexapro), 120, 127
Esmolol (Brevibloc), 102, 207
Esomeprazole (Nexium), 281
Essential tremor, treatment of, 143
Estazolam (ProSom), 147
Esterified estrogens (Menest), 312
Esters
  benzocaine, 182
  chloroprocaine (Nesacaine), 181
  cocaine, 182
  procaine (Novacain), 181
  tetracaine (Pontocaine), 181
Estradiol, 312
Estrogen preparations
  conjugated estrogens (Premarin), 312
  esterified estrogens (Menest), 312

estradiol, 312
estropipate (Ogen), 312
ethinyl estradiol, 312
mestranol, 312
Estrogens, 343
Estropipate (Ogen), 312
Eszopiclone (Lunesta), 153
Etanercept (Enbrel), 354
Ethacrynic Acid (Edecrin), 222
Ethanol, 383
Ethinyl estradiol, 312
Ethosuximide (Zarontin), 159
Ethotoin (Peganone), 161
Ethyl chloride, 185
Etidronate (Didronel), 305
Etomidate (Amidate), 190
Etonogestrel (Implanon, Nexplanon), 315
Etoposide (VP-16, VePesid), 339
Etravirine (Intelence), 57
Everolimus (Afinitor, Zortress), 347
Ewing's sarcoma, 324
Exemestane (Aromasin), 345
Extended spectrum penicillins, 21–22
  amoxicillin (Amoxil, Trimox), 17, 21
  ampicillin (Ampicin), 17, 21
  carbenicillin (Geocillin), 17, 22
  piperacillin (Pipracil), 17, 22
  ticarcillin (Ticar), 17, 22
Extrapyramidal syndrome (EPS), 110
Eye, pharmacology of
  clinically important structures and receptors, 108
  eye conditions, cholinergic and adrenergic drugs for, 104
  eye diseases, drugs for treatment of
    acetylcholine (Miochol-E), 105
    apraclonidine (Iopidine), 107
    atropine (Isopto Atropine), 106

betaxolol (Betoptic), 107
brimonidine (Alphagan), 106
carbachol (Isopto Carbachol, Miostat), 105
carteolol (Ocupress, 107
cyclopentolate (Cyclogyl), 106
dipivefrin (Propine), 107
echothiophate Iodide (Phospholine Iodide), 105
epinephrine (Epifrin, Glaucon), 106
homatropine (Isopto Homatropine), 106
levobunolol (Betagan), 107
metipranolol (Optipranolol), 107
phenylephrine (Neosynephrine), 106
pilocarpine (Isopto Carpine, Pilopine HS), 105
timolol (Timoptic), 107
tropicamide (Mydriacyl), 106
  receptor mechanisms, 105
Ezetimibe (Zetia), 250
Ezogabine (Potiga), 159

F

Facilitated diffusion, 7
Factor Xa inhibitors
  fondaparinux (Arixtra), 256
  rivaroxaban (Xarelto), 256
Famciclovir (Famvir), 54
Famotidine (Pepcid), 279
Febuxostat (Uloric), 370
Felbamate (Felbatol), 157
Felodipine (Plendil, Renedil), 213
Fenofibrate (Tricor, Antara, Fenoglide, Lipofen, Triglide), 251
Fenofibric acid (Fibricor, Trilipix), 251
Fentanyl (Actiq, Abstral Lazanda, Subsys Onsolis, Fentora, Duragesic), 165
Fentanyl (Sublimaze), 191
Feverfew, 390
Fexofenadine (Allegra), 380

Fibric acid derivatives, 251
  fenofibrate (Tricor, Antara, Fenoglide, Lipofen, Triglide), 251
  fenofibric acid (Fibricor, Trilipix), 251
  gemfibrozil (Lopid), 251
Fidaxomicin (Dificid), 39
Filgrastim (Neupogen), 362
Finasteride (Proscar, Propecia), 320
Fingolimod (Gilenya), 360
First-order elimination, 10
  vs. zero-order elimination, 10
Flecainide (Tambocor), 236
Floxuridine (FUDR), 332
Fluconazole (Diflucan), 63
Flucytosine (Ancobon), 65
Fludarabine (Fludara, Oforta), 331
Fludrocorticosone (Florinef), 300
Flumazenil (Romazicon), 383
Fluoroquinolones, 41
  antimicrobial action of, 46
  fourth-generation
    gemifloxacin (Factive), 46
    moxifloxacin (Avelox), 46
  second-generation
    ciprofloxacin (Cipro), 45
    norfloxacin (Noroxin), 45
    ofloxin (Floxin), 45
  third-generation
    levofloxacin (Levaquin), 46
5-fluorouracil (Adrucil), 331
Fluoxetine (Prozac), 120
Fluoxymesterone (Androxy), 318
Fluphenazine (Prolixin, Permitil), 113
Flurazepam (Dalmane), 148
Flurbiprofen (Ansaid), 374
Flutamide (Eulexin), 344
Fluticasone (Flovent), 273
Fluvastatin (Lescol), 250
Fluvoxamine (Luvox), 120

Folic acid antagonist
  methotrexate (Rheumatrex, Trexall), 333
  pemetrexed (Alimta), 333
Follicle-stimulating hormone (FSH), 292–293
Follitropin Alfa (Gonal-F), 296
Follitropin Beta (Follistim), 296
Fomepizole (Antizol), 383
Fondaparinux (Arixtra), 256
Formoterol (Foradil, Perforomist), 97, 272
Fosamprenavir (Lexiva), 59
Foscarnet (Foscavir), 52
Fosfomycin (Monurol), 34
Fosinopril (Monopril), 215
Fosphenytoin (Cerebyx), 160
Frovatriptan (Frova), 174
Fungal cyclic peptide antibiotic
  cyclosporine (Neoral, Gengraf, Sandimmune), 352
  tacrolimus-FK-506 (Prograf, Hecoria), 353
Furosemide (Lasix), 222, 246

G

Gabapentin (Neurontin, Gralise), 158
Galantamine (Razadyne), 145
Gallium nitrate (Ganite), 306
Ganciclovir (Cytovene), 53
Ganglionic blockers
  classification of, 93
  depolarizing
    nicotine (Nicoderm, Nicotrol, Nicotrol inhaler, Nicorette), 94
  nondepolarizing
    mecamylamine (Inversine), 94
    trimethaphan (Arfonad), 94
Garlic, 390
Gastrointestinal drugs
  antacids and proton pump inhibitors, 280–281

  antiemetics, 282–283
  bismuth subsalicylate (Pepto Bismol, Bismatrol, Kaopectate), 285
  chenodiol (Chenodal), 286
  H₂-receptor antagonists
    cimetidine (Tagamet), 279
    famotidine (Pepcid), 279
    nizatidine (Axid), 279
    ranitidine (Zantac), 279
  laxatives, 284
  mesalamine (Asacol, Pentasa, Rowasa, Canasa, Apriso, Lialda), 286
  misoprostol (Cytotec), 285
  octreotide (Sandostatin), 286
  sites of action of drugs to treat peptic ulcer disease, 287
  sucralfate (Carafate), 285
  terms to learn, 278
  ursodiol (Actigall), 286
Gastroparesis, definition of, 278
Gemcitabine (Gemzar), 332
Gemfibrozil (Lopid), 251
Gemifloxacin (Factive), 46
General anesthetic drugs
  classification of, 186
  inhaled
    desflurane (Suprane), 187
    enflurane (Ethrane), 188
    halothane (Fluothane), 188
    isoflurane (Forane, Terrell), 187
    nitrous oxide, 188
    sevoflurane (Ultane, Sojourn), 187
  intravenous nonopioids
    dexmedetomidine (Precedex), 190
    etomidate (Amidate), 190
    ketamine (Ketalar), 189
    methohexital (Brevital), 189
    midazolam (Versed), 189
    pentobarbital (Nembutal), 189

propofol (Diprivan, Fresenius Propoven), 190
  remifentanil (Ultiva), 192
  thiopental, 189
intravenous opioids, 191
  alfentanil (Alfenta), 191
  meperidine (Demerol), 192
  morphine (Duramorph, Astramorph, Infumorph), 191
  remifentanil (Ultiva), 192
  sufentanil (Sufenta), 191
nonanesthetic drugs used during, 191
Generalized (grand mal) seizures, 162
Gentamicin, 35
Gestational trophoblastic neoplasms, 324
Giant cell tumors, 324
Ginger, 390
Gingko biloba, 390
Ginseng, 391
Glimepiride (Amaryl), 309
Glipizide (Glucotrol), 309
Glossitis, definition of, 388
Glucocorticoids, 353
  prednisone (Deltasone), 345
Glucosamine, 391
Glyburide (DiaBeta, Glynase, PresTab), 309
Glycoprotein IIb/IIIa receptor antagonists
  abciximab (Reopro), 259
  eptifibatide (Integrilin), 259
  tirofiban (Aggrastat), 259
Goldenseal, 391
Golimumab (Simponi), 355
Gonadotropin-releasing hormone (GnRH), 292–293
Gonadotropin-releasing hormone analogs
  goserelin (Zoladex), 343
  histrelin (Supprelin LA, Vantas), 343
  leuprolide (Lupron, Eligard), 343
  triptorelin (Trelstar), 343
Goserelin (Zoladex), 295, 319, 343

Gout, drugs for treatment of, 367–369
  allopurinol (Zyloprim), 370
  colchicine, 369
  febuxostat (Uloric), 370
  indomethacin (Indocin), 369
  mechanism of action of drugs, 371
  probenecid (Benemid, Probalan), 370
  rasburicase (Elitek), 370
G6PD deficiency, 15
Graded dose-response curve, 4–5
  characteristics of, 2
  definition of, 2
Granisetron (Granisol, Sancuso), 282
Gray baby syndrome, 15
Griseofulvin, 65
Growth hormone (GH), 292–293
Growth hormone-releasing hormone (GHRH), 292–293
Guaifenesin (Mucinex, Robitussin), 269
Guanabenz (Wytensin), 203
Guanadrel (Hylorel), 204
Guanethidine (Ismelin), 202
Guanfacine (Intuniv, Tenex), 130, 203
Guanosine analogs, 50
Gynecomastia, definition of, 278

H

Half-life, equation for, 11
Hallucinogens
  lysergic acid diethylamide (LSD), 132
  phencyclidine (PCP, wet), 132
Halogenated hydrocarbons
  desflurane (Suprane), 187
  enflurane (Ethrane), 188
  halothane (Fluothane), 188
  isoflurane (Forane, Terrell), 187
  nitrous oxide, 188
  sevoflurane (Ultane, Sojourn), 187

Haloperidol (Haldol), 113
Halothane (Fluothane), 188
H_1 blockers (Antihistamines)
  classification of, 378
  first-generation, 379–380
    chlorpheniramine (Chlor-Trimeton), 379
    clemastine (Tavist), 380
    dimenhydrinate (Dramamine), 379
    diphenhydramine (Benadryl), 379
    hydroxyzine (Atarax, Vistaril), 379
    meclizine (Antivert), 379
    promethazine (Phenergan), 380
    tripelennamine (Triplen, Pelamine), 379
  second generation, 380
    azelastine (Astelin, Astepro), 380
    cetirizine (Zyrtec, Aller-Relief), 380
    desloratidine (Clarinex), 380
    fexofenadine (Allegra), 380
    levocetirizine (Xyzal), 380
    loratidine (Claritin, Alavert, Tavist ND), 380
Heparin, 255
Herbal remedies
  aloe vera, 389
  capsicum/cayenne, 389
  cascara sagrada, 389
  chondrotin, 389
  cranberry, 389
  echinacea, 390
  feverfew, 390
  garlic, 390
  ginger, 390
  gingko biloba, 390
  ginseng, 391
  glucosamine, 391
  goldenseal, 391
  honey (medihoney), 391
  kava, 391
  ma-huang (Ephedra), 392
  melatonin, 392

Herbal remedies (*continued*)
  milk thistle, 392
  S-adenosylmethionine (SAM-e), 392
  saw palmetto, 393
  soy, 393
  St. John's wort, 393
  valerian, 393
  yohimbe, 393
Heroin, 132
Heterocyclics antidepressants
  bupropion (Wellbutrin, Zyban, Budeprion, Forfivo, Aplenzin), 119
  mirtazapine (Remeron), 119
  trazadone (Oleptro), 119
Hirsutism, 350
Histrelin (Supprelin LA, Vantas), 343
Histrelin (Vantas, Supprelin), 295
HMG-CoA reductase inhibitors, 251
  atorvastatin (Lipitor), 250
  fluvastatin (Lescol), 250
  lovastatin (Mevacor, Altoprev), 250
  pitavastatin (Livalo), 250
  pravastatin (Pravachol), 250
  rosuvastatin (Crestor), 250
  simvastatin (Zocor), 250
Hodgkin's lymphoma, 324
Homatropine (Isopto Homatropine), 106
Honey (Medihoney), 391
Hormonal anticancer drugs
  aromatase Inhibitors
    anastrozole (Arimidex), 345
    exemestane (Aromasin), 345
    letrozole (Femara), 345
  classification of, 342
  glucocorticoids
    prednisone (Deltasone), 345
  gonadotropin-releasing hormone analogs
    goserelin (Zoladex), 343
    histrelin (Supprelin LA, Vantas), 343

leuprolide (Lupron, Eligard), 343
    triptorelin (Trelstar), 343
  sex hormone antagonists
    flutamide (Eulexin), 344
    tamoxifen (Soltamox), 344
    toremifene (Fareston), 344
  sex hormones
    androgens, 343
    estrogens, 343
    progestins, 343
H_2-receptor antagonists
  cimetidine (Tagamet), 279
  famotidine (Pepcid), 279
  nizatidine (Axid), 279
  ranitidine (Zantac), 279
$5\text{-HT}_{1B/1D}$ receptor agonists
  almotriptan (Axert), 174
  eletriptan (Relpax), 174
  frovatriptan (Frova), 174
  naratriptan (Amerge), 173
  rizatriptan (Maxalt), 173
  sumatriptan (Imitrex, Alsuma, Sumavel), 173
  zolmitriptan (Zomig), 173
Huntington's disease, treatment of, 143
Hydralazine (Apresoline, NovoHylazin, Nu-Hydral), 211, 247
Hydrochlorothiazide (HCTZ), 221
Hydrochlorothiazide (HCTZ, Microzide), 246
Hydrocortisone (Cortef, A-Hydrocort), 298
Hydromorphone (Dilaudid, Exalgo), 164
Hydroxocobalamin (Cyanokit), 384
Hydroxyprogest erone (Makena), 315
Hydroxyzine (Atarax, Vistaril), 379
Hydroxyzine (Vistaril), 127
Hyperprolactinemia, definition of, 290
Hypertensive emergency, definition of, 199
Hypertensive urgency, definition of, 199
Hyperthyroidism, medications for
  methimazole (Tapazole), 303

potassium iodide (Lugol's Solution, Strong Iodide solution), 303
propylthiouracil (PTU), 303
radioactive sodium iodide (I^{131}, Hicon), 303
Hypertrichosis, definition of, 199
Hypogonadotropichypogonadism, definition of, 290
Hypothalamic and pituitary hormones
  endogenous, 293
  exogenous, 293–297
    bromocriptine (Parlodel, Cycloset), 296
    chorionic gonadotropin (Novarel, Pregnyl), 296
    corticotropin (ACTH, Acthar), 295
    corticotropin-releasing hormone, 295
    desmopressin (DDAVP, Stimate), 297
    follitropin alfa (Gonal-F), 296
    follitropin beta (Follistim), 296
    goserelin (Zoladex), 295
    histrelin (Vantas, Supprelin), 295
    leuprolide (Lupron, Eligard), 295
    nafarelin (Synarel), 295
    octreotide (Sandostatin), 294
    oxytocin (Pitocin), 297
    pramipexole (Mirapex), 296
    protirelin (Thyrel TRH), 294
    ropinirole (Requip), 297
    somatotropin, 294
    tesamorelin (Egrifta), 294
    thyrotropin alfa (Thyrogen), 294
    urofollitropin (Bravelle), 296
    vasopressin (Pitressin), 297
  hypothalamic-pituitary hormonal axis, 292
Hypothyroidism, medications for
  desiccated thyroid (Armour Thyroid, Nature-Throid, Westhroid), 302
  levothyroxine (Levothroid, Levoxyl, Synthroid Tirosint, Unithroid), 302
  liothyronine (Cytomel, Triostat), 302
  liotrix (Thyrolar), 302

I

Ibandronate (Boniva), 305
Ibuprofen (Advil, Motrin), 175
Ibuprofen (Motrin, Advil), 374
Ibutilide (Corvert), 238
Idarubicin (Idamycin), 336
Ifosfamide (IFEX), 327
Iloperidone (Fanapt), 115
Imipenem (Primaxin), 32
Imipramine (Tofranil), 118
Immune globulin intravenous, 358
Immunomodulators
    classification of, 351
    immunostimulants, 362–363. *See also*
        Immunostimulants
    immunosuppressants, 352–361. *See also*
        Immunosuppressants
    terms to learn, 350
Immunostimulants
    aldesleukin (Proleukin), 362
    filgrastim (Neupogen), 362
    interferon-α-2b (Intron A), 363
    interferon alfacon-1 (Infergen), 363
    interferon-β-1b (Betaseron, Extavia), 363
    interferon-γ-1b (Actimmune), 363
    pegylated-α-2b (Peglntron, Redipen, Sylatron), 363
    pegylated interferon-α-2a (Pegasys), 363
    sargramostim (Leukine), 362
Immunosuppressants
    antibody
        abatacept (Orencia), 360
        alemtuzmab (Campath, Lemtrada), 360
        anakinra (Kineret), 360
        antilymphocyte globulin-lymphocyte immune
            globulin (Atgam), 358
        basiliximab (Simulect), 358
        belatacept (Nulojix), 360

belimimab (Benlysta), 359
fingolimod (Gilenya), 360
immune globulin intravenous, 358
muromonab-CD3 (Orthoclone OKT3), 359
natalizumab (Tysabri), 360
ofatumumab (Arzerra), 359
rituximab (Rituxan), 359
secukinumab (Cosentyx), 359
teriflunomide (Aubagio), 360
tocilizumab (Actemra), 358
ustekinumab (Stelara), 359
anti TNF-α agents
    adalimumab (Humira), 355
    certolizumab pegol (Cimzia), 355
    etanercept (Enbrel), 354
    golimumab (Simponi), 355
    infliximab (Remicade), 355
    thalidomide (Thalomid), 354
cytotoxic agents
    azathioprine (Imuran, Azasan), 355
    cyclophosphamide (Cytoxan), 356
    methotrexate (Trexall, Rheumatrex), 356
enzyme inhibitors
    apremilast (Otezla), 357
    leflunomide (Arava), 357
    mycophenolate Mofetil (Cellcept, Myfortic), 357
    tofacitinib (Xeljanz), 357
fungal cyclic peptide antibiotic
    cyclosporine (Neoral, Gengraf, Sandimmune),
        352
    tacrolimus-FK-506 (Prograf, Hecoria), 353
glucocorticoid
    prednisone, 353
macrolide antibiotics
    sirolimus (Rapamune), 352
sites of action, 361
Inamrinone (Inocor), 242
Indacaterol (Arcapta), 272
Indapamide, 221, 245

Indinavir (Crixivan), 58
Indomethacin (Indocin), 369, 375
Inert binding site, definition of, 2
Infantile spasms, 161, 163
Inflammation, drugs for treatment of
    analgesics, 370–375. *See also* Analgesics
    drugs for gout, 367–369
        allopurinol (Zyloprim), 370
        colchicine, 369
        febuxostat (Uloric), 370
        indomethacin (Indocin), 369
        mechanism of action of, 366
        probenecid (Benemid, Probalan), 370
        rasburicase (Elitek), 370
    H_1 blockers (Antihistamines)
        classification of, 378
        first-generation, 379–380
        second generation, 380
    prostaglandin analogs
        PGE_2 analog, 368
        PGE_1 analogs, 367
        PGI_2 analog, 366
    terms to learn, 366
Infliximab (Remicade), 355
Inhalation adminstration route, 8
Inhibitor of 5′-lipoxygenase, 275
Insulin
    determir, 307
    glargine, 307
    glulisine, 307
    lispro, 307
    NPH, 307
    regular, 307
Insulin aspart (Novolog), 307
Insulin determir, 307
Insulin glargine (Lantus), 307
Insulin glulisine (Apidra), 307
Insulin lispro (Humalog), 307
Interferon-α-2b (Intron A), 363

Interferon alfa-2a, 51
Interferon alfa-2b (Intron-A), 51
Interferon alfacon-1 (Infergen), 51, 363
Interferon alfa-n3 (Alferon N), 51
Interferon-β-1b (Betaseron, Extavia), 363
Interferon-γ-1b (Actimmune), 363
Interferons
   interferon alfa-2a, 51
   interferon alfa-2b (Intron-A), 51
   interferon alfacon-1 (Infergen), 51
   interferon alfa-n3 (Alferon N), 51
Intramuscular (IM) adminstration route, 8
Intravenous (IV) adminstration route, 8
Intravenous nonopioids
   dexmedetomidine (Precedex), 190
   etomidate (Amidate), 190
   ketamine (Ketalar), 189
   methohexital (Brevital), 189
   midazolam (Versed), 189
   pentobarbital (Nembutal), 189
   propofol (Diprivan, Fresenius Propoven),
      190
   remifentanil (Ultiva), 192
   thiopental, 189
Intravenous opioids
   alfentanil (Alfenta), 191
   fentanyl (Sublimaze), 191
   meperidine (Demerol), 192
   morphine (Duramorph, Astramorph, Infumorph),
      191
   remifentanil (Ultiva), 192
   sufentanil (Sufenta), 191
Intrinsic sympathomimetic activity (ISA),
   80
Iodoquinol (Yodoxin), 69
Ipratropium (Atrovent), 92, 273
Irbesartan (Avapro), 217
Irinotecan (Camptosar), 340
Irreversible antagonist, definition of, 2

Isocarboxazid (Marplan), 122
Isoflurane (Forane, Terrell), 187
Isoproterenol, 96
Isosorbide dinitrate (Isordil, IsoDitrate, Dilatrate), 225,
   247
Isosorbide mononitrate (Imdur), 225
Isradipine, 213
Ixabepilone (lxempra), 347

K

Kanamycin, 36
Kaposi's sarcoma, definition of, 290
Kava, 391
Kawasaki disease, 350
K_d, definition of, 2
Ketamine (Ketalar), 189
Ketoconazole, 64
Ketorolac (Toradol), 375

L

LABA. *See* Long-acting β-agonists (LABA)
Labetalol (Trandate), 103, 207
Lacosamide (Vimpat), 161
Lactulose (Enulose, Constulose, Generlac, Kristalose),
   284
Lamivudine (Epivir), 56
Lamotrigine (Lamictal), 161
Lansoprazole (Prevacid), 281
Lassa fever, 15
Laxatives
   bisacodyl (Dulcolax, Correctol), 284
   docusate (Colace), 284
   lactulose (Enulose, Constulose, Generlac, Kristalose),
      284
   methylcellulose (Citrucel), 284
   polycarbophil (FiberCon, Fiber-Lax, Fiber-Tabs,
      Equalactin), 284

   polyethylene Glycol (Miralax), 284
   psyllium (Metamucil), 284
   senna (Ex-Lax, Senokot), 284
LD_{50}, definition of, 2
Leflunomide (Arava), 357
Lennox–Gastaut syndrome, 163
Lennox-Gastaut syndrome, definition of, 137, 161
Letrozole (Femara), 345
Leukotriene receptor antagonist
   montelukast (Singulair), 275
   zafirlukast (Accolate), 275
Leuprolide (Lupron, Eligard), 295, 319, 343
Levalbuterol (Xopenex), 271
Levetiracetam (Keppra), 157
Levobunolol (Betagan), 107
Levocetirizine (Xyzal), 380
Levodopa (Larodopa), 140
Levodopa/Carbidopa (Sinemet, Parcopa), 141
Levofloxacin (Levaquin), 46
Levonorgestrel, 315
Levonorgestrel (Mirena), 315
Levorphanol, 164
Levothyroxine (Levothroid, Levoxyl, Synthroid
   Tirosint, Unithroid), 302
Lidocaine (Xylocaine), 183, 235
Linezolid (Zyvox), 40
Liothyronine (Cytomel, Triostat), 302
Liotrix (Thyrolar), 302
Lipid solubility, definition of, 80
Lisdexamfetamine (Vyvanse), 129
Lisinopril (Prinivil, Zestril), 215, 244
Lithium (Lithobid), 123
Loading dose, 12
Local anesthetics and adjunctive drugs
   amides and other nonesters
      articaine-epinephrine (Articadent, Orabloc,
         Septocaine, Zorcaine), 184
      bupivacaine (Marcaine, Sensorcaine), 183
      epinephrine, 185

ethyl chloride, 185
lidocaine (Xylocaine), 183
mepivacaine (Carbocaine), 183
prilocaine (Citanest), 184
ropivacaine (Naropin), 184
classification of, 180
esters
benzocaine, 182
chloroprocaine (Nesacaine), 181
cocaine, 182
procaine (Novacain), 181
tetracaine (Pontocaine), 181
overview, 180
Lomustine (CeeNU), 327
Long-acting β-agonists (LABA)
arformoterol (Brovana), 272
formoterol (Foradil, Perforomist), 272
indacaterol (Arcapta), 272
salmeterol (Serevent), 272
Loop diuretics
bumetanide (Bumex), 222, 246
ethacrynic acid (Edecrin), 222
furosemide (Lasix), 222, 246
torsemide (Demadex), 222, 246
Loperamide (Imodium), 167
Lopinavir and ritonavir (Kaletra), 59
Loratidine (Claritin, Alavert, Tavist ND), 380
Lorazepam (Ativan), 126, 147, 156
Losartan (Cozaar), 216
Lovastatin (Mevacor, Altoprev), 250
Low-molecular-weight heparins
dalteparin (Fragmin), 255
enoxaparin (Lovenox), 255
Loxapine (Loxitane), 113–114
Lupus-like syndrome, 199
Luteinizing hormone (LH), 292–293
Lysergic aciddiethylamide (LSD), 132

M

Macrolide antibiotics, 352
Macrolides, 38–39
azithromycin (Zithromax), 39
clarithromycin (Biaxin), 38
erythromycin (Erythrocin), 38
fidaxomicin (Dificid), 39
Magnesium hydroxide (Phillips' Milk of Magnesia), 280
Ma-huang (Ephedra), 392
Maintenance dose, 12
Malathion (Ovide), 89
Malignant hypertension, definition of, 80
Malignant osteopetrosis, 350
Mannitol (Osmitrol), 224
Marijuana (Mary Jane, Weed, Pot), 131
Mast cell stabilizer
cromolyn sodium (Gastrocrom), 274
nedocromil (Tilade), 274
Mazzotti reaction, 15
Mecamylamine (Inversine), 94
Mechlorethamine (Mustargen), 326
Meclizine (Antivert), 379
Medroxyprogest erone (Depo Provera), 315
Medroxyprogest erone (Provera), 315
Mefloquine, 68
Megaloblastic anemia, definition of, 388
Megestrol (Megace), 316
Meglitinide derivatives
nateglinide (Starlix), 310
repaglinide (Prandin), 310
Melatonin, 392
Melphalan (Alkeran), 327
Memantine (Namenda), 145
Membrane stabilizing activity (MSA), 80
Meperidine (Demerol), 192
Meperidine (Demerol, Meperitab), 165
Mephobarbital (Mebaral), 149

Mepivacaine (Carbocaine), 183
Mercaptopurine-6-MP (Purinethol), 330
Meropenem (Merrem), 32
Mesalamine (Asacol, Pentasa, Rowasa, Canasa, Apriso, Lialda), 286
Mestranol, 312
Metabolism, 9
Metaproterenol, 271
Metaproterenol (Metaprel, Alupent), 97
Metaxalone (Skelaxin), 179
Metformin (Glucophage), 310
Methadone (Dolophine, Methadose), 164
Methamphetamine (crystal meth), 133
Methamphetamine (Desoxyn), 129
Methemoglobinemia, 15
Methimazole (Tapazole), 303
Methocarbamol (Robaxin), 179
Methohexital (Brevital), 151, 189
Methotrexate (Rheumatrex, Trexall), 333
Methotrexate (Trexall, Rheumatrex), 356
Methsuximide (Celontin), 159
Methyclothiazide, 221
Methylcellulose (Citrucel), 284
Methyldopa, 202
Methyldopa (Aldomet), 218
3,4-methylenedioxy-N-methylamphetamine (MDMA, Ecstasy), 133
Methylphenidate (Concerta, Ritalin,Daytrana, Metadate, Methylin, Quillivant), 129
Methylphenidate (Ritalin, Metadate,Daytrana, Concerta), 97
Methyl-salicylate (Ben-Gay), 373
Methyltestosterone (Android, Testred, Methitest), 316
Methyl xanthine, 273
Metipranolol (Optipranolol), 107
Metoclopramide (Reglan), 283
Metolazone (Zaroxolyn), 221, 246
Metoprolol, 245

Metoprolol (Lopressor, Toprol), 206, 229
Metoprolol (Toprol XL,Lopressor), 102
Metronidazole (Flagyl, Metro), 68
Metyrapone (Metopirone), 300
Metyrosine (Demser), 101, 204
Mexiletine, 235
Micafungin (Mycamine), 62
Miconazole (Monistat, Oravig), 64
Midazolam (Versed), 146, 189
Mifepristone (Mifeprex, Korlym), 317
Miglitol (Glyset), 310
Migraines, drugs for treatment of
    abortive antimigraine drugs
        caffeine and ergotamine (Cafergot, Migergot),
            172
        ergots, 172
        5-HT$_{1B/1D}$ receptor agonists, 173–174
    prophylactic migraine drugs
        amitriptyline (Elavil), 175
        cyproheptadine (Periactin), 175
        ibuprofen (Advil, Motrin), 175
        propranolol (Inderal), 175
Migraines, drugs for treatment of
    classification, 169
Milk thistle, 392
Milrinone, 242
Mineralocorticoid agonist, 300
Mineralocorticoid antagonists
    eplerenone (Inspra), 300
    metyrapone (Metopirone), 300
    spironolactone (Aldactone), 300
Minimum alveolar concentration (MAC), definition of,
    137
Minocycline (Minocin), 37
Minoxidil, 211
Miosis, definition of, 80
Mirtazapine (Remeron), 119
Misoprostol (Cytotec), 285, 367
Mitomycin (Mutamycin), 337

Mitoxantrone (Novantrone), 337, 346
Moclobemide (Manerix), 122
Moexipril (Univasc), 215
Mometasone (Asmanex), 274
Monoamine oxidase (MAO) inhibitors
    isocarboxazid (Marplan), 122
    moclobemide (Manerix), 122
    phenelzine (Nardil), 122
    rasagiline (Azilect), 122
    selegiline (Eldepryl, Emsam, Zelapar), 122
    tranylcypromine (Parnate), 122
Monobactam, 33
Montelukast (Singulair), 275
Mood disorder, medications for, 128
Mood stabilizing agents
    carbamazepine (Tegretol, Carbatrol, Epitol, Equetro),
        124
    lithium (Lithobid), 123
    valproate (Depakene, Depacon, Depakote, Stavzor),
        124
Morphine (Duramorph, Astramorph, Infumorph),
    191
Morphine (MS Contin, Duramorph, Kadian, Avinza,
    Infumorph, Astramorph), 164
Moxifloxacin (Avelox), 46
Multiple myeloma, 324
Muromonab-CD3 (Orthoclone OKT3), 359
Muscarinic antagonists
    classification of, 90
    ipratropium (Atrovent), 273
    quaternary amines, 92
        ipratropium (Atrovent), 92
        propantheline (Pro-Banthine), 92
    tertiary amines, 91
        atropine (Sal-Tropine, Isopto Atropine), 91
        scopolamine (Isopto Hyoscine, Hyoscine),
            91
    tiotropium (Spiriva), 273
Myasthenia gravis, definition of, 80

Mycophenolate Mofetil (Cellcept, Myfortic), 357
Mydriasis, definition of, 80
Myoclonic seizures, 163

N

Nabilone (Cesamet), 283
N-Acetylcysteine/NAC (Mucomyst, Acetadote),
    383
Nadolol (Corgard), 103, 207, 230
Nafarelin (Synarel), 295
Nafcillin, 17, 20
Naftifine (Naftin), 63
Nalbuphine (Nubain), 167
Naloxone (Narcan), 168, 384
Naltrexone (ReVia, Vivitrol), 168
Naphazoline (Privine), 269
Naproxen (Naprosyn), 375
Naratriptan (Amerge), 173
Natalizumab (Tysabri), 360
Nateglinide (Starlix), 310
Nebivolol (Brevibloc), 206
Nebivolol (Bystolic), 102
Nedocromil (Tilade), 274
Nelarabine (Arranon), 331
Nelfinavir (Viracept), 58
Neomycin (Neo-Fradin), 36
Neostigmine (Prostigmin, Bloxiverz), 89
Netilmicin (Netromycin), 36
Neuraminidase inhibitors
    oseltamivir, 51
    zanamivir (Relenza), 51
Neuroblastoma, 324
Neuroleptic malignant syndrome (NMS), 110
Neurologic function, drugs affecting
    Alzheimer's disease, 144–145. See also Alzheimer's
        disease, drugs for
    antiepileptic drugs, 154–163, 176–179
    general anesthetics, 186–193

local anesthetics and adjunctive drugs, 180–185
migraines, 171–175. *See also* Migraines, drugs for treatment of
movement. *See* Parkinson's disease, drugs for
neuromuscular blockers, 194–196
opioids, 164–170
sedatives and hypnotics, 146–153
terms to learn, 137
Neuromuscular blockers
  depolarizing
    succinylcholine (Anectine, Quelicin), 195
  nondepolarizing
    atracurium, 196
    cisatracurium (Nimbex), 196
    doxacurium (Nuromax), 196
    pancuronium, 196
    rocuronium, 196
    vecuronium, 196
  overview, 194
Neuronal blockers
  metyrosine (Demser), 101
  reserpine, 101
Neutropenia, 382
Nevirapine (Viramune), 57
Niacin (Niaspan, Niacor), 249
Nicardipine (Cardene), 213, 229
Nicotine, 133
Nicotine (Nicoderm, Nicotrol, Nicotrol inhaler, Nicorette), 94
Nicotinic acid, 249, 251
Nifedipine (Adalat, Afeditab, Procardia, Nifediac, Nifedical), 213, 229
Nilutamide (Nilandron), 319
Nisoldipine (Sular), 213
Nitazoxanide (Alinia), 69
Nitrates
  isosorbide dinitrate (Isordil, IsoDitrate, Dilatrate), 247
  nitroprusside (Nitropress), 247

Nitrofurantoin (Macrobid), 47
Nitroglycerin (Nitro-Bid, Nitro-Dur, Minitran, Nitro-Time, Nitrolingual, NitroMist, Nitronal, Nitrostat, Rectiv), 210
Nitroglycerin (Nitro-Bid, Nitro-Dur, Minitran, Nitrolingual, NitroMist, Rectiv,Nitronal, Nitrostat), 225
Nitroprusside (Nitropress), 210, 247
Nitrous oxide, 188
Nizatidine (Axid), 279
NMS. *See* Neuroleptic malignant syndrome (NMS)
Non-β_2-adrenergic agonists
  aerosol corticosteroids
    beclomethasone (QVAR), 274
    budesonide (Pulmicort), 274
    ciclesonide (Alvesco), 274
    fluticasone (Flovent), 273
    mometasone (Asmanex), 274
  inhibitor of 5'-lipoxygenase
    zileuton (Zyflo), 275
  leukotriene receptor antagonist
    montelukast (Singulair), 275
    zafirlukast (Accolate), 275
  mast cell stabilizer
    cromolyn sodium (Gastrocrom), 274
    nedocromil (Tilade), 274
  methyl xanthine
    theophylline (Elixophyllin, Theo-24, Theochron), 273
  muscarinic antagonist
    ipratropium (Atrovent), 273
    tiotropium (Spiriva), 273
Non-β-lactams, 34
  bacitracin, 34
  cycloserine (Seromycin), 34
  fosfomycin (Monurol), 34
  vancomycin (Vancocin), 34
Noncatecholamines
  albuterol (Proventil, Ventolin), 97

amphetamine-dextroamphetamine (Adderall), 97
bitolterol (Tornolate), 97
ephedrine, 97
formoterol (Foradil, Perforomist), 97
metaproterenol (Metaprel, Alupent), 97
methylphenidate (Ritalin, Metadate, Daytrana, Concerta), 97
pirbuterol (Maxair), 97
salmeterol (Serevent), 97
terbutaline (Brethine), 97
Nondihydropyridine calcium channel blockers
  diltiazem (Cardizem, Dilacor, Diltzac, Matzim, Taztia, Tiazac), 228
  verapamil (Calan, Isoptin, Verelan), 228
Non-Hodgkin's lymphoma, 324
Non-nucleoside reverse transcriptase inhibitors
  delavirdine (Rescriptor), 57
  efavirenz (Sustiva), 57
  etravirine (Intelence), 57
  nevirapine (Viramune), 57
  rilpivirine (Edurant), 57
Nonselective α-adrenergic blockers
  definition of, 80
  phenoxybenzamine (Dibenzyline), 204
  phentolamine (Regitine, Rogitine), 204
Nonselective β-blockers, definition of, 80
Nonsteroidal anti-inflammatory drugs (NSAIDs)
  diflunisal (Dolobid), 374
  flurbiprofen (Ansaid), 374
  ibuprofen (Motrin, Advil), 374
  indomethacin (Indocin), 375
  ketorolac (Toradol), 375
  mechanism of action, 377
  naproxen (Naprosyn), 375
  piroxicam (Feldene), 375
  sulindac (Clinoril), 375

Nonsulfonylureas, 310–311
  biguanide, 310
  α-glucosidase inhibitor
    acarbose (Precose), 310
    miglitol (Glyset), 310
  meglitinide derivatives
    nateglinide (Starlix), 310
    repaglinide (Prandin), 310
  thiazolidinediones, 311
    pioglitazone (Actos), 311
    rosiglitazone (Avandia), 311
Norepinephrine (Levophed), 96
Norethindrone (Aygestin, Camila, Errin, Heather,
    Jolivette, Nor-QD, Nora-BE, Micronor), 316
Norfloxacin (Noroxin), 45
Nortriptyline (Pamelor), 118
NPH insulin, 307
NSAIDs. See Nonsteroidal anti-inflammatory drugs
    (NSAIDs)
Nucleoside analogues
  acyclovir (Zovirax), 53
  famciclovir (Famvir), 54
  ganciclovir (Cytovene), 53
  penciclovir (Denavir), 54
  trifluridine (Viroptic), 54
  valcyclovir (Valtrex), 53
  valganciclovir (Valcyte), 53
Nucleoside reverse transcriptase inhibitors
  abacavir (Ziagen), 56
  adefovir (Hepsera), 56
  didanosine/DDI (Videx), 55
  emtricitabine (Emtriva), 55
  entecavir (Baraclude), 56
  lamivudine (Epivir), 56
  stavudine (Zerit), 55
  tenofovir (Viread), 55
  zidovudine/AZT (Retrovir), 55
Nucleotide analogue, 54
Nystatin (Nyamyc), 61

O

Obsessive compulsive disorder (OCD), 110
OCD. See Obsessive compulsive disorder (OCD)
Octreotide (Sandostatin), 286, 294
Ofatumumab (Arzerra), 359
Ofloxin (Floxin), 45
Olanzapine (Zyprexa), 115
Oligospermia, definition of, 290
Omeprazole (Prilosec), 281
Oncologic drugs
  alkylating drugs, 326–329
  antimetabolites, 330–333
  antitumor antibiotics, 334–337
  cell cycle phases, 325
  chemotherapeutic drugs, 346–348
  hormonal anticancer drugs, 342–345
  plant alkaloids, 338–341
  terms to learn, 324
Ondansetron (Zofran, Zuplenz), 282
Opiates, 132
Opioids, 164–170
  alfentanil (Alfenta), 167
  classification of, 165
  fentanyl (Actiq, Abstral Lazanda, Subsys Onsolis,
    Fentora, Duragesic), 167
  hydromorphone (Dilaudid, Exalgo), 166
  levorphanol, 166
  mechanism of action, 164
  meperidine (Demerol, Meperitab), 167
  methadone (Dolophine, Methadose), 166
  mixed agonist/antagonists
    buprenorphine (Buprenex, Butrans Subutex), 169
    buprenorphine and naloxone (Suboxone,
      Zubsolv), 169
    butorphanol (Stadol), 169
    nalbuphine (Nubain), 169
    pentazocine (Talwin), 169

moderate to weak opioid agonists
  codeine, 168
  dextromethorphan (Delsym, Robitussin DM), 168
  difenoxin (Motofen), 168
  diphenoxylate (Lomotil), 168
  loperamide (Imodium), 169
  oxycodone (Oxycontin, Oxecta, Roxicodone), 168
morphine (MS Contin, Duramorph, Kadian, Avinza,
    Infumorph, Astramorph), 166
opioid antagonists
  naloxone (Narcan), 170
  naltrexone (ReVia, Vivitrol), 170
oxymorphone (Opana), 166
remifentanil (Ultiva), 167
sufentanil (Sufenta), 167
summary of, 164
Oral (PO) adminstration route, 8
Oral diabetic drugs
  classification of, 308
  nonsulfonylureas, 310–311
    biguanide, 310
    α-glucosidase inhibitor, 310
    meglitinide derivatives, 310
    thiazolidinediones, 311
  sulfonylureas, 309
    first-generation, 309
    second-generation, 309
Organophosphates
  echothiophate (Phospholine iodide), 89
  malathion (Ovide), 89
  parathion, 89
  sarin, 89
  soman, 89
  tabun, 89
Orphenadrine (Norflex), 179
Orthostatic hypotension, 366
Orthostatic tremor, treatment of, 143
Oseltamivir, 51
Osmotic diuretics, 224

Oxacillin (Bactocill), 17, 20
Oxandrolone (Oxandrin), 318
Oxazepam (Serax), 146
Oxcarbazepine (Trileptal, Oxtellar), 160
Oxycodone (Oxycontin, Oxecta, Roxicodone), 166
Oxygen, 383
Oxymetazoline (Afrin), 268
Oxymorphone (Opana), 164
Oxytetracycline (Terramycin), 37
Oxytocin, 292–293
Oxytocin (Pitocin), 297

P

Paclitaxel (Taxol), 341
Paliperidone (Invega), 115
Palonosetron (Aloxi), 282
Pamidronate (Aredia), 305
Pancuronium, 196
Pantoprazole (Protonix), 281
Papilledema, definition of, 388
Parathion, 89
Paresthesias, 382
Parkinson's disease, drugs for
    anticholinergics
        benztropine (Cogentin), 139
    antiviral
        amantadine, 139
    classification, 138
    MAO B inhibitors
        rasagiline (Azilect), 139
        selegiline (Emsam, Eldepryl, Zelapar), 139
    second-line drugs for
        carbidopa (Lodosyn), 141
        entacapone (Comtan), 141
        levodopa (Larodopa), 140
        levodopa/Carbidopa (Sinemet, Parcopa), 141
        tolcapone (Tasmar), 141

third-line drugs for
    apomorphine (Apokyn), 142
    bromocriptine (Parlodel, Cycloset), 142
    pramipexole (Mirapex), 142
    ropinirole (Requip), 142
    rotigotine (Neupro), 142
Paromomycin, 36
Paromomycin (Humatin), 69
Paroxetine (Paxil), 120
Partial agonist, definition of, 2
Partial seizures, 162
Passive diffusion, 7
PDE3 inhibitors
    inamrinone (Inocor), 242
    milrinone, 242
Pegylated-α-2b (Peglntron, Redipen, Sylatron), 363
Pegylated interferon-α-2a (Pegasys), 363
Pellagra, definition of, 388
Pemetrexed (Alimta), 333
Penbutolol (Levatol), 207
Penciclovir (Denavir), 54
Penicillamine (Cuprimine, Depen), 386
Penicillin G (Pentids, Pfizerpen), 17, 19
Penicillins
    β-lactamase-resistant, 19–20
        cloxacillin, 17
        dicloxacillin, 17, 20
        nafcillin, 17, 20
        oxacillin (Bactocill), 17, 20
    classification of, 18
    combination preparations
        amoxicillin and clavulinic acid (Augmentin), 23
        ampicillin and sulbactam (Unasyn), 23
        piperacillin and tazobactam (Zosyn), 23
        ticarcillin and clavulinic acid (Timentin), 23
    extended spectrum, 21–22
        amoxicillin (Amoxil, Trimox), 17, 21
        ampicillin (Ampicin), 17, 21

carbenicillin (Geocillin), 17, 22
        piperacillin (Pipracil), 17, 22
        ticarcillin (Ticar), 17, 22
    overview, 17
    penicillin G (Pentids, Pfizerpen), 17, 19
    penicillin V (Pen-Vee K, V-cillin), 17, 19
Penicillin V (Pen-Vee K, V-cillin), 17, 19
Pentamidine (Pentam, Nebupent), 69
Pentazocine (Talwin), 167
Pentobarbital (Nembutal), 151, 189
Pentostatin (Nipent), 331
Peptide antibiotics
    bleomycin (Blenoxane), 335
    dactinomycin (Cosmegen), 335
Perampanel (Fycompa), 159
Perindopril (Aceon), 215
Perphenazine, 113
Pervasive developmental disorder, medications for, 128
pH
    definition of, 2
    equation for, 11
Pharmacodynamics
    definition of, 2
    dose-response curve
        comparison of, 5
        graded, 4–5
        quantal, 4–5
        time action, 4–5
    response curves
        agonist, 6
        antagonist, 6
Pharmacokinetics
    administration, 8. *See also* Administration route
    binding, 8
    definition of, 2
    distribution, 8
    dosing, 12
    drug movement within body, 7

Pharmacokinetics (*continued*)
  drug solubility, 7
  elimination
    first-order, 10
    zero-order, 10
  equations, 11
  metabolism, 9
  therapeutic values, 11
Pharmacologic antagonist, definition of, 2
Pharmacology, definition of, 3
Phencyclidine (PCP, wet), 132
Phenelzine (Nardil), 122
Phenobarbital (Luminal), 150, 155
Phenothiazines, 113
Phenoxybenzamine (Dibenzyline), 100, 204
Phentolamine, 100
Phentolamine (Regitine, Rogitine), 204
Phenylephrine, 96
Phenylephrine (Neo-Synephrine), 106, 269
Phenylephrine (Sudafed PE), 268
Phenytoin (Dilantin, Phenytek), 160, 235
Pheochromocytoma, definition of, 80, 199
Physiologic antagonist, definition of, 3
Physostigmine, 88
Physostigmine (Antilirium, Eserine), 383
Pilocarpine (Isopto Carpine, Pilopine HS), 105
Pilocarpine (Isopto Carpine, Salagen), 87
Pimozide (Orap), 113
Pindolol, 103, 208, 230
Pioglitazone (Actos), 311
Piperacillin (Pipracil), 17, 22
Piperacillin and tazobactam (Zosyn), 23
Pirbuterol (Maxair), 97, 271
Piroxicam (Feldene), 375
Pitavastatin (Livalo), 250
pK_a, definition of, 3
Plant alkaloids
  action of mechanism, 338
  camptothecins

irinotecan (Camptosar), 340
  topotecan (Hycamtin), 340
classification of, 338
podophyllotoxins
  etoposide (VP-16, VePesid), 339
  teniposide (Vumon), 340
taxanes
  docetaxel (Taxotere, Docefrez), 341
  paclitaxel (Taxol), 341
vinca alkaloids
  vinblastine (Velban, Velsar), 339
  vincristine (Vincasar), 339
  vinorelbine (Navelbine), 339
Plasma binding, definition of, 80
Plicamycin (Mithracin, Mithramycin), 306
PMDD. *See* Premenstrual dysphoric disorder
  (PMDD)
Pneumothorax, definition of, 137
Podophyllotoxins
  etoposide (VP-16, VePesid), 339
  teniposide (Vumon), 340
Polycarbophil (FiberCon, Fiber-Lax, Fiber-Tabs,
  Equalactin), 284
Polyenes
  amphotericin B, 61
  nystatin (Nyamyc), 61
Polyethylene Glycol (Miralax), 284
Posaconazole (Noxafil), 64
Positive inotropric drugs
  digoxin (Lanoxin, Digox), 241
  dobutamine, 242
  dopamine (Intropin), 242
  inamrinone (Inocor), 242
  milrinone, 242
Posttraumatic stress disorder (PTSD), 110
Postural (orthostatic) hypotension, definition of,
  80
Potassium iodide (Lugol's solution, Strong Iodide
  solution), 303

Potassium-sparing diuretics
  amiloride (Midamor), 223
  eplerenone (Inspra), 223, 243
  spironolactone (Aldactone), 223, 243
  triamterene (Dyrenium), 223
Potency, definition of, 3
PPIs. *See* Proton pump inhibitors (PPIs)
Pralidoxime (2-PAM, Protopan), 384
Pramipexole (Mirapex), 142, 296
Prasugrel (Effient), 260
Pravastatin (Pravachol), 250
Prazosin (Minipress), 101, 205
Prednisone, 298, 353
Prednisone (Deltasone), 345
Pregabalin (Lyrica), 158
Premenstrual dysphoric disorder (PMDD), 110
PRH. *See* Prolactin-releasing hormone (PRH)
Prilocaine (Citanest), 184
Primaquine, 68
Primidone (Mysoline), 155
Probenecid (Benemid, Probalan), 370
Procainamide, 234
Procaine (Novacain), 181
Procarbazine (Matulane, Natulan), 329
Prochlorperazine (Compazine, Compro), 282
Progesterone preparations
  etonogestrel (Implanon, Nexplanon), 315
  hydroxyprogest erone (Makena), 315
  levonorgestrel, 315
  levonorgestrel (Mirena), 315
  medroxyprogest erone (Depo Provera), 315
  medroxyprogest erone (Provera), 315
  megestrol (Megace), 316
  norethindrone (Aygestin, Camila, Errin, Heather,
    Jolivette, Nor-QD, Nora-BE, Micronor), 316
Progestins, 343
Prolactin (PRL), 292–293
Prolactin-inhibiting hormone (PIH, dopamine),
  292–293

Prolactin-releasing hormone (PRH), 292–293
Promethazine (Phenergan), 283, 380
Propafenone (Rythmol), 236
Propantheline (Pro-Banthine), 92
Prophylactic migraine drugs
    amitriptyline (Elavil), 175
    cyproheptadine (Periactin), 175
    ibuprofen (Advil, Motrin), 175
    propranolol (Inderal), 175
Propofol (Diprivan, Fresenius Propoven), 190
Propofol-related infusion syndrome, definition of, 137
Propranolol (Hemangeol, Inderal, InnoPran), 208, 230
Propranolol (Inderal), 175, 218
Propranolol (Inderal LA), 103
Propylthiouracil (PTU), 303
Prostaglandin analogs
    PGE_2 analog, 368
    PGE_1 analogs, 367
    PGI_2 analog, 366
Protamine sulfate, 263, 384
Protease inhibitors
    atazanavir (Reyataz), 58
    darunavir (Prezista), 59
    fosamprenavir (Lexiva), 59
    indinavir (Crixivan), 58
    lopinavir and ritonavir (Kaletra), 59
    nelfinavir (Viracept), 58
    ritonavir (Norvir), 58
    saquinavir (Invirase), 58
    tipranavir (Aptivus), 59
Protirelin (Thyrel TRH), 294
Proton pump inhibitors (PPIs)
    dexlansoprazole (Kapidex), 281
    esomeprazole (Nexium), 281
    lansoprazole (Prevacid), 281
    omeprazole (Prilosec), 281
    pantoprazole (Protonix), 281
    rabeprazole (AcipHex), 281
Pseudoephedrine (Sudafed), 268

Psychiatric medications
    antidepressants, 116–122
    antipsychotics, 112–115
    anxiolytics, 125–127
    for disorders diagnosed in childhood, 128–130
    drugs of abuse, 131–133
    mood stabilizing agents, 123–124
    terms to learn, 110–111
Psychotic disorder, medications for, 128
Psyllium (Metamucil), 284
PTSD. See Posttraumatic stress disorder (PTSD)
PTU. See Propylthiouracil (PTU)
Purine antagonists
    cladribine (Leustatin), 330
    clofarabine (Clolar), 330
    fludarabine (Fludara, Oforta), 331
    mercaptopurine-6-MP (Purinethol), 330
    nelarabine (Arranon), 331
    pentostatin (Nipent), 331
    thioguanine-6-TG (Tabloid), 330
Pyridostigmine (Mestinon, Regonol), 89
Pyrimethamine (Daraprim), 70
Pyrimidine analog, 65
Pyrimidine antagonists
    azacitidine (Vidaza), 333
    capecitabine (Xeloda), 332
    cytosine arabinoside-ara-C-cytarabine (Cytosar), 331
    decitabine (Dacogen), 332
    floxuridine (FUDR), 332
    5-fluorouracil (Adrucil), 331
    gemcitabine (Gemzar), 332
Pyrimidines, 41

Q

Quantal dose-response curve, 4–5
    characteristics of, 4
    definition of, 3

Quaternary alcohols
    donepezil (Aricept), 88
    edrophonium (Enlon, Tensilon), 88
    tacrine (Cognex), 88
Quaternary amines, 92
    ipratropium (Atrovent), 92
    propantheline (Pro-Banthine), 92
Quazepam (Doral), 148
Quetiapine (Seroquel), 115
Quinapril (Accupril), 215, 244
Quinidine, 67, 234
Quinidine syncope, definition of, 199
Quinine (Qualaquin), 67
Quinolones. See Fluoroquinolones
Quinupristin and dalfopristin (Synercid), 40

R

Rabeprazole (AcipHex), 281
Radioactive sodium iodide (I^{131}, Hicon), 303
Raloxifene (Evista), 304, 313
Ramelteon (Rozerem), 153
Ramipril (Altace), 215, 244
Ranitidine (Zantac), 279
Rasagiline (Azilect), 122, 137
Rasburicase (Elitek), 370
Raynaud's disease, definition of, 80
Receptor, definition of, 3
Receptor site, definition of, 3
Recombinant human factor IX (BeneFIX, Rixubis), 262
Recombinant human factor VIIa (NovoSeven RT), 262
Recombinant human factor VIII (AdvateHelixate FS, Kogenate FS, Recombinate,Xyntha, Xyntha Solofuse), 262
Rectal adminstration route, 8
Remifentanil (Ultiva), 165, 192
Renal dose, 11

Repaglinide (Prandin), 310
Reproductive hormones, drugs affecting
  antiandrogen drugs
    bicalutamide (Casodex), 319
    dutasteride (Avodart), 320
    enzalutamide (Xtandi), 319
    finasteride (Proscar, Propecia), 320
    goserelin (Zoladex), 319
    leuprolide (Lupron, Eligard), 319
    nilutamide (Nilandron), 319
    site of action, 321
    spironolactone (Aldactone), 320
  antiestrogen drugs
    clomiphene (Clomid, Serophene), 313
    raloxifene (Evista), 313
    tamoxifen (Soltamox), 313
  antiprogesterone drug
    mifepristone (Mifeprex, Korlym), 317
  estrogen and progesterone combinations
    biphasic combination, 314
    ethinyl estradiol and levonorgestrel, 314
    ethinyl estradiol and norethindrone, 314
    monophasic combination, 314
    triphasic combination, 314
  estrogen preparations
    conjugated estrogens (Premarin), 312
    esterified estrogens (Menest), 312
    estradiol, 312
    estropipate (Ogen), 312
    ethinyl estradiol, 312
    mestranol, 312
  progesterone preparations
    etonogestrel (Implanon, Nexplanon), 315
    hydroxyprogest erone (Makena), 315
    levonorgestrel, 315
    levonorgestrel (Mirena), 315
    medroxyprogest erone (Depo Provera), 315
    medroxyprogest erone (Provera), 315
    megestrol (Megace), 316

    norethindrone (Aygestin, Camila, Errin, Heather, Jolivette, Nor-QD, Nora-BE, Micronor), 316
  testosterone preparations
    fluoxymesterone (Androxy), 318
    methyltestosterone (Android, Testred, Methitest), 318
    oxandrolone (Oxandrin), 318
    testosterone cypionate (Depo-Testosterone), 318
    testosterone enanthate (Delatestryl), 318
Reserpine, 101
Reserpine (Serpasil), 203
Respiratory drugs
  asthma drugs, 270–276. See also Asthma drugs
  cold medications. See also Cold medications
  terms to learn, 266
Response curves
  agonist, 6
  antagonist, 6
Reteplase (Retavase), 258
Reye's syndrome, 199
Rhabdomyolysis, definition of, 199
Ribavirin, 50
Rilpivirine (Edurant), 57
Rimantadine (Flumadine), 50
Risedronate (Actonel, Atelvia), 305
Risperidone (Risperdal), 114
Ritonavir (Norvir), 58
Rituximab (Rituxan), 348, 359
Rivaroxaban (Xarelto), 256
Rivastigmine (Exelon), 145
Rizatriptan (Maxalt), 173
Rocuronium, 196
Ropinirole (Requip), 142, 297
Ropivacaine (Naropin), 184
Rosiglitazone (Avandia), 311
Rosuvastatin (Crestor), 250
Rotigotine (Neupro), 142
Rufinamide (Banzel), 161

S

SABA. See Short-acting β-agonists (SABA)
SAD. See Seasonal affective disorder (SAD)
S-Adenosylmethionine (SAM-e), 392
Salicylic acid, 373
Salmeterol (Serevent), 97, 272
30S antibacterial agents
  aminoglycosides, 35–36
    amikacin, 36
    gentamicin, 35
    kanamycin, 36
    neomycin (Neo-Fradin), 36
    netilmicin (Netromycin), 36
    paromomycin, 36
    streptomycin, 35
    tobramycin (Tobi), 35
  tetracyclines, 37
    demeclocycline (Declomycin), 37
    doxycycline (Vibramycin), 37
    minocycline (Minocin), 37
    oxytetracycline (Terramycin), 37
    tetracycline (Sumycin), 37
50S antibacterial agents
  chloramphenicol, 39
  clindamycin (Cleocin), 39
  linezolid (Zyvox), 40
  macrolides, 38–39
    azithromycin (Zithromax), 39
    clarithromycin (Biaxin), 38
    erythromycin (Erythrocin), 38
    fidaxomicin (Dificid), 39
  quinupristin and dalfopristin (Synercid), 40
Saquinavir (Invirase), 58
Sargramostim (Leukine), 362
Sarin, 89
Saw palmetto, 393
Scopolamine, 283

Scopolamine (Isopto Hyoscine, Hyoscine), 91
Seasonal affective disorder (SAD), 110
Secobarbital (Seconal), 150
Secukinumab (Cosentyx), 359
Sedatives and hypnotics
  barbiturates
    amobarbital (Amytal), 149
    butabarbital (Butisol), 149
    mephobarbital (Mebaral), 149
    methohexital (Brevital), 151
    pentobarbital (Nembutal), 151
    phenobarbital (Luminal), 150
    secobarbital (Seconal), 150
    thiopental, 150
  benzodiazepines
    alprazolam (Xanax), 146
    chlordiazepoxide (Librium), 147
    clonazepam (Klonopin), 147
    clorazepate (Tranxene), 148
    diazepam (Valium, Diastat), 148
    estazolam (ProSom), 147
    flurazepam (Dalmane), 148
    lorazepam (Ativan), 147
    midazolam (Versed), 146
    oxazepam (Serax), 146
    quazepam (Doral), 148
    temazepam (Restoril), 147
    triazolam (Halcion), 146
  buspirone (Buspar), 152
  chloral hydrate, 152
  eszopiclone (Lunesta), 153
  ketamine (Ketalar), 189
  ramelteon (Rozerem), 153
  zaleplon (Sonata), 153
  zolpidem (Ambien, Edluar, Intermezzo, Zolpimist), 152
Selective α-adrenergic blockers
  definition of, 81
  doxazosin (Cardura), 205

prazosin (Minipress), 205
  terazosin (Hytrin), 205
Selective β-adrenergic blockers, definition of, 81
Selective estrogen receptor modulators
  raloxifene (Evista), 304
  tamoxifen (Nolvadex), 304
Selective serotonin reuptake inhibitors (SSRIs)
  citalopram (Celexa), 120
  escitalopram (Lexapro), 120, 126
  fluoxetine (Prozac), 120
  fluvoxamine (Luvox), 120
  paroxetine (Paxil), 120
  sertraline (Zoloft), 120
  vilazodone (Viibryd), 120
Selegiline (Emsam, Eldepryl, Zelapar), 122, 137
Senna (Ex-Lax, Senokot), 284
Serotonin norepinephrine reuptake inhibitors
  desvenlafaxine (Pristiq), 121
  duloxetine (Cymbalta), 121, 127
  venlafaxine (Effexor), 121, 127
Serotonin syndrome, 110
Sertraline (Zoloft), 120
Sevoflurane (Ultane, Sojourn), 187
Sex hormone antagonists
  flutamide (Eulexin), 344
  tamoxifen (Soltamox), 344
  toremifene (Fareston), 344
Sex hormones
  androgens, 343
  estrogens, 343
  progestins, 343
Short-acting β-agonists (SABA)
  albuterol (AccuNeb, ProAir, Vospire, Proventil, Ventolin), 271
  levalbuterol (Xopenex), 271
  metaproterenol, 271
  pirbuterol (Maxair), 271
  terbutaline, 271
SIADH, definition of, 291

Silodosin (Rapaflo), 101
Simvastatin (Zocor), 250
Sirolimus (Rapamune), 352
Sjögren's syndrome, definition of, 81
Sodium bicarbonate (Brioschi), 280
Sodium fluoride, 306
Sodium thiosulfate (All packaged as cyanide), 383
Soman, 89
Somatostatin, 292–293
Somatotropin, 294
Sorbitol, 284
Sotalol (Betapace), 237
Sotalol (Betapace, Sorine), 103
Soy, 393
Spare receptors, definition of, 3
Spironolactone (Aldactone), 223, 243, 300, 320
SSRIs. *See* Selective serotonin reuptake inhibitors (SSRIs)
St. John's wort, 393
Status epilepticus, 161, 163
Stavudine (Zerit), 55
Steatorrhea, definition of, 291
Stevens-Johnson syndrome, 15
Stimulants
  caffeine, 133
  cocaine (crack, coke), 133
  methamphetamine (crystal meth), 133
  3,4-methylenedioxy-N-methylamphetamine (MDMA, Ecstasy), 133
  nicotine, 133
Strabismus, definition of, 137
Streptomycin, 35
Streptozocin (Zanosar), 328
Subcutaneous (SC) adminstration route, 8
Sublingual adminstration route, 8
Succimer/DMSA (Chemet), 385
Succinylcholine (Anectine, Quelicin), 195
Sucralfate (Carafate), 285

Sufentanil (Sufenta), 165, 191
Sulfadiazine, 43
Sulfisoxazole, 43
Sulfonamides, 41
   antibacterial synergy of, 42
   sulfadiazine, 43
   sulfisoxazole/erythromycin, 43
   trimethoprim/sulfamethoxazole, 43
Sulfonylureas
   first-generation
      chlorpropamide (Diabinese), 309
      tolazamide (Tolinase), 309
      tolbutamide (Orinase), 309
   second-generation
      glimepiride (Amaryl), 309
      glipizide (Glucotrol), 309
      glyburide (DiaBeta, Glynase, PresTab),
         309
Sulindac (Clinoril), 375
Sumatriptan (Imitrex, Alsuma, Sumavel),
   173
Sumycin, 37
Superinfection, 15
Sympathetic antagonists
   clonidine (Catapres), 218
   methyldopa (Aldomet), 218
   propranolol (Inderal), 218
Sympathomimetics
   catecholamines, 95–96
      dobutamine, 96
      dopamine, 95
      epinephrine (Adrenalin, Epipen), 96
      isoproterenol, 96
      norepinephrine (Levophed), 96
      phenylephrine, 96
   classification of, 95
   dobutamine, 242
   dopamine (Intropin), 242
   effects on organ systems, 98

noncatecholamines
   albuterol (Proventil, Ventolin), 97
   amphetamine-dextroamphetamine (Adderall),
      97
   bitolterol (Tornolate), 97
   ephedrine, 97
   formoterol (Foradil, Perforomist), 97
   metaproterenol (Metaprel, Alupent), 97
   methylphenidate (Ritalin, Metadate, Daytrana,
      Concerta), 97
   pirbuterol (Maxair), 97
   salmeterol (Serevent), 97
   terbutaline (Brethine), 97
Systemic decongestants
   chlorpheniramine (Chlor-Trimeton), 268
   diphenhydramine (Benadryl), 268
   phenylephrine (Sudafed PE), 268
   pseudoephedrine (Sudafed), 268
Systemic lupus erythematous, 382

T

Tabun, 89
Tacrine (Cognex), 88, 145
Tacrolimus-FK-506 (Prograf, Hecoria), 353
Tamoxifen (Nolvadex), 304
Tamoxifen (Soltamox), 313, 344
Tamsulosin (Flomax), 101
Tardive dyskinesia (TD), 111
Taxanes
   docetaxel (Taxotere, Docefrez), 341
   paclitaxel (Taxol), 341
TD. See Tardive dyskinesia (TD)
Temazepam (Restoril), 147
Temozolomide (Temodar), 329
Tenecteplase (TNKase), 258
Teniposide (Vumon), 340
Tenofovir (Viread), 55
TENS. See Toxic epidermal necrolysis (TENS)

Terazosin (Hytrin), 101, 205
Terbinafine (Lamisil, Terbinex), 62
Terbutaline, 271
Terbutaline (Brethine), 97
Teriflunomide (Aubagio), 360
Tertiary amines, 91
   atropine (Sal-Tropine, Isopto Atropine), 91
   scopolamine (Isopto Hyoscine, Hyoscine), 91
Tesamorelin (Egrifta), 294
Testosterone cypionate (Depo-Testosterone), 318
Testosterone enanthate (Delatestryl), 318
Testosterone preparations
   fluoxymesterone (Androxy), 318
   methyltestosterone (Android, Testred, Methitest),
      318
   oxandrolone (Oxandrin), 318
   testosterone cypionate (Depo-Testosterone), 318
   testosterone enanthate (Delatestryl), 318
Tetracaine (Pontocaine), 181
Tetracyclines, 37
   demeclocycline (Declomycin), 37
   doxycycline (Vibramycin), 37
   minocycline (Minocin), 37
   oxytetracycline (Terramycin), 37
   Sumycin, 37
Thalidomide (Thalomid), 354
Theophylline (Elixophyllin, Theo-24, Theochron), 273
Therapeutic index (TI$_{50}$), 11
   definition of, 3
Therapeutic values, 11
Therapeutic window, 11
Thiazide diuretics
   chlorothiazide (Diuril), 221, 246
   chlorthalidone, 221, 246
   hydrochlorothiazide (HCTZ), 221
   hydrochlorothiazide (HCTZ, Microzide), 246
   indapamide, 221, 247
   methyclothiazide, 221
   metolazone (Zaroxolyn), 221, 246

Thiazolidinediones, 311
 pioglitazone (Actos), 311
 rosiglitazone (Avandia), 311
Thioguanine-6-TG (Tabloid), 330
Thiopental, 150, 189
Thioridazine (Mellaril), 113
Thiotepa, 329
Thrombolytics
 alteplase (Activase), 258
 reteplase (Retavase), 258
 tenecteplase (TNKase), 258
 urokinase (Kinlytic), 258
Thrombotic thrombocytopenic purpura, definition of, 199
Thyroid drugs
 hyperthyroidism
  methimazole (Tapazole), 303
  potassium iodide (Lugol's Solution, Strong Iodide solution), 303
  propylthiouracil (PTU), 301
  radioactive sodium iodide (I^{131}, Hicon), 303
 hypothyroidism
  desiccated thyroid (Armour Thyroid, Nature-Throid, Westhroid), 302
  levothyroxine (Levothroid, Levoxyl, Synthroid Tirosint, Unithroid), 302
  liothyronine (Cytomel, Triostat), 302
  liotrix (Thyrolar), 302
 overview, 301
Thyroid-stimulating hormone (TSH), 292–293
Thyrotropin Alfa (Thyrogen), 294
Thyrotropin-releasing hormone (TRH), 292–293
Tiagabine (Gabitril), 155
Ticarcillin (Ticar), 17, 22
Ticarcillin and clavulinic acid (Timentin), 23
Tic disorders, medications for, 128
Ticlopidine, 260
Time action dose-response curve, 4–5
Timolol, 208

Timolol (Blocadren), 103
Timolol (Timoptic), 107
Tinidazole (Tindamax), 69
Tinnitis, 366
Tinnitis, definition of, 199
Tiotropium (Spiriva), 273
Tipranavir (Aptivus), 59
Tirofiban (Aggrastat), 259
Tizanidine (Zanaflex), 179
Tobramycin (Tobi), 35
Tocilizumab (Actemra), 358
Tofacitinib (Xeljanz), 357
Tolazamide (Tolinase), 309
Tolbutamide (Orinase), 309
Tolcapone (Tasmar), 141
Tolerance, definition of, 199
Tolvaptan (Samsca), 224
Topical adminstration route, 8
Topical decongestants
 naphazoline (Privine), 269
 oxymetazoline (Afrin), 268
 phenylephrine (Neo-Synephrine), 269
Topiramate (Topamax, Topiragen, Trokendi), 157
Topotecan (Hycamtin), 340
Toremifene (Fareston), 344
Torsade de pointes, definition of, 199
Torsemide (Demadex), 222, 246
Torticollis, definition of, 388
Tourette's syndrome
 definition of, 81
 treatment of, 143
Toxic epidermal necrolysis (TENS), 111
Toxicology
 chelators
  deferoxamine (Desferel), 386
  dimercaprol (BAL), 385
  edetate calcium disodium (EDTA, Endrate, Versenate), 385

  penicillamine (Cuprimine, Depen), 386
  succimer/DMSA (Chemet), 385
 terms to learn, 382
 treatment of specific poisons
  amyl nitrite and sodium nitrite, 383
  atropine, 384
  digoxin-specific antibodies (Digibind), 383
  ethanol, 383
  flumazenil (Romazicon), 383
  fomepizole (Antizol), 383
  hydroxocobalamin (Cyanokit), 384
  N-acetylcysteine/NAC (Mucomyst, Acetadote), 383
  naloxone (Narcan), 384
  oxygen, 383
  physostigmine (Antilirium, Eserine), 383
  pralidoxime (2-PAM, Protopan), 384
  protamine sulfate, 384
  sodium thiosulfate, 383
Trachoma, 15
Trandolapril (Mavik), 216, 245
Transdermal adminstration route, 8
Tranylcypromine (Parnate), 122
Trastuzumab (Herceptin), 348
Trazadone (Oleptro), 119
Triamcinolone (Kenalog, Aristospan), 299
Triamterene (Dyrenium), 223
Triazolam (Halcion), 146
Tricyclic amines
 amantadine, 50
 rimantadine (Flumadine), 50
Tricyclic antidepressants
 amitriptyline (Elavil), 118
 clomipramine (Anafranil), 118
 desipramine (Norparmin), 118
 doxepin (Silenor), 118
 imipramine (Tofranil), 118
 nortriptyline (Pamelor), 118

Trifluoperazine (Stelazine), 113
Trifluridine (Viroptic), 54
Trigeminal neuralgia, 111
Trimethaphan (Arfonad), 94
Trimethoprim (TMP), 44
    antibacterial synergy of, 42
Trimethoprim/sulfamethoxazole (Bactrim),
        43, 70
Tripelennamine (Triplen, Pelamine),
        379
Triptorelin (Trelstar), 343
Tropicamide (Mydriacyl), 106
Typical antipsychotics, 113–114
    butyrophenones, 113
    chlorpromazine (Thorazine), 113
    dibenzoxazepine, 113–114
    diphenylbutylpiperidinesd, 113
    fluphenazine (Prolixin, Permitil),
        113
    haloperidol (Haldol), 113
    loxapine (Loxitane), 113–114
    perphenazine, 113
    phenothiazines, 113
    pimozide (Orap), 113
    thioridazine (Mellaril), 113
    trifluoperazine (Stelazine), 113

U

Urofollitropin (Bravelle), 296
Urokinase (Kinlytic), 258
Ursodiol (Actigall), 286
Ustekinumab (Stelara), 359
Uterine fibroids, definition of, 291

V

Valcyclovir (Valtrex), 53
Valerian, 393

Valganciclovir (Valcyte), 53
Valproate (Depacon, Depakene, Stavzor),
        158
Valproate (Depakene, Depacon, Depakote, Stavzor),
        124
Valrubicin (Valstar), 337
Valsartan (Diovan), 216
Valsartan (Dlovan), 245
Vancomycin (Vancocin), 34
Vasodilators
    arterial and venous, 208–209
        hydralazine (Apresoline, Novohylazin,
            Nu-Hydral), 247
    classification of, 209
    hydralazine (Apresoline, NovoHylazin, Nu-Hydral),
        211
    minoxidil, 211
    nitroglycerin (Nitro-Bid, Nitro-Dur,Minitran,
        Nitro-Time, Nitrolingual, NitroMist, Nitronal,
        Nitrostat, Rectiv), 210
    nitroprusside (Nitropress), 210
Vasopressin, 292–293
Vasopressin (Pitressin), 297
Vasopressin receptor antagonists
    conivaptan (Vaprisol), 224
    tolvaptan (Samsca), 224
Vecuronium, 196
Venlafaxine (Effexor), 121, 127
Verapamil (Calan, Isoptin), 239
Verapamil (Calan, Isoptin, Verelan),
        212, 228
Vigabatrin (Sabril), 155
Vilazodone (Viibryd), 120
Vinblastine (Velban, Velsar), 339
Vinca alkaloids
    vinblastine (Velban, Velsar), 339
    vincristine (Vincasar), 339
    vinorelbine (Navelbine), 339
Vincristine (Vincasar), 339

Vinorelbine (Navelbine), 339
Virilization, definition of, 291
Vitamin K (Mephyton), 263
Vitamins
    A, 395
    B_1 (thiamine), 395
    B_2 (riboflavin), 395
    B_3 (niacin), 395
    B_5 (pantothenic acid), 395
    B_6 (pyridoxine), 395
    B_7 (biotin), 396
    B_9 (folic acid), 396
    B_{12} (cobalamin), 396
    C (ascorbic acid), 396
    D, 396
    E, 396
    K, 396
    water soluble and fat soluble, 394
Volume of distribution (V_d), 11
Voriconazole (Vfend), 65

W

Warfarin (Coumadin, Jantoven), 254
Wernicke-Korsakoff syndrome, 111
West's syndrome, definition of, 137
Wilms' tumor, 324
Wilson's disease, 382
Wolff-Parkinson-White syndrome,
        199

X

Xerosis, definition of, 388
Xerostomia, definition of, 81

Y

Yohimbe, 393

Z

Zafirlukast (Accolate), 275
Zaleplon (Sonata), 153
Zanamivir (Relenza), 51

Zero-order elimination, 10
    vs. first-order elimination, 10
Zidovudine/AZT (Retrovir), 55
Zileuton (Zyflo), 275
Ziprasidone (Geodon), 115
Zoledronic acid (Reclast, Zometa), 305

Zollinger-Ellison syndrome, definition of, 278
Zolmitriptan (Zomig), 173
Zolpidem (Ambien, Edluar, Intermezzo, Zolpimist), 152
Zonisamide (Zonegran), 159